Implementing
Early Intervention

•

edited by

Carol Tingey, Ph.D.
Utah State University
Early Intervention
Research Institute

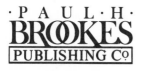

·P A U L·H·
BROOKES
PUBLISHING C⁰

Baltimore • London • Toronto • Sydney

Paul H. Brookes Publishing Co.
Post Office Box 10624
Baltimore, Maryland 21285-0624

Copyright © 1989 by Paul H. Brookes Publishing Co., Inc.
All rights reserved.

Typeset by Brushwood Graphics, Inc., Baltimore, Maryland.
Manufactured in the United States of America by
The Maple Press Company, York, Pennsylvania.

Library of Congress Cataloging in Publication Data
Implementing early intervention.

   Bibliography: p.
   Includes index.
   1. Handicapped children—Services for—United States.   2. Handicapped
children—Care—United States.   I. Tingey, Carol, 1933–   .
HV888.5.I46   1988   362.4'088054   88-14515
ISBN 1-55766-005-0 (pbk.)

Contents

•

Contributors

●

W. Steven Barnett, Ph.D.
Early Intervention Research Institute
Developmental Center for
  Handicapped Persons
Utah State University
Logan, UT 84322-6580

James A. Blackman, M.D., M.P.H.
Department of Pediatrics
247 HS
University of Iowa
Iowa City, IA 52242

Philippa H. Campbell, Ph.D.
Family Child Learning Center
Children's Hospital Medical Center
  of Akron
281 Locust Street
Akron, OH 44308

Glendon Casto, Ph.D.
Early Intervention Research Institute
Developmental Center for
  Handicapped Persons
Utah State University
Logan, UT 84322-6580

Wendy B. Doret, Ph.D.
Association for Children with Down
  Syndrome
2616 Martin Avenue
Bellmore, NY 11710

Colette M. Escobar, M.S.
Early Intervention Research Institute
Developmental Center for
  Handicapped Persons
Utah State University
Logan, UT 84322-6580

Barbara Davis Goldman, Ph.D.
Frank Porter Graham Child
  Development Center
University of North Carolina at
  Chapel Hill
Chapel Hill, NC 27514

Jean W. Gowen, Ph.D.
Family, Infant, and Preschool
  Program
Western Carolina Center
Morganton, NC 28655

Mary Ann Hanson, M.A.
Gila River Indian Community
Special Services Program
P.O. Box 69
Sacaton, AZ 85247

Kathryn Haring, Ph.D.
California Research Institute
San Francisco State University
14 Tapia Drive
San Francisco, CA 94132

Norris G. Haring, Ed.D.
110 Miller Hall, DQ-05
University of Washington
Seattle, WA 98195

DeAnna Horstmeier, Ph.D.
Ohio Resource Center for Low
  Incidence and Severe Handicaps
470 Glenmont Avenue
Columbus, OH 43214

Mark S. Innocenti, M.S.
Early Intervention Research Institute
Developmental Center for
  Handicapped Persons
Utah State University
Logan, UT 84322-6580

Nancy M. Johnson-Martin, Ph.D.
Duke University Medical Center
CHILD Project
2213 Elba Street
Durham, NC 27705

John Killoran, M.Ed.
Services for At-Risk Students
Utah State Office of Education
250 East 500 South
Salt Lake City, UT 84111

Helen Mitchell, Ph.D.
Early Intervention Research Institute
Developmental Center for
    Handicapped Persons
Utah State University
Logan, UT 84322-6580

Adrienne L. Peterson, R.P.T., M.S.
MAPPS Project
Utah State University
Logan, UT 84322-6580

Robert K. Rittenhouse, Ph.D.
Education of Hearing-Impaired
    Children
2801 South University
The University of Arkansas
Little Rock, AR 72204

Roberta Rosenblum, M.S.P.D.
Association for Children with Down
    Syndrome
2616 Martin Avenue
Bellmore, NY 11710

Fredda Stimell, M.S.W.
Association for Children with Down
    Syndrome
2616 Martin Avenue
Bellmore, NY 11710

Carol Tingey, Ph.D.
Early Intervention Research Institute
Developmental Center for
    Handicapped Persons
Utah State University
Logan, UT 84322-6580

Richard A. van den Pol, Ph.D.
COTEACH Preschool Program
University of Montana
Missoula, MT 59812

Karl R. White, Ph.D.
Early Intervention Research Institute
Developmental Center for
    Handicapped Persons
Utah State University
Logan, UT 84322-6580

Preface

•

Current interest in early intervention for infants and young children with handicaps or those children who are at risk for handicapping conditions has been stimulated by the passage of Public Law 99-457, which consists of a series of amendments to Public Law 93-380, the Education of the Handicapped Act Amendments of 1974. The law requires a statewide system that includes:

... (1) a definition of the term "developmentally delayed" that will be used by the State in carrying out programs under this part.

(2) timetables for ensuring that appropriate early intervention services will be available to all handicapped infants and toddlers in the State before the beginning of the fifth year of a State's participation under this part,

(3) a timely, comprehensive, multidisciplinary evaluation of the functioning of each handicapped infant and toddler in the State and the needs of the families to appropriately assist in the development of the handicapped infant or toddler,

(4) for each handicapped infant and toddler in the State, an individualized family service plan in accordance with section 677, including case management services in accordance with such service plan,

(5) a comprehensive child find system, consistent with Part B, including a system for making referrals to service providers that includes timelines and provides for the participation by primary referral sources,

(6) a public awareness program focusing on early identification of handicapped infants and toddlers,

(7) a central directory which includes early intervention services, resources, and experts available in the State and research and demonstration projects being conducted in the State,

(8) a comprehensive system of personnel development,

(9) a single line of responsibility in a lead agency designated or established by the Governor. . . . (Public Law 99-457, Section 676, Paragraph b)

Public Law 99-457 was passed in order to ensure that:

Each handicapped infant or toddler and the infant or toddler's family shall receive—

(1) a multidisciplinary assessment of unique needs and the identification of services appropriate to meet such needs, and

(2) a written individualized family service plan developed by a multidisciplinary team, including the parent or guardian. . . . (Public Law 99-457, Section 677, Paragraph a)

Early intervention is by no means a new concept, philosophy, or service. Services in some form for infants and their families have been part of American society from the beginning of the century; however, early services may bear little resemblance to what is offered today. The concepts, philosophies, and agencies involved in today's services have historical roots in what might be called the growth of more sophisticated public understanding and concern for the needs of children.

In the early 1900s, Public Health Services were expanded by the addition of the Maternal and Child Health Services specialization. Services of this department focused on decreasing childhood stress by reducing the incidence of communicable diseases and situations that contributed to infant death. With the increasing interest in the health of young children, President Theodore Roosevelt convened the first White House Conference that formed a Children's Bureau. Later, the White House Conference of 1930 on Child Health and Protection gathered information to support the need of federally financed programs for "crippled children."

In the mid-1930s, legislation, incorporated into the Social Security Act of 1935, designated state grant programs for Maternal and Child Health Services, Crippled Children's Services, and Child Welfare Services. Crippled Children's Services were funded to locate children with handicaps; and to diagnose, hospitalize, conduct corrective surgery, and provide postoperative care for such children. The mission of finding and treating young children to prevent them from spending their youth and adult years with handicapping conditions became the philosophy of American society.

The Crippled Children's Services expanded to treat conditions such as cystic fibrosis, neurological defects, and inborn errors of metabolism. In the 1950s, a focus was created within the Maternal and Child Health Services to provide assistance to children with mental retardation.

As is the case with most human services, as soon as there were indications that the procedures needed to protect the individual's health were in place, interest in the child's social and emotional climate increased. The effect of maternal deprivation, as shown in various studies, and the growth of orphans who had been placed in the individual care of interested adults in the 1930s were key issues of interest to social workers, psychologists, and educators just prior to World War II (Skeels, 1938; Skeels & Fillmore, 1937). However, these educational services were diverted during the war. It was not until after the country began recovering from the economic strains of the war that the need to enhance optimal development by providing educationally oriented services for young children again became the focus of public interest.

It was at this time that the United States Office of Education began funding model programs for early intervention. These services were operated through public health and educational agencies. The White House Conference of 1962 used the published reports of the Children's Bureau to show that there was a relationship between mental retardation and premature birth, brain damage, low income, and inadequate prenatal care. President John F. Kennedy's personal interest in the needs of persons with handicaps was soon translated into public policy. Soon afterward, funding for exemplary services to young children with handicaps was established.

The establishment of a comprehensive system of neonatal intensive care units was authorized by Congress in 1973 along with family planning, dental services, and surgery for infants with congenital anomalies. With this authorization, such services became part of the State Public Health Services' plan. Continuation of service to children with handicaps was then ensured.

In the early 1980s, interest in the needs and rights of infants and young children with handicaps was shown in the Baby Doe case (*American Academy of Pediatrics v. Heckler,* 1983). In this case, it was argued that the infant had the right to optimal care even if the parents did not want to provide it. This established a public commitment to recognize and provide for the needs of infants and young children even when parental care was discontinued. During this century, the interest of committed professionals and parents has focused on the multitude of needs of infants and young children. Specialization in developmental practices has become part of the training of educators, psychologists, physical and occupational therapists, speech/language therapists, nurses, nutritionists, and medical personnel. Presently, almost all of these professions offer some training or internship in treatment of infants and young children and their families in specific areas of expertise.

The implementation of Public Law 99-457 can now move forward with a host of knowledge from a variety of fields, including the common sense of experienced parents and careproviders of these children. However, the challenge still remains of how to evaluate and organize the known information into a format that can serve each infant adequately and nonobtrusively. If this can be done, each child and family can be served on an individual level using resources to pinpoint specific needs.

This book is written as a guide for planners and serviceproviders as they negotiate their way through the variety of practical considerations that are important to the quality of services that are being provided in early intervention programs.

Implementing Early Intervention is divided into four sections, the first of which highlights the "Best Practices" in the field. This section comprises Chapters 1 and 2 that discuss what is known about early intervention and who is eligible for such services. Chapter 1 is a summary of existing programs and provides information that is derived from research conducted to determine the effectiveness of various programs. Chapter 2 explains the process of identifying infants and young children who need early intervention and offers suggestions that can be used to determine each child's difficult areas of development.

The second section, Chapters 3–7, highlights the various "Administrative Concerns" that early intervention programs encounter as they provide services to children with handicaps. Chapter 3 gives a thorough description of the costs involved in early intervention, and provides assistance to program planners in the area of funds allocation. It offers various outlooks on how programs can accommodate the needs of children and their families. In keeping with financial matters, Chapter 4 proposes suggestions on how to implement interagency agreements, and how to recruit and train volunteers. By implementing the assistance of volunteers, services to these children can be increased. Staff development is discussed in Chapter 5. This chapter presents examples for staff of how to continue to provide quality service to children with handicaps and their families, and how to combat staff "burnout" with fresh attitudes. When staff volunteers are operating effectively, it shows. Chapter 6 offers guidance on the topic of evaluation by providing a variety of perspectives on this subject. In evaluating a program, the issue of mainstreaming should also be discussed. The need for young children with handicaps to have the opportunity to associate with nonhandicapped children—mainstreaming—is approached in Chapter 7.

Section III includes an in-depth look at "Implementing Specific Interventions." These six chapters highlight the various facets of a child's development. Each child begins formal schooling, or early intervention, with an evaluation. The early intervention program designs services to meet the specific needs of each individual child. How such plans can be devised and how instruction can simultaneously meet the needs of several children are discussed in Chapter 8. One of the skills that a child should develop in the early years is language competence. This process is very complex; however, Chapter 9 provides suggestions on how parents and teachers can assist in this process. Along with language learning comes motor learning. Chapter 10 details the child's early posture and movement skills and deficits, and offers solutions on how to adapt the child's physical environment to meet his or her specific motor abnormalities. Cognitive development is discussed in Chapter 11 as it outlines methods for increasing the child's basic understanding of his or her surrounding environment. As important as achieving cognitive development, a child must also obtain social skills. How the child with handicaps can learn to become more socially competent is discussed in Chapter 12. Self-care skills are highlighted in Chapter 13 as its authors describe various methods of teaching children with handicaps to take care of their personal needs.

The last section of *Implementing Early Intervention,* Chapters 14–16, details "Related Concerns" of operating an early intervention program. The first chapter of this section describes the health needs of children with handicaps and the various problems that are encountered when providing services. Although few people consider spanking children as a method of "controlling" them, some techniques are needed to manage children. Chapter 15 offers management techniques used to train children in formal settings while keeping the typical informal ambience of a preschool setting. Since the passage of Public Law 99-457, parents are taking a more active role in their child's intervention. Chapter 16 describes the recent increase in family participation and offers suggestions on how to meet the needs of the entire family.

Public officials, professionals from different fields, and families with at-risk children are all watching early intervention projects and hoping for development miracles that erase the effects of the potential handicap. Although from the start we know that this will not be possible for all children, if we plan, implement, and continue to evaluate, life will be richer for the children and families served by early intervention programs.

REFERENCES

American Academy of Pediatrics v. Heckler, 561 F. Supp. 395 (District of Columbia 1983).

Skeels, H. M. (1938). Mental development of children in foster homes. *Journal of Consulting Psychology, 2,* 33–43.

Skeels, H. M., & Fillmore, E. A. (1937). Mental development of children from underpriviledged homes. *Journal of Genetic Psychology, 50,* 427–439.

Acknowledgments

•

It is always amazing to me how much time it takes to organize thoughts on paper. I thank my professional colleagues for taking the time to share the history of their own professional experiences. I also wish to thank Lance Mortensen and Beccie Brown for finding and refinding references; Deb Peck for creating and recreating charts and tables; and Mary Ellen Heiner and Debbie Risk for typing and retyping chapters.

*This volume is dedicated
to all of the infants
and their families
who unexpectedly find
that they need someone
who can make an educated guess
about their future by having
a more complete understanding
of the past. . . .*

Implementing
Early Intervention

●

BEST PRACTICES
IN EARLY
INTERVENTION

———————— • ————————

Knowledge of the success of yesterday is essential to effective planning for today. Study of the ideas and elements of the pioneer early intervention activities is a prerequisite to the creation of more comprehensive services for young handicapped children and their families. However, even when the system is in place, one of the essential concerns is who is in need of such services and who is not. Eligibility criteria is determined by state regulations defined through the state advisory committee and interpreted by each local serviceprovider. Identification procedures and process will vary in different settings and will undoubtedly be refined and rerefined as practitioners gain more experience. However, the process must always be slowly and cautiously repeated anew as each infant is individually and meticulously observed.

Chapter 1

What Is Known
about Early Intervention

Karl R. White and Glendon Casto

●

In the fall of 1986, Congress passed, and the President signed into law, a landmark piece of legislation for handicapped children. Officially known as Public Law 99-457, the Education of the Handicapped Act Amendments of 1986, this legislation created a series of incentives and sanctions that will substantially expand the provision of early intervention programs to handicapped infants, toddlers, and preschoolers. Thus, in a single stroke, Congress accomplished what advocates, parents, administrators, and researchers have worked toward for decades—the wider availability of appropriate early intervention services for handicapped children.

Although the passage of Public Law 99-457 generated renewed public interest concerning services provided to young children and their families, early intervention is not a new idea. Before the passage of Public Law 99-457, limited services had been available for infants and young children and their families for some time, but such services were not universally available. The nature and extensiveness of available services depended primarily on where a child resided, and the economic conditions surrounding the family. With the passage of Public Law 99-457, however, such services will become more widely available, and discussions about early intervention will appropriately shift to identifying what types of intervention are most effective for each child.

Research findings have historically played a central role in discussions about early intervention services. Hundreds of studies have been conducted.

Work reported in this chapter was carried out in part with funds from the U.S. Department of Education (Contract #s 300-82-0367 and 300-85-0173) to the Early Intervention Research Institute at Utah State University.

The purpose of this chapter is to summarize what has been learned from that research, identify some of the questions that remain unanswered, point out some of the difficulties of using research to address the concerns of policymakers and practitioners, and suggest the areas where research can provide answers in the future.

WHO SHOULD PARTICIPATE IN EARLY INTERVENTION?

What sorts of questions regarding early intervention exist? Perhaps the most basic question is who should be eligible for early intervention services under Public Law 99-457. The framers of this important piece of legislation left this decision to state and local decisionmakers. Should it be environmentally at-risk children, medically at-risk children, or children with established handicaps? If at-risk children are to be served, how *at-risk* do they need to be? For example, even though low birthweight and premature babies constitute a population that has frequently been the target of early intervention services (Bennett, 1984), longitudinal data now available indicate that in the absence of *any* early intervention services, more than 90% of these children will be indistinguishable from their normal birthweight peers by the time they reach school age (McCormick, 1985; Phillip, Little, Polivy, & Lucey, 1981). So how should *at risk* be defined?

Do such questions about whom to serve extend to children with established handicaps? Once again, the answer is not so clear. How delayed do children have to be before they are considered handicapped? What about children with mild to moderate articulation problems? Will these problems grow worse or resolve themselves in the absence of intervention? What about learning disabled and hyperactive children? Are early intervention services under Public Law 99-457 appropriate for such children? As one considers further the issue of which children should be served, it becomes clear that the question is not easily answered. Many opinions are available, but very few data are accessible to help determine answers (see Chapter 2).

WHAT IS EARLY INTERVENTION?

Even the term *early intervention* means very different things to different people. For example, early intervention services provided in the past have ranged from spinning a child with cerebral palsy in a chair for a few seconds at a time to obtain vestibular nerve stimulation (e.g., Sellick & Over, 1980), to 40 hours per week of multidisciplinary efforts that begin at birth and last through the time the child starts school (e.g., Ramey, Bryant, Sparling, & Wasik, 1985). The term includes home-based visits that utilize parents as the primary interveners, medically oriented intervention in neonatal intensive care units, consultation in day care centers, and educationally oriented center-based programs. Early intervention can cost anywhere from a few hundred dollars to tens of thousands of dollars per child per year. The variety of activities and programs that have been included under the designation of early intervention is staggering. This diversity is one of the reasons why it is so important to step back from our perceptions of early intervention and consider, together, what is known about this topic.

Since the 1960s, there have been literally hundreds of studies conducted on the effectiveness of early intervention. Results of those studies have been used to support a wide variety of firmly entrenched options. Almost everyone in the education and rehabilitation fields agrees that early intervention is effective. For example, a report from the Office of Special Education and Rehabilitative Services to Congress stated that:

> Studies of the effectiveness of preschool education for the handicapped have demonstrated beyond doubt the economic and educational benefits for programs of young handicapped children. In addition, the studies have shown that the earlier intervention is started, the greater is the ultimate dollar savings and the higher the

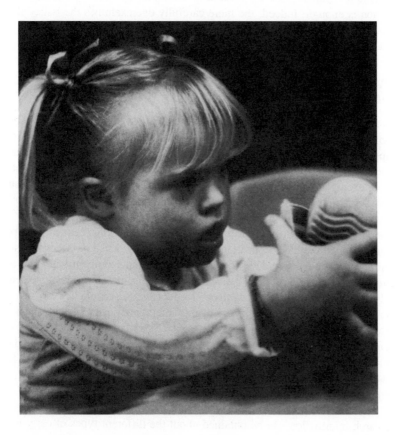

rate of educational attainment by handicapped children. (Office of Special Education and Rehabilitative Services, 1985, p. 211)

However, there are other issues about which there is not unanimous agreement. For example, some people are certain that home-based programs are the most cost-beneficial way to provide early intervention services. Others see that center-based classrooms are far more effective for the same groups of children. Depending on where a family with a handicapped child lives, it might receive transdisciplinary services, interdisciplinary services, or services from only one discipline. Such distinctions translate into very different types of services for children. In one town, parents may be told to leave the provision of therapy to trained professionals, while in another area they may be encouraged to provide most of the therapy services themselves. Even in settings where all of the services are provided in center-based programs, it is unclear about what sort of training is necessary for the most effective provision of services. Do interventionists need to be certified or can paraprofessionals provide services that are equally as good? Furthermore, although almost everyone agrees that more intervention is better, there is a great deal of disagreement abut how much intervention is enough. Indeed, the more carefully one examines the issues about what constitutes appropriate intervention services, the more difficult it is to find clear answers.

PROGRAMS APPROVED BY THE
JDRP AS EXAMPLES OF VARIATION

As an example of the diversity that exists within the field of early intervention, consider the programs receiving federal funds since 1968 from the Handicapped Children's Early Education Program (HCEEP). More than 400 early intervention programs designed to demonstrate and disseminate information about exemplary practices have been sponsored by HCEEP. Research results from some of these HCEEP projects were submitted to the Joint Dissemination Review Panel (JDRP). The JDRP is an interagency panel established by the federal government in 1975 for the purpose of determining if educational programs from all fields of education have sufficient evidence of effectiveness to justify incuding them in an official government publication entitled *Programs that Work* (National Diffusion Network, 1983). This material was published to help share successful ideas with other educators. Each application was reviewed by at least seven members of this interagency panel. It was then approved for national dissemination if the panel concluded that the project had demonstrated educationally significant effects, based on reliable and valid data, obtained using well-documented and replicable procedures (Fang, 1981; Tallmadge, 1977). It was also contingent on whether projects were willing to help train others to use the techniques.

Given the rigorous evaluation to which JDRP subjects projects, valuable research information can be obtained about the different types of early intervention programs. Indeed, Odom and Fewell (1983, p. 445) concluded that JDRP projects "were among the best the field has to offer." Given the criteria considered by the JDRP, the systematic evaluation process to which all JDRP approved projects are subjected, and the widespread perception that JDRP approved projects are of an exemplary nature (Datta, 1977), it would appear that a careful examination of the projects that have been approved by JDRP would provide some of the most valuable information about what types of early intervention programs are most effective.

Tables 1.1 and 1.2 contain information about the HCEEP funded programs that have been certified by the JDRP for national validation. A careful examination of these programs reveals great diversity. For example, some of these programs are home-based, some are center-based, and some are both home- and center-based programs. Validated programs include those that intervened with very young children, as well as older preschoolers. Some of the programs were as short as 14 weeks, and some lasted for almost 2½ years. Some home-based programs visited families once per week, others as infrequently as once per month. Some of the center-based programs are full-day and some are half-day, some are 3 days per week, some are 5 days per week. Interestingly, the results for the various programs are not dramatically different, in spite of the great degree of variation among them.

What does all of this say about early intervention? So far at least, it has been found that a variety of different programs result in similar benefits for handicapped children. This conclusion is consistent with the committee report to Public Law 99-457 that states:

> The committee also wishes to observe that there are currently a variety of effective special education models for serving handicapped children age 3–5 being utilized across the country. Based on the unique needs of the particular child, these models range from part-day home-based to part- or full-day center-based. (Congressional Report No. Public Law 99-860, p. 20)

The excerpt from the committee report emphasizes that the key to improving the provision of early intervention services is to focus more attention on deciding what types of programs are best for each child. This, of course, requires that activities and results of programs initiated are systematically documented. Public Law 99-457 could be seen as an invitation to engage in documentation of systematic variations in services. If such systematic variation could be accompanied by objective research and evaluation data, a dramatic increase in what is known about early intervention services could result during the next few years.

DIMENSIONS ALONG WHICH
EARLY INTERVENTION PROGRAMS CAN VARY

Obviously, early intervention programs can vary along many different dimensions. Past research provides some insight about each of these dimensions, but a great deal of work remains to be done before it can be definitively stated which

Table 1.1. Descriptions of selected early intervention projects approved by the JDRP

Project name and location	Organization of services	In-service offered	Description of program
Rutland Center Project Athens, GA	A center-based project for preschoolers with severe emotional problems	Variety	Behavior/socialization/preacademic curriculum, assume disturbed, follow normal development, mainstreaming component.
PEECH Project Champaign, IL	A center-based program for children and families—½ day, 5 days per week	12–14/2 or 3 hr. workshop; fees	Manuals on classroom planning, family involvement manuals, normal children integrated, paraprofessionals trained to teach, lending library for families.
Peoria 0–3 Project Peoria, IL	A home-based program for children and their families	2–3 day initial, 4–6 day follow-up; fees	OT/PT/speech/social work and developmental specialist, design weekly lessons taken to home, continuous monitoring of child progress, parent discussion groups.
ERIN Project Dedham, MA	Curriculum/assessment to use for home- or center-based individual instruction	5-day on-site visit, fees	Teaching adult organizes materials and environment to meet individual child goals. Self-help/developmental concept and academic readiness curriculum suggests home and classroom modifications.
High/Scope Project Ypsilanti, MI	Piagetian theory center-based intervention program	At center or on location; fees	Needs/interests of children assessed. Teachers support children's decisions. Room arrangement/schedule designed to stimulate. Materials available for purchase in connection with training paid by those receiving training.
Regional Demonstration Program Yorktown Heights, NY	A center-based inter-disciplinary team intervention program	1–2 days and follow-up; fees	Language intervention and positive reinforcement, diagnostic/ prescriptive teaching, verbal/ perceptual/motor/ cognition. Manuals describing interactive teaching, transdisciplinary team, parent involvement available at cost.
Teaching Research Project Monmouth, OR	Home- and center-based individualized skills instruction program for moderately/severely handicapped	5-days and follow-up; fees	Trained volunteers give care and feedback to children and record progress. Teacher uses data to plan next day's teaching. Generalization of skills to other settings stressed. Some instructional programs selected by parent and teacher to be taught at home. Teachers learn to manage inappropriate behavior.

Project	Description	Training	Details
MAPPS Project Logan, UT	A home- or center-based program for children in remote areas	1–2 days; fees	Curriculum & monitoring system for receptive and expressive language, motor development, self-help, preacademic skills, and social/emotional development (manual $48). Assessment for curriculum placement. Curriculum appropriate for parent or preschool use.
SKI*HI Project Logan, UT	A home-based diagnostic and intervention program	Fees	Screening, audiological, diagnostic assessment services suitable for state or regional service. Curriculum for home program for hearing aid, communication, auditory, total communication, and language. Psychological, emotional, and child-development support provided for parents in home.
Down Syndrome Project Seattle, WA	0–18 months parent training; 18 months–6 yrs., classroom		Systematic instruction (assessing, establishing goals and objectives, planning, implementing, and evaluating program). Criterion-referenced assessment in motor/cognitive/communication/social/self-help. Parent training in center, birth–18 months, less parent involvement as child enters classroom program at 18 months. Parent training then on as-needed basis.
Communication Project Seattle, WA	A home- and center-based program for communicatively disordered	2 days; fees	Serves children with language problems who do not have hearing loss. Trains classroom teachers and speech/language clinicians in management of communication behavior. Decision making and classroom management training. Data collection procedures.
Portage Project Portage, WI	A home teaching program for the multi-categorical handicapped	3 days; fees	Home teacher works with parent weekly to choose child goals and to plan how to teach developmental skills. Can also be used in connection with classroom. Instructional materials prepared and available for purchase.

Table 1.2. HCEEP projects approved for national dissemination by the joint dissemination review panel

Project	Primary handicap of children	Ages served	Sample size	Duration (weeks)
Home-Based				
Macomb 0–3 Project, IL	Combination	0–3	34	77
Peoria 0–3 Project, IL	Combination	0–3	77	52
UNISTAPS Project, MN	Hearing-impaired	0–5	25	39
Central Institute Project, MO	Hearing-impaired	0–4	29	154
DEBT Project, TX	Combination	0–2	103	65
PEECH Project, IL	Combination	1/2–6	98	189
SKI*HI Project, UT	Hearing-impaired	0–6	40	43
C.P. Project, WI	Orthopedically impaired	0–3	36	39
Portage Project, WI	Combination	0–6	57	39
Center-Based				
Rutland Center, GA	Emotionally	2–8	49	22
PEECH Project, IL	Combination	3–5	37	30
High/Scope Project, MI	Combination	4–6	16	39
Regional Demo. Project, NY	Combination	3–5		
Chapel Hill Project, NC	Combination	4–6	90	34
Good Samaritan Hospital	Multiple handicapped	0–6	28	39
Down Syndrome Project, WA	Mentally retarded	0–6	66	39
Combined Home-Center				
ERIN Project, MA	Combination	2–7	25	26
Preschool/Families Project, ND	Combination	0–6	35	30
Teaching Research Project, OR	Combination	1–8	20	—
MAPPS Project, UT	Combination	0–5	120	77
Communication Project, WA	Speech/language	0–6	39	43

type of program is most effective for each child and each family. Listed below are some of the key dimensions of early intervention that are still open to question.

Setting of program   Whether the program takes place in a home-based, center-based, or combination of home- and center-based setting will determine a great deal about what type of intervention services are offered. Related to the issue of program setting is whether the services are provided in an integrated (with other nonhandicapped children) or self-contained setting. Furthermore, there is a great deal of variation within each of these categories. For example, a center-based setting might occur in conjunction with a day care program, educationally based classroom-type setting, or a clinic setting in a hospital (see Chapter 7).

Instructional Grouping   What proportion of the intervention is delivered in large groups versus small groups, versus one-on-one time with the child (see Chapter 8)? Related to this are questions about how much of the intervention time is *engaged learning time,* versus transition versus custodial time (see Chapter 15).

Duration/Intensity of Services   How often are services provided (e.g., number of sessions per month), how long does each session last, and what is the expected duration of services? This dimension raises issues about the relative effectiveness of massed versus distributed learning. Another important question is related to the percentage of time that scheduled services are actually provided.

Staffing   What type of staff is necessary for an appropriate early intervention service? Should these services be carried out by certified, noncertified, or even paraprofessional staff? How many disciplines should be represented (e.g., occupational therapists, behavioral therapists, nutritionists, physicians, music therapists, adaptive physical education teachers, and so on) (see Chapters 5 and 8)?

Type of Services   Related to the type of staff available are additional questions about the configuration and availability of services. For example, does the program provide routine medical/health care, major medical health care, swimming, psychological services for the family, and so on (see Chapter 3)? Furthermore, are these services available to all those who need them, only available to children and families who have the most urgent needs, available through referral to other agencies and programs, or not available at all (see Chapter 4)?

Family Involvement   Even though Public Law 99-457 stipulates that early intervention should be family-focused, there is a great deal of disagreement about what constitutes family involvement. Are parents expected to act as interventionists, or are services provided to assist family members in learning to cope with and manage a handicapped child? To what degree do parents become involved in program governance and educational planning for their child, and is there access to respite care? Moreover, to what degree are various options available directly from the program, or by referral to other programs, and how extensively are these options utilized by parents (see Chapter 16)?

Philosophical Orientation   Undergirding all of the dimensions outlined above is the philosophical orientation that guides the early intervention program. Figure 1.1 summarizes some of the key dimensions along which programs vary with respect to philosophical orientation.

Obviously, early intervention programs can vary in many dimensions. Research is only beginning to provide answers about which dimensions are important and which programs are best for each child.

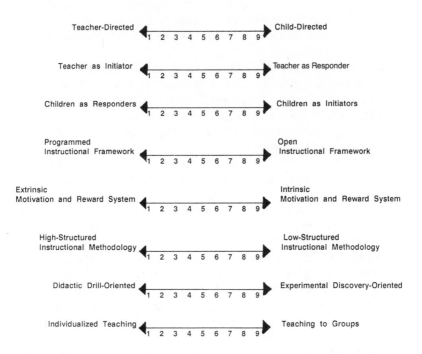

Figure 1.1. Components of philosophical orientation that vary among intervention programs.

ECONOMIC CONCERNS

In a time of shrinking resources for social service programs in general, additional questions are raised by the tremendous variation in early intervention costs. Surprisingly, very little effort has been devoted to analyzing the costs of early intervention services. The Early Intervention Research Institute at Utah State University, Logan, Utah, suggests that costs should be considered simultaneously with effects in drawing conclusions about which early intervention programs are most appropriate for each child (Barnett, 1986; Barnett & Escobar, 1987; White, in press). However, very few data are available at this point to draw conclusions about the relative cost-effectiveness of different early intervention alternatives (see Chapter 3).

The questions would be much less difficult if resources for providing early intervention programs were unlimited. However, in a time of finite or even shrinking resources for early intervention programs, costs are becoming more and more important. Consider the information shown in Table 1.3, which indicates that different types of early intervention programs can have dramatically different annual costs per child. The costs range from a low of $1,370 per year

Table 1.3. Estimated costs associated with serving 20 children in various types of early intervention programs

Alternative	Teachers	Aides	Home or visits	Therapy and support services	Administration	Supplies	Child transportation	Staff transportation	Technical assistance	Assess/ diagnosis	Building	Total	Cost per child
Home-Based 1 x month	—	—	14,667	6,000	840	500	—	2,400	600	2,000	400	27,407	$ 1,370
Home-Based 4 x month	—	—	44,000	6,000	4,200	500	—	9,600	600	2,000	1,200	68,100	3,405
Center-Based 5 x week (full day; mild/moderate)	52,800	24,000	—	6,000	4,400	4,500	16,000	—	600	2,000	8,000	119,300	5,965
Center-Based 5 x week (½ day; severe)	26,400	12,000	—	6,000	4,200	500	16,000	—	600	2,000	4,000	74,700	3,735
Center-Based 5 x week (full day; severe)	105,600	48,000	—	8,000	8,400	4,500	16,000	—	600	2,000	8,000	201,100	10,055
Center- and Home-Based 5 days/week and 4 x month (full day; severe)	105,600	48,000	26,400	8,000	12,600	4,500	16,000	9,600	600	2,000	9,200	242,500	12,125

per child, to a high of $11,825 per year per child. A specific location could vary the prices of the calculated figures. Given a finite budget, decisions about what type of program is offered may affect the number of children to whom services are provided. Financial assistance from the federal government will remain a relatively small amount of the total funding, since Public Law 99-457 is only authorized to provide a maximum of $1,000 per child. Many expect the actual financial assistance to be much lower (see Chapter 4 for other methods of program expansion).

THE ROLE OF RESEARCH IN DESIGNING EARLY INTERVENTION PROGRAMS

Research is the scientific search for answers to questions. At first glance, the current situation seems like an ideal opportunity for research to illuminate the complex and often contradictory variables that must be considered in deciding what types of early intervention programs to provide. Research does have an important role to play. But before deciding where research could be most helpful, it is important to step back and realize that hundreds of research studies have already been conducted. However, these studies have not been too successful in resolving many of the same issues that are now being faced.

There are at least three reasons that past research has been unsuccessful in resolving many of these issues. Understanding those reasons will explain why past research has not been conclusive and to plan the direction of future research. First, it is important to realize that a number of variables contribute to decisions about whether or not to provide early intervention programs. This was pointed out in 1981, in a report from the National Academy of Sciences, which concluded:

> As the growth in public programs that benefit children has accelerated, questions about how those services can be provided most equitably and efficiently have become more insistent. Controversies among elected officials, practitioners, and parents concerning public policies affecting children have become more intense and widespread. Because these issues are both value laden and political, they will not be resolved by research alone. (p. 2)

The point made by the National Academy of Sciences should be clear. Research is not required on whether someone ought to have enough food to eat or whether there ought to be neonatal intensive care units. Such decisions are made based on societal values, and a sense of obligation to fellow human beings. Once such decisions have been made, research can address how well services are being provided or the relative effectiveness of various alternatives. However, research should not be used as a tool to decide whether or not to provide such services.

Fortunately, the passage of Public Law 99-457 eliminates concern about whether or not early intervention services should be offered. The law points the way to the more fruitful and important debate — what is the most cost-effective way to provide early intervention services to each child?

A second reason why past research has had limited impact is that research has often been implemented to defend or to refute an existing position. Funding patterns, at the time, provided only enough resources for program evaluation, not for true comparison (see Chapter 6).

A third factor that has limited the use of past research is that those concerned about the welfare of young children tend to be optimists, and, consequently, often interpret data more optimistically than deserved. Indeed, many of the statements that are made about early intervention efficacy have been based more on optimism than fact. For example, when President Lyndon Johnson signed the Head Start Act into law, he said, "As a result of Head Start, 30 million man-years, the combined life span of these youngsters, will be spent productively and rewardingly, rather than wasted in tax-supported institutions or welfare supported lethargy." Even to those who support Head Start programs, it must be clear that Head Start has not had the far-reaching impact predicted by President Johnson. The same is true of many of the other statements made about the effectiveness of early intervention programs. It would be nice if early intervention programs could enroll children with established handicaps, and graduate them without any handicaps. The fact that early intervention, even if effective, cannot do this for the wide majority of enrolled children does not mean that it is not a worthwhile endeavor. However, the contribution of research to improving early intervention programs can only be realized if the findings of research are interpreted realistically and objectively.

In summary, research will be most useful in contributing to the improvement of early intervention programs if it: 1) focuses on the correct question (what type of early intervention is best for which children?), 2) is used objectively to investigate alternative types of intervention programs, and 3) is interpreted realistically instead of being used to support hopes that may be unrealistic.

A BRIEF SUMMARY OF EARLY INTERVENTION RESEARCH FINDINGS

Since the early 1980s, the Early Intervention Research Institute at Utah State University, Logan, Utah, has collected more than 2,000 different articles that have addressed the effectiveness of early intervention programs. Many of these articles are program descriptions, philosophical statements, or did not actually report data. However, approximately 600 different articles that reported the results of more than 400 studies of early intervention research have been systematically analyzed and summarized. Each of these articles was carefully coded as to the type of intervention provided, the nature of participating children and families, the type of experimental design utilized, the outcomes measured, and the results. Although space does not permit a complete discussion of this effort (see Casto & Mastropieri, 1986; Casto, White, & Taylor, 1983; White & Casto, 1985, for more complete discussions), it is useful to consider briefly some of the major conclusions of that analysis.

First, the analysis underscores the fact, noted earlier in this chapter, that early intervention is a multifaceted undertaking. The term is used to refer to such a wide variety of interventions, with such dramatically different groups of children, that research results can be, and often are, misleading. Children who participate in intervention programs range from low birthweight infants with no discernible delays to profoundly retarded deaf-blind infants and preschoolers who, heretofore, have often spent their lives in custodial institutions. Frequently, applied interventions range from rocking low birthweight babies on waterbeds in neonatal intensive care units, to comprehensive interdisciplinary, educational, psychological, and medical intervention services beginning at birth and lasting through the preschool years. The annual cost of early intervention programs per child ranges from a few hundred dollars to tens of thousands of dollars. Given this range in terms of type and comprehensiveness of intervention programs, and the variety of populations of children served, it is easy to see how simple answers to the questions, *Is early intervention effective?* and/or *What kind of early intervention is best?* can be incomplete and misleading.

A second conclusion that can be drawn from the analysis of existing literature is that a lot of the previously completed research does not meet rigid criteria for scientific research (cf., Bricker, Bailey, & Bruder, 1984; Dunst & Rheingrover, 1981; Simeonsson, Cooper, & Scheiner, 1982, for similar conclusions). Most of the more scientific studies have been done with disadvantaged children, but there are some studies with handicapped and at-risk children.

The area about which we know the most concerning the efficacy of early intervention is with disadvantaged children. Based on dozens of studies of reasonably fair methodological quality, it is clear that well-conducted intervention programs produce substantial immediate effects as measured by child progress. Typically obtained effects are of the magnitude of eight points on an IQ test, or one year's worth of reading gain at the second grade, or movement from the 10th to the 22nd percentile on a test of motor functioning or self-concept. These are substantial gains that are clinically significant by any standards. The evidence for immediate gains of this magnitude for disadvantaged children, as can be determined, holds up across different types of interventions, conducted in different settings, by different types of interveners. There is some, but not conclusive evidence that more comprehensive programs of longer duration and more highly-structured programs are more effective. However, there are no data that either confirm or refute many other commonly held positions such as earlier intervention being better, or that programs that involve parents are more effective than programs that do not.

Although there is abundant evidence for substantial immediate effects with disadvantaged children, the evidence concerning long-term benefits is more equivocal. Considering only those studies that compared children who received intervention to children in a randomly assigned control group, the majority of the studies demonstrate very small residual effects 4 years after intervention is completed. However, there are several notable exceptions to this trend. One is the Perry Preschool Project (Berrueta-Clement, Schweinhart, Barnett, Epstein, & Weikart, 1984), an exceptionally well-designed and executed study that shows dramatic increases in high school graduation rates, employment, and reduction in crime and teenage pregnancies, as a result of early intervention programs.

For handicapped children, the data are less clear-cut, and there are much less data available. Based on approximately a dozen carefully designed studies, there is evidence of similar, but slightly smaller, effects for handicapped children (e.g., six points on an IQ test or movement from the 10th to the 19th percentile in terms of language or motor functioning). These types of gains have been found for children with various handicapping conditions and with interventions that focus on diverse therapies such as motor functioning, cognitive stimulation, and language. At the present time, there is no evidence from well-designed studies, either pro or con, concerning the long-term effects of early intervention for handicapped children.

The most striking and important conclusion from the Early Intervention Research Institute analysis of previous research is that, as mentioned previously, far too little research has been devoted to the questions of what type of intervention is best with which children. The majority of previously conducted research has focused on the more general question of whether or not early intervention should be provided, rather than more specific questions concerning the relative effectiveness and cost-effectiveness of one type of intervention versus another type. There need no longer be any question about whether or not early intervention should be provided. The real issue is what type of intervention is best?

WHAT ANSWERS ARE NEEDED FOR THE FUTURE?

In an enlightened society, answering certain questions provides a data base that generates new questions. Certain questions always appear more vital and more timely. Today's early intervention research questions concern issues such as:

When should intervention begin?
What type of parental involvement is optimal?
How intense should intervention programs be?
How can we effectively assess child and family needs?
What training is needed for professionals?
How can professionals learn to work together?

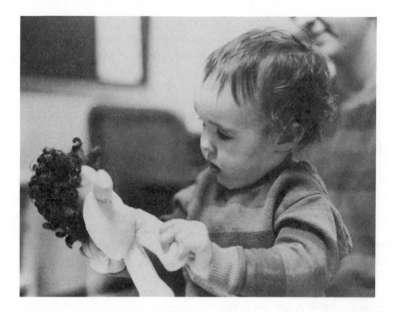

Tomorrow's research will focus, most probably, on more refined questions coming from what is learned while looking for answers to today's questions. Certainly, there will be research after tomorrow's research. But those needing to implement programs today cannot wait for answers to today's research, because children and their families need services now. This book is a representation of what is known today that can be used today . . . and hopefully tomorrow. . . .

SUMMARY

This chapter shows how the passage of Public Law 99–457 will alter the focus of future early intervention research. Instead of asking whether intervention is effective, future research will focus on what type of intervention is best for which children. This chapter highlights how the benefits of previous early intervention research has been limited by the types of questions addressed, the purpose for which it was conducted, and the way in which it was interpreted. In the future, research can play an increasingly important role by focussing on the effects and costs of alternative types of intervention services.

STUDY QUESTIONS

1. What early intervention services are available for families in your state/ community?

2. Which agencies provide services to families of handicapped infants and preschoolers. How long have the agencies been providing these services?

3. How many children are served in your state/community and what kind of problems do these children have?

4. What is the philosophy/goal of the various serviceproviders?

REFERENCES

Barnett, W. S. (1986). Methodological issues in economic evaluation of early intervention programs. *Early Childhood Research Quarterly, 1,* 249–268.

Barnett, W. S., & Escobar, C. M. (in press). The economics of early intervention for handicapped children: What do we really know? *Journal of the Division for Early Childhood.*

Bennett, F. C. (1984). Neurodevelopmental outcome of low birthweight infants. In V. C. Kelley (Ed.), *Practice of pediatrics* (pp. 1–24). New York: Harper & Row.

Berrueta-Clement, J. R., Schweinhart, L. J., Barnett, W. S., Epstein, A. S., & Weikart, D. P. (1984). *Changed lives: The effects of the Perry Preschool Program on youths through age 19* (Monograph No. 8). Ypsilanti, MI: High/Scope Press.

Bricker, D., Bailey, E., & Bruder, M. B. (1984). The efficacy of early intervention and the handicapped infant: A wise or wasted resource. In R. Wolriach & D. Routh (Eds.), *Advances in developmental and behavioral pediatrics: A research annual* (Vol. 5, pp. 373–423). Greenwich, CT: JAI Press.

Casto, G., & Mastropieri, M. A. (1986). The efficacy of early intervention programs for handicapped children: A meta-analysis. *Exceptional Children, 52,* 417–424.

Casto, G., White, K. R., & Taylor, C. (1983). An Early Intervention Research Institute: Efficacy and cost studies in early intervention. *Journal of the Division of Early Childhood, 7,* 5–17.

Congressional Report. (1987). *Report accompanying the Education of the Handicapped Act Amendments of 1986* (House of Representatives Report No. 99–860). Washington, DC: National Center for Clinical Infant Programs.

Datta, L. (1977). The external implications of an internal review of effectiveness: The DHEW Education Division's Joint Dissemination Review Panel (ERIC Document Reproduction Service No. ED 156–217). *Education Division's Joint Dissemination Review Panel: Three papers.* New York: EPIE Institute.

Dunst, C. J., & Rheingrover, R. M. (1981). An analysis of the efficacy of infant intervention programs with organically handicapped children. *Evaluation and Program Planning, 4,* 287–323.

Fang, W. L. (1981). *The Joint Dissemination Review Panel: Can approved submittals be distinguished from rejected ones on the basis of presented evidence of effectiveness related to cognitive objectives?* Doctoral dissertation, University of Virginia, Charlottesville.

McCormick, M. C. (1985). The contribution of low birthweight to infant mortality and childhood morbidity. *New England Journal of Medicine, 312,* 82–90.

National Academy of Sciences. (1981). *Services for children: An agenda for research.* Washington, DC: National Academy Press.

National Diffusion Network. (1983). *Educational programs that work.* San Francisco: Far West Laboratory for Educational Research and Development.

Odom, S. L., & Fewell, R. R. (1983). Program evaluation in early childhood special education: A meta-evaluation. *Educational Evaluation and Policy Analysis, 5,* 445–460.

Office of Special Education and Rehabilitative Services. (1985). *Seventh annual report to Congress on the implementation of the education of the handicapped act.* Washington, DC: U.S. Department of Education.

Philip, A. G. S., Little, G. A., Polivy, D. R., & Lucey, J. F. (1981). Neonatal mortality risk for the '80s: The importance of birthweight/gestational age groups. *Pediatrics, 68,* 122–130.

Ramey, C. T., Bryant, D., Sparling, J. J., & Wasik, B. H. (1985). Educational interventions to enhance intellectual development: Comprehensive day care versus family education. In S. Harel & N. J. Anastasiow (Eds.), *The at-risk infant* (pp. 75–85). Baltimore: Paul H. Brookes Publishing Co.

Sellick, K. J., & Over, R. (1980). Effects of vestibular stimulation on motor development of cerebral-palsied children. *Development Medicine in Child Neurology, 22,* 475–483.

Simeonsson, R. J., Cooper, D. H., & Scheiner, A. P. (1982). A review and analysis of the effectiveness of early intervention programs. *Pediatrics, 69,* 635.

Tallmadge, G. K. (1977). *Ideabook: The Joint Dissemination Review Panel.* Washington, DC: U.S. Office of Education.

White, K. R. (in press). Cost analysis in family support programs. In H. Weiss & F. Jacobs (Eds.), *Evaluating family programs.* Hawthorne, NY: Aldine.

White, K. R., & Casto, G. (1985). An integrative review of early intervention efficacy studies with at-risk children: Implications for the handicapped. *Analysis and Intervention in Developmental Disabilities, 5,* 7–31.

Chapter 2

Determining Eligibility for Specialized Intervention

Assessment in Handicapped Infants and Toddlers

Robert K. Rittenhouse and Helen Mitchell

●

Determining the eligibility criteria for early intervention services will be an ongoing challenge for planners and implementors of early intervention services in each state with the passing of Public Law 99-457. Obviously, no state will be willing to provide intensive services to infants and families who do not require specialized services, but in order to determine which children and families may benefit from each of the various services, the wisdom of several professions will be required. For example, medical personnel may know more about the effects of birth defects than other professionals, psychologists may be better able to measure cognitive ability, and social workers may be more equipped to determine the effects of the child's home life unlike other professionals. In each state and community, this professional judgment must be applied to local circumstances and to the needs of the patrons of the community. Complicating the early identification of children who are handicapped or at-risk is the interventionists' lack of confidence in any single measure that has been proven to work.

In spite of the fact that predictions made during the early developmental period about the child's future capabilities may not hold the scientific rigor that would be desired, there are some guidelines for identification of infants and toddlers that would benefit from additional services.

The process of determining eligibility for specialized intervention beings with public awareness of the importance of services and community screening procedures that are designed to identify the infants and toddlers that need a formal assessment.

WHAT IS ASSESSMENT?

The assessment of handicapped toddlers has come to mean a rather formal and sophisticated activity that has been described as "Normed or statistically valid tests that follow standardized procedures used to determine the developmental progress. . . " (p. 4). This is no small task indeed! When W. H. Auden proclaimed that "No statistic can ever compete with the single intuitive glance" (p. 1), he had something much less complicated, and far more individualized in mind (Rittenhouse, 1977). The complex nature of child development suggests that certainty about the diagnostic findings made through clinical assessment is neither warranted nor helpful. Although the kind of information obtained from such evaluation is important to better understand the toddler and how to help him or her grow mentally and emotionally, the information that is obtained using *clinically accepted* practices must be supplemented. Clinical procedures miss much of what happens when a human being interacts with another person or with his or her environment, and when these experiences are internalized. Through extensive observation, interview, and actual interaction, one is able to begin (and only begin) to assess the abilities of the handicapped toddler.

While this chapter describes some of the many diagnostic avenues available to parents of handicapped toddlers, and since clinical data are important to have, practical suggestions for using other nonstandardized means to arrive at a *diagnosis* are also described. Diagnosis appears in italic because the actual diagnosis is never really made. Human development involves innumerable processes and changes, making the *diagnosis* merely a momentary description. The deaf, blind, or retarded toddler, diagnosed as disabled, does not benefit from a label defined by statistical averages. Labeling a child as such may limit his or her potential, which in turn may lead to unrealistically low expectations in the adults who serve the child. This chapter describes children, birth through the early developmental years, and covers child behaviors recognizable to almost everyone.

PROBLEMS IN ASSESSMENT

Methods and tests used to assess handicapped toddlers have been widely criticized due to their small number and the lack of sensitivity to human development. Nevertheless, there is a need to identify and use statistically valid and appropriate assessment measures in order to identify which children need assistance and the extent to which early intervention can help the toddler and his or her family. In the not so distant past, the benefits of early assessment focused on the toddler's IQ and disregarded developmental and emotional domains

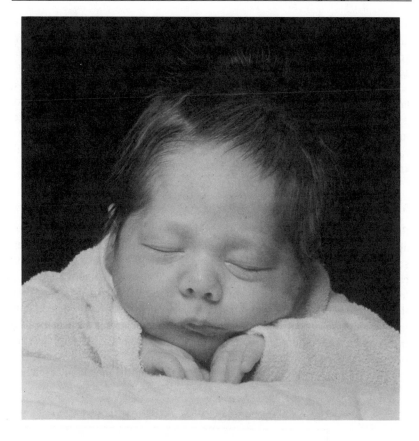

as well as the adaptability of the family. The use of IQ tests and other norm-referenced measures in favor of criterion-referenced tests are now being questioned as valid means for measuring the value of early intervention (Shonkoff, 1983). Whereas norm-referenced tests compare a toddler's performance to a statistical average or scale of what others have done, the criterion-referenced test indicates what one must do to master a particular skill and/or if the skill has been mastered (Mott et al., 1987). (See Chapter 6 for a discussion of criterion-referenced and norm-referenced tests.)

In addition to using instruments that provide more constructive information, early intervention assessment emphasizes the entire family unit and its influence on the toddler's development. These instruments are commonly referred to as *family measures* (Mott et al., 1987) (see Chapters 6 and 16). The result of this current review or approach to assessment has been (at least on the surface) to include and even emphasize the dynamic relationship between a toddler and his environment, particularly, and usually, his family environment. Even though this new approach is very significant, it is not without limitations.

These limitations are just as significant as the new direction assessment has taken. The principal problem of accurately describing the effect that early intervention has (or does not have) on the toddler and his family still remains. This awareness of test limitations has led to the inclusion of nonstandardized methods for obtaining information. Some such methods include parent interviews, home visits, observation, and other more personal means in assessment programs. These methods are elaborated on later in the chapter. Generally speaking, assessment can be seen as medical or behavioral, and standardized or clinical, as seen in Figures 2.1 and 2.2. It is also true that various professionals will emphasize different types of assessment, as shown in Figure 2.3.

MEDICAL ASSESSMENT

Parents, educational diagnosticians, and interventionists learn a great deal about handicapped toddlers from the family pediatrician and other medical personnel who come into contact with the child. From diagnosis to rehabilitative care, it is probably the pediatrician and the medical staff to whom the parents look first for guidance. While there has been concern about the estranged relationship that exists between physicians and educators, much has also been written about the major contributions that the field of medicine has made in the lives of handicapped toddlers and their families. The challenge is to improve the process and content of the communication.

There are several prenatal and neonatal medical-diagnostic interventions

	MEDICAL	BEHAVIORAL
Standard	Prenatal *Amnio* *CUB* *Ultrasound* Postnatal *LBW* *Apgar* *PKU*	Denver Battelle Bayley
Clinical	Sensory Brazelton	Ambulation Reflex Videoevaluation Behavioral samples

Figure 2.1. Assessment by professionals.

	MEDICAL	BEHAVIORAL
Standard	temperature weight height alertness	response to interview questions parent-child interactions
Clinical	food intake sleep patterns skin color posture	child play daily care games

Figure 2.2. Observation by parents.

that are used to identify abnormalities that might affect the child's developmental potential. For further reference, *Human Development*, by Diane Papalia and Sally Olds (1986), offers a more detailed explanation of these medical evaluations.

DISCIPLINE	ASSESSMENT
ob/gyn	prenatal
pediatrician	neonatal and post-birth health
nurse	health
audiologist	hearing
speech pathologist	speech and language
physical therapist	ambulation
occupational therapist	functional movement (e.g., self-care, feeding)
psychologist	cognitive fuctioning/social interaction
teacher	learning
parents	daily routines

Figure 2.3. Specific assessments by various disciplines.

Prenatal Assessment

Chromosomal Abnormalities Each cell contains 46 chromosomes that collectively provide direction for physical characteristics and development. When chromosomal development does not proceed normally, abnormalities may develop. Some chromosomal defects are inherited and some are adventitious, occurring during the development of the fetus. Down syndrome, the most common chromosomal disorder, is caused by an extra chromosome 21, or the dislocation of a part of that chromosome onto another chromosome. This disorder occurs once in every 900 live births and usually causes developmental delay.

Prospective parents may benefit from genetic counseling if they have any concerns about one or both of their family histories, or if they are anticipating parenting when one or both of the parents is over the age of 35. The genetic counselor may be a pediatrician, the family doctor, or a genetic specialist.

To the trained eye, physical appearance can give a clue to certain genetic abnormalities. Complete family histories are taken, as well as a medical exam. There are also sophisticated laboratory examinations that can be performed when appropriate. These include amniocentesis, chorionic villus biopsy, ultrasound, maternal blood test, fetoscopy, and electronic fetal monitoring.

Amniocentesis The detection of some kinds of birth defects is now possible through a procedure called *amniocentesis*. At approximately the 15th week of pregnancy, a sample of the amniotic fluid is drawn and analyzed. While it is not possible to detect all defects, this procedure is extremely accurate in identifying nearly 100 inborn errors of metabolism, spina bifida, and anencephaly (a rare defect in which all or part of the brain is missing). It is considered to be a relatively safe procedure as well (Golbus, 1979).

Chorionic Villus Biopsy Chorionic villus biopsy is similar to amniocentesis in that it takes an embryo sample (in this case, tissue from the embryo membrane environment) and analyzes it for the presence of several conditions. CVB is performed earlier than amniocentesis and the test results are available faster. It is also a highly safe procedure.

Ultrasound A picture or sonogram of the fetus can be obtained by directing high-frequency sound waves into the abdomen. The picture can help to detect irregularities, but the procedure itself is only recommended if there are specific medical indications of an abnormality, as there are possible harmful side effects (National Institute of Health, 1984).

Maternal Blood Test Between the 14th and 20th week of pregnancy, a maternal blood test can be performed (and usually is) to indicate whether there is a need for further examinations, such as amniocentesis or ultrasound.

Fetoscopy Fetoscopy is a procedure that helps to diagnose several disorders through direct contact with the fetus. A tiny *telescope* is inserted into the uterus, or blood may be drawn from the fetus.

Electronic Fetal Monitoring   The heartbeat of the unborn child can be monitored, and the ongoing results can reveal fetal irregularities. While providing valuable information, it has risks for both the mother and the fetus.

While test results do not provide absolute possibilities, they do provide the parents with mathematical probability for producing a handicapped child. Specific information concerning genetic diseases can be obtained by writing to the National Clearinghouse for Human Genetic Diseases of the Department of Human Services. The clearinghouse address is: 805 15th Street, Suite 500, P.O. Box 28612, Washington, D.C. 20050.

NEONATAL ASSESSMENT

A number of tests are available soon after birth, and some of these are performed routinely by the hospital before the baby leaves the hospital. Some of these tests provide only indications that the newborn may be at-risk, while others are more definitive.

Low Birthweight

Babies who weigh less than 3 pounds at birth are especially at-risk. They account for about two-thirds of the babies who die in the first month of life (U.S. Department of Health and Human Services, 1980). These babies are commonly called *preemies*. However, some low birthweight babies go the full gestational term and they are called *small-for-date* babies. These babies are significantly less likely to have a handicap than premature babies.

Apgar Scale

The Apgar test is administered at 1 minute after birth and again at 5 minutes after birth, and includes five basic, nonintrusive observations that can be made by the attending nurse. Infants receive a rating of 0, 1, or 2 on each observation, with the highest overall score being 10. Ninety percent of normal infants score 7 or better. A score below 7 means that the baby needs help to establish breathing. A score of 5 or less means that the baby is at-risk and needs immediate life-saving treatment.

The Apgar score at birth is thought to be statistically related to later development in the baby. Low-Apgar babies are more likely to be motorically and cognitively delayed than normal Apgar babies and also are more likely to have neurological, hearing, and vision disorders (Mahoney, 1984; Serunian & Broman, 1975).

The Apgar Scale is named after its developer, Dr. Virginia Apgar (1953), and can be used when highlighting the five medical observations that are made: appearance (color), pulse (heart rate), grimace (reflex irritability), activity (muscle tone), and respiration (breathing). Table 2.1 describes the Apgar rating scale.

Table 2.1. Apgar Rating Scale

Observation	Rating		
	0	1	2
Appearance (color)	Blue, pale	Body pink, extremities blue	Entirely pink
Pulse (heart rate)	Absent	Slow (<100)	Rapid (>100)
Grimace (reflex irritability)	No response	Grimace	Coughing, crying, sneezing
Activity (muscle tone)	Limp	Weak, inactive	Strong, active
Respiration (breathing)	Absent	Irregular, slow	Good, crying

Brazelton Neonatal Behavioral Assessment Scale

The Brazelton Neonatal Behavioral Assessment Scale (BNBAS) takes about 30 minutes to perform and is also given soon after birth. This test measures how the newborn responds to his or her environment by assessing alertness and cuddliness; reflex, muscle tone, and hand-mouth activity; self-control over crying (how well the baby quiets himself after crying); and the startle reflex (Brazelton, 1973).

Phenylketonuria Exam

Phenylketonuria (PKU) is a metabolic disorder and it, along with several others, can be detected immediately after birth through a screening test. Upon detection, a special diet is begun, and the effect of PKU (mental retardation) is curbed. While PKU is rare (1 case in 14,000 live births), as are other metabolism disorders, hospitals routinely screen for them. However, parents are advised to check with their hospital if there is concern.

Sensory Exams

Observational exams are performed in the hospital to determine the relative status of the newborn's hearing and vision. After the first few hours of birth, the newborn begins to respond differentially to visual and auditory stimuli. These responses can be observed through heart rate measures and body movements.

While these observations are routinely made in most hospitals, parents can also observe the child for the medical conditions described, and ask the pediatrician to repeat observations that may have borderline results. Although these physical symptoms may indicate medical problems, they do not necessarily also indicate problems in psychological development.

BEHAVIORAL ASSESSMENT

It is not uncommon for handicaps to go undetected by pediatricians during the prenatal and neonatal stages as well as while the baby is developing. This is because the tests that were described earlier can be either misinterpreted or mishandled, and also because symptoms of handicaps often do not emerge until after the newborn leaves the hospital. Parents and other immediate care-providers can identify areas of concern not noticed by medical evaluators. When a handicap does emerge, the pediatrician may not detect it unless the mother reports possible irregularities. Therefore, parents should observe their baby at home for abnormal physical responses to environmental stimulation. For example, a baby who does not flinch or jerk when a loud noise occurs may be hearing-impaired and should be examined more closely. Careful observation by parents is helpful. Later in this chapter, *games* and activities that can be used at home to help observe the developing baby's progress are given. Early emerging behavioral signs are also evident in motor development.

Motor Development

Basic motor skills in healthy babies do not need to be taught; they emerge normally as long as the baby is in an environment that provides him or her with freedom of movement. As the baby learns a new skill on his or her own, he or she practices it independently until he or she is good enough to go on to the next preordered motor behavior. These skills become part of the baby's repertoire of motor skills that develop into complex physical abilities that provide the baby with more opportunity for learning. Theories of child development are based on the infant's early motor skills, including Piaget's description of sensorimotor intelligence discussed later in this chapter (see also Chapter 11 for a discussion of Piaget's work).

Infants have reflex behaviors that are not as purposeful or thought-through as learned motor skills and tend to disappear as the neurologically healthy baby develops. The complete absence of these reflex behaviors or their prolonged maintenance can be an indication of mental retardation, brain damage, or a neurological disorder. Table 2.2 presents reflex behaviors that are present in healthy babies, the stimulation that the mother can provide to provoke them, and the approximate age at which they tend to disappear (see Chapter 10 for a more complete discussion of motor development).

A parent who has concerns about his or her new baby, either because of a low Apgar score or for some other reason, can be taught to stimulate these reflexes from the baby and chart the responses. Any irregularities or perceived irregularities should be reported to the pediatrician along with the documented observation.

All healthy babies reach motoric milestones that parents can observe and monitor. These behavioral milestones are particularly important indications during the child's first year. Although the normal range is indeed wide, with no real *average* baby, research indicates that there are *average ages* at which babies reach normally occurring motor milestones (Behrman & Vaughan, 1983). Table 2.3 (pp. 31–32) shows seven basic motor skills learned by the

Table 2.2. Reflex behaviors of healthy babies

Reflex	Stimulation	Behavior	Age of dropping out
Placing	Backs of feet drawn against edge of flat surface (e.g., kitchen table)	Pulls foot away	1 month
Grasping	Palm of hand stroked	Makes a strong fist and can actually hold onto something, such as Dad's finger, sufficiently tight enough to be raised	2 months
Tonic neck	Lay down on back	Head turns to one side or the other, extends arms and legs on one side and flexes opposite limbs	2 months
Walking	Hold under arm with bare feet touching flat surface	Makes step-like movement that looks like actual walking	2 months
Startle	Sudden and unexpected noise such as a loud bang or being dropped on bed	Will extend legs, arms and fingers, arch back and draw back head	3 months
Swimming	Place in water face down	Will make well-coordinated swimming movements	6 months
Babinski	Stroke bottom of foot	Toes will fan out, foot will twist in	6–9 months
Rooting	Stroke cheek with finger or nipple	Head will turn and mouth will open, sucking movements will begin	9 months

developing baby and the average age at which he or she begins to master them (see Chapter 10 for description of motor skills intervention).

Cognitive Assessment

Developing babies show other signs of intelligence in addition to the basic motor abilities just described. Their thinking or cognitive abilities are overt, and to one who observes, they become increasingly more complex. At about 18 months to 2 years, they begin to talk or use language. Language is a highly complex system of symbols used to represent thinking or ideas. In toddlers, this is part of normal development, just as natural as learning to walk (see Chapter 9 for a discussion of language intervention). When language fails to develop normally, parents should be concerned as problems may be present. Again, the key to *assessment* is the observant family who knows what to look for and who reports irregularities to the pediatrician, or in the case of young toddlers, to the pediatrician and the special education department at the local school.

Intelligence is an elusive quality; in babies and toddlers, it is especially

Table 2.3. Basic motor skills learned by the developing baby

Motor skill	Behavior	Average age learned
Head control	The baby will turn his or her head from side to side and lift it enough to turn himself or herself. The baby will first lift his or her head while on his or her stomach. After mastering this skill, he or she will hold his or her head up independently while being held, and finally while on his or her back.	Birth–3 months
Rolling over	The baby will first begin to purposefully roll over from stomach to back and later from back to stomach. There are times when the baby will accidentally roll over before the skill is actually learned.	5–6 months
Sitting	The baby will first sit alone with assistance from mother in assuming the correct position. Later, the baby will get himself or herself into a sitting position independently. The act of learning to sit comes through repetition. The baby will either get up from a lying position or plop down from a standing position.	6–9 months
Pre-walking locomotion	The baby intentionally gets around before he or she actually learns to walk, and does this in a number of ingenious ways. He or she wriggles on his or her belly and pulls with his or her arms; he or she scoots in a sitting position; he or she *bear walks* on all fours; and he or she creeps or crawls on his or her hands and knees.	7–10 months
Standing	With a helping hand, the baby can stand long before he or she does so independently. Having had this experience, he or she will quickly hold onto a piece of furniture and after a few months pull himself or herself up. Finally, he or she can stand alone without any physical support other than his or her own two little legs.	8–14 months
Manipulation	The baby goes through a whole array of manipulative behaviors in a sequence from simple (grasping a moderate-sized object at 4 months) to complex (placing 6 cubes neatly on top of the other at 2 years). After learning to grasp a moderately sized object, the baby learns to transfer it to the other hand. Soon thereafter, he or she can hold a tiny object (like a pea) but can't coordinate his or her fingers well enough for a couple of months to pick it up. Six months later, the baby can pick up the pea and put it into a container and turn it over. At about this time, the baby can coordinate his or her fingers well enough to begin piling stackable objects such as cubes on top ot each other so that over approximately a 9-month period, he or she gets pretty good at this, finally stacking them 6 cubes high.	4 months–2 years

(continued)

Table 2.3. *(continued)*

Motor skill	Behavior	Average age learned
Walking	A month after first standing alone, the baby will unsuccessfully attempt to walk. Within a few days, he or she is walking (although shakily), and the milestone that all parents hope for has fortunately arrived in the healthy baby. As with the emerging manipulative skills, there are an array of complex walking skills that begin at 9–11 months when the baby walks with assistance, to standing on one foot at age 3 years. Soon after walking and practicing with help, the baby begins to walk alone (usually around 15 months). Three months later, the baby begins to attempt running, which usually takes about 6 months to master.	9 months to 4 years
	At about the time the baby is beginning to attempt running, he or she begins to walk upstairs one foot after the other on the same step. By the time he or she is a toddler (age 3 years), he or she uses alternating feet, and a year later, he or she is walking down the stairs by himself or herself.	

difficult to define and measure (see Chapter 11 for a discussion of cognitive development). In later development, language is fairly easily recognized even though it can be difficult to characterize or evaluate. There are a number of infant and child developmental scales that are reasonably sensitive to normal language development. Three of the more widely accepted ones are described in this chapter. For the family who wants to make at-home observations of their children, there is a framework for monitoring the developing baby's progress. This framework comes from the theory of Jean Piaget. Piaget's belief, which is now almost universally accepted, was that toddlers, children, and, to some extent, adolescents, actually rationalize about their own world differently than do adults. This belief, seemingly unquestioned by most on the surface, is commonly rejected in practical situations. For example, the question, "Is a rock alive?" would seem to have but one plausible answer. However, for Piaget, it could have many answers depending on the rationale of the person answering the question. While most psychologists were interested in the rightness or wrongness of an answer, Piaget was interested only in the rationale. From careful observations and countless experiments, he redefined intelligence.

Piaget's theory is reported in many sources, including some 50 books written by him. However, John Flavell's book *Cognitive Development* (1977) is an especially clear and accurate summary. The first two stages of Piaget's four-stage theory are the sensorimotor stage and the pre-operational stage. The sensorimotor stage involves the developing baby in increasingly complex interactions with his or her environment. This stage is concluded at about age 2 years when the toddler comes to realize that things such as toys, brothers and sisters, and family dog (e.g., people and things that he or she has come to know) exist even though he or she may not hear or see them. This ability to internalize or to know that there is a permanence or stability to his or her environment, provides the foundation on which language develops. The toddler need not see Spot to say "Spot"; he or she can call for Spot because he or she has come to know that Spot exists even though he or she does not see him. Table 2.4 shows the six substages of Piaget's sensorimotor stage and the approximate ages at which they emerge.

The next stage of development, called the pre-operational stage by Piaget, is marked by the full emergence of language. Apart from the child's newfound speech, thinking at this stage is also unique. Table 2.5 shows the key points of this stage. (Chapter 11 on cognitive development provides an expanded description of all of Piaget's stages.)

Thinking also becomes more complex, and even though the developing toddler tends to be bound to the here and now for most of his or her understanding, he or she is able to engage in conversations about familiar events and things that are not visually present. While the baby usually does not utter his or her first word until a year or older, a number of language or prelanguage behaviors begin to emerge before that initial utterance (see Chapter 9 for a more in-depth discussion of language development). Table 2.6 sequences prelanguage and language development in normally developing babies and toddlers.

There are a number of tests used to assess the abilities of babies and toddlers. They are commonly used for either screening or assessment purposes.

Standardized Assessment

Assessment is the process of obtaining an objective measure of a sample of an individual's performance on a given type of task. This sample is then compared with a criterion for performance or with other individuals' performances on the same tasks in order to *assess* the individual's status or progress in a given area. The Bayley Scales of Infant Development and the Battelle Developmental Inventory are commonly used assessment devices. The Bayley covers the chronological period from birth to 30 months and is largely a motor cognitive and language test. The Battelle has been standardized on handicapped infants and toddlers and has adaptations that make the testing of handicapped children reliable. The Battelle, introduced in 1984, is being used in a major longitudinal research study of early intervention in handicapped children ages birth to 5 years being conducted by Utah State University (White, 1985). It assesses development across five developmental areas, including language, cognitive, motor, social, and adaptive. The Battelle also includes techniques for data gathering through observation and parent interviews as well as the direct testing of the baby or toddler. Table 2.7 (p. 36) is a listing of some widely used tests developed for use with infants and toddlers.

Before concluding this section on developmental milestones and tests used

Table 2.4. Substages of Piaget's sensorimotor stage

Substage	Behavior	Age
Use of reflexes	The baby only exercises his or her reflexes through repeated, jerking movements in an effort to gain control over them.	Birth–1 month
Reactions to behaviors	At this stage, the baby will repeat an action that led to pleasure but that occurred by accident. For example, the baby who is exercising may accidentally put his or her hand in his or her mouth and then intentionally suck as such stimulation is pleasurable.	1–4 months
Repetition of pleasurable behaviors	The developing baby shows more interest in his or her environment and more purpose to his or her behavior. He or she will now repeat actions that bring about interesting results. For example, he or she may continue to hit at an overhead crib toy because each time he strikes it, it moves, and he or she finds pleasure in it. At this substage also, the baby will begin to search visually and physically for partially visible toys or objects that he or she has been playing with. The little toy elephant that gets pushed partially under the playpen blanket is still the same little toy elephant, and he or she will look at it and try to retrieve it.	4–8 months
Coordination of various behaviors	The developing baby is now able to coordinate rather effectively two or more learned behaviors and do so in a purposeful, goal-directed manner. A toy that he or she was playing with earlier and now spots across the room can be gotten by locating it visually, crawling to it, and picking it up. The baby can now do a particular behavior well. Also, at this substage, the baby will search for an object that has completely disappeared; however, if he or she does not find it where he or she thought it disappeared to, he or she will not look anywhere else.	8–12 months
Creative manipulation of behaviors	The baby now begins to experiment with his or her environment by varying his or her learned behaviors in interactive situations. The baby begins to explore the *possibilities* of his or her environment by doing new things with old things. The toy elephant is now stood on its head or is placed on top of the toy horse. The search for the elusive object becomes more persistent, although the baby will not search for it in a place that he or she has not seen it placed. For example, if the toy elephant slipped under the blanket and then as the baby went to get it, was pushed under further, the pursuit will continue. However, if mom or dad intervened and put it back with the other toys unbeknownst to the baby, pursuit of it ceases.	12–18 months
Mental representation	This final substage marks the emergence of language or speech in the toddler. The stability of the environment is now permanent and is reflected in the toddler's pursuit of his or her favorite things. The toddler can and does ask questions such as, "Mommy, where's Daddy?" The toddler now understands why certain things happen and can even appreciate his or her own actions. Imitative behavior emerges at this stage, even when the person he or she may be imitating is not present.	Beyond 18 months

Table 2.5. Key points of Piaget's pre-operational stage

Behavior	Age
Begins to play with objects in meaningful way (e.g., will put a cup on a saucer and pretend to stir)	21–24 months
Will move objects to represent real-life relationships (e.g., will take doll and make it pick up the cup and drink)	2½–3 years
Pretend play starts to emerge and people will be invented	3–4 years
Will dress up in adult clothes	4–5 years

to measure them, a sequence of early hearing and vision achievements is presented. These two senses play an important role in the life of the infant and toddler who is confronting his or her world, reacting to it, doing things to it, organizing it, and adapting to it. When one, or both of them, is impaired,

Table 2.6. Language milestones

Behavior	Age
Will move his or her body in the same rhythm as the adult speech he or she hears.	Birth
Distinguishes certain speech sounds that sound familiar (e.g., "Dad" versus "glad").	1 month
Baby begins to coo.	6 months
He or she will make sounds when being fed.	3 months
He or she begins to laugh.	4 months
Begins to link specific acts to words (e.g., if someone is putting on his or her coat to leave, the baby will say "bye-bye").	10–12 months
Utters first word.	1 year
Can say 10 words.	15–16 months
He or she will respond to limited commands (e.g., "Give Mommy the cookie").	16–18 months
He or she can say 50 words.	20 months
He or she can now put two words together.	20–24 months
He or she will begin to answer routine questions (e.g., "What is your name?").	21 months
He or she can say 272 words.	2 years
He or she can provide yes/no answers to questions about his or her environment (e.g., "Is Daddy sleeping?").	2 years
Word combinations begin to emerge.	2–2½ years
He or she can say 446 words.	2½ years
Can appropriately respond to "what" questions (e.g., "What is this?" [book]).	2½ years
Can answer "who" questions.	3 years
He or she produces "d'want" questions (e.g., "D'want me to go home?").	3 years
Can respond to "how" questions.	3½ years
He or she can say 896 words.	3½ years
Understands location words (e.g., "in," "on").	4 years
Can respond to "how much" questions.	4 years
He or she can say 1,540 words.	4 years

Table 2.7. Selected infant and preschool tests

Test	Age range	Test type	Areas assessed
Uzgiris-Hunt Ordinal Scales of Psycholog-ical Development (Uzgiris & Hunt, 1975)	0–2 years	Provides description of cogni-tive development based on Piagetian theory.	Sensorimotor development
Bayley Scales of In-fant Development (Bayley, 1968)	0–30 months	Evaluates infant developmen-tal status (standardized).	Cognitive func-tioning, motor skills, social behavior
Battelle Developmen-tal Inventory (New-borg, Stock, Wnek, Guidubaldi, & Suinicki, 1984)	0–8 years	Nationally standardized screening and diagnostic test. Determines strengths and weaknesses in five areas.	Personal social, adaptive, motor, communication, cognitive
Developmental Test of Visual-Motor Inte-gration (Beery & Buktenica, 1967)	2–15 years	Evaluates ability to integrate visual perception and motor behavior.	Integration of vi-sual perception and motor behavior
Goldman Fristoe Test of Articulation (Gold-man & Fristoe, 1986)	4–8 years	Measures discrimination abil-ity through response to tape-recorded stimulus.	Discrimination of speech sounds
Receptive-Expressive Emergent Language Scale (REEL) (Bzock & League, 1971)	0–3 years	Measures early language through parent interview. Yields Receptive Language, Expressive Language Age, and Combined Language Age scores.	Receptive language, expressive language
Peabody Picture Vo-cabulary Test (PPVT) —Revised (Dunn, 1981)	2½–18 years	Measures receptive vocab-ulary through pointing task.	Receptive vocabulary
McCarthy Scales of Children's Abilities (McCarthy, 1972)	2½–18 years	Determines general intel-lectual level, strengths, and weakness.	Verbal, percep-tual-perfor-mance, quan-titative, general cognitive, mem-ory, motor

developmental progress is often slowed. Table 2.8 gives a list of hearing and visual milestones and the age at which they begin to appear.

IMPLEMENTING SCREENING PROCEDURES IN THE COMMUNITY

Let us suppose there is a need to identify the children in a class of 30 who may have difficulty in development. To identify the children with the difficulties, an

Table 2.8. Hearing and visual milestones

Behavior	Age
HEARING MILESTONES	
Will tighten eyelids in response to sharp/loud sounds.	Birth
Will stop movements in response to sharp sound.	1 month
Will stop whimpering when a soothing voice is nearby, although will not stop if it is feeding time.	1 month
May cry or otherwise show alarm (e.g., quiver or blink eyes) when startled by a sudden loud noise.	1–3 months
Will smile when talked to or smiled at.	6 weeks–4 months
Will stop whimpering or will smile at the sound of mother's soothing voice.	3 months
Will turn head toward a sound that is coming from the side and at eye level (but not up or down).	4–7 months
Will stop what he or she is doing when he or she hears "no, no."	7–9 months
Will imitate "oh, oh."	7–9 months
Begins to respond to "bye-bye" in conjunction with his or her name (e.g., "bye-bye, _____").	9 months
Can differentiate between his or her mother's voice and a strange voice.	9 months
Can distinguish between speech and nonspeech sounds.	11–14 months
Locates sounds from any angle.	21–24 months
VISION MILESTONES	
Indifferent to faces.	Birth
Will look at a bright light over a dim light.	Birth
Begins to show color preference.	2 weeks
Tends to look at the top of things (e.g., a fruit jar or a milk bottle).	3 weeks
Will turn head and eyes toward light.	1 month
Will close eyelids tightly if a light is shone directly into eyes.	1 month
Will focus on things within reach.	2–3 months
Will look at rattle in his or her hand.	3 months
Will smile at the whole face, but not partial (e.g., Daddy playing peek-a-boo).	5–6 months

individual development test could be arranged for every child in the class. However, this would be costly and time consuming. A more efficient way of identifying children who might need extra help would be to give them a screening test. *Screening* is the process of selecting children for a major, thorough assessment by giving them a short test beforehand, thus eliminating those children who are not in need of complete assessment. A screening test simply answers the question, "Who are the individuals who may have problems and who are in need of a more thorough assessment?" The Denver Developmental Screening Test (DDST) is a good example of a widely used screening test. The DDST is a norm-referenced screening test for infants and children birth to 6 years old. It is used to detect developmental gross motor, fine motor, language, and personal-social delays and reports testing results as age equivalent scores. Psychometric data are available as well.

Child Find and Referral

Case-finding is the first step in locating infants and other preschoolers who require early intervention. Case-finding activities are designed to get agencies and individuals to refer at-risk infants and preschoolers for further study.

Case-finding involves a campaign to develop community awareness, and it requires setting up a system for referral of children, getting referrals, and canvasing the community for children who need screening. Recruitment of infants is best done through contact with pediatricians, public health nurses, intensive care units, and parent groups. Recruitment of preschoolers should be done through nursery schools, day care settings, and through public awareness activities. However, it may be more efficient to screen a number of children on the same day since all children are in need of screening as soon as they indicate an interest in a particular school. The screening process needs to be an ongoing activity and available for any child soon after the child's potential problem is identified.

Recommended Procedures

The National Program for Early and Periodic Screening, Diagnosis, and Treatment (EPSDT) suggests that screening should evaluate children from several key perspectives that affect development: biological, psychological, family context, and environmental and social/cultural variables unique to each child. Using this comprehensive approach, a screening program recommended by Peterson (1987) would include:

Pediatric examination

Developmental history obtained through interview of the parent(s) or primary caregiver, and possible use of a checklist or questionnaire to gather specific facts about the developmental history

Parental or primary caregiver input regarding special problems or concerns about the child

Evaluation of child's general developmental status using a screening instrument

Specialized developmental reviews (as determined by the services available, the child population, and the individual subject) in four domains: 1) physical status; 2) psychological/developmental status; 3) family status; and 4) environmental, social/cultural status. The psychological/developmental domain may include a review of cognitive development, emotional development, speech and language development, auditory perception, visual perception, self-help and adaptive skills, and motor development.

Trained Personnel

The screening process requires trained personnel including a developmental pediatrician, a pediatric nurse, and individuals from other disciplines (e.g., physical therapists, speech therapists, early childhood special educators, and psychologists). Once assembled, the screening team is trained in the assessment process and knows exactly what each team member does.

Parents should also be briefed about the screening process and be asked to participate, due to their wealth of observational information about their child.

After the Screening

Those children who are identified as requiring further study following the screening are referred to interdisciplinary teams for additional observation. A

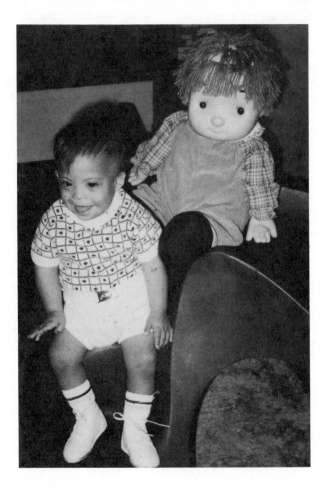

brief report is written on all of the children who participate in the screening. The assessment report is sent to the referring agency as well as to the parents.

PARENT OBSERVATIONS

A vital part of the referral process is informed parent observation. The most important thing that parents can do if they are concerned that their baby may be having developmental problems is to observe him or her in interaction with the environment and report those observations to the family pediatrician or the local special education program. Hearing losses or vision problems are probably the easiest handicaps to detect. However, these handicaps often go unnoticed if parents fail to recognize and report the signs. Two simple parent *tests* are offered in Figure 2.4 as examples of activities that can be used at home to keep track of the developing baby's progress, along with charts that can be used to trace developmental growth.

These activities can be modified to accommodate individual family situations. Figures 2.5 through 2.10 are forms that can be used at home to record the infant's or toddler's progress. The forms allow for 5 days of observation, since any child might be tired or uncooperative if measures are taken at only one time. For full descriptions of the behaviors, the reader is referred to the earlier detailed developmental charts in this chapter.

---

1. Obtain three distinct noisemakers (a small drum, a whistle, and clackers) and make noises with them at different distances and from different locations, and observe your baby's response.

   a. Baby winced. _____
   b. Baby turned in the direction of sound. _____
   c. Baby ignored sound. _____

2. Obtain a small toy that can be easily scooted across the floor. Engage the baby with it. While the baby is lying face up in the crib or playpen or being held on the floor by someone, slowly move or scoot it from side to side. Observe baby's response.

   a. Baby followed it. _____
   b. Baby saw and reached for it. _____
   c. Baby ignored it. _____

Figure 2.4. Parent tests for checking baby's developmental progress.

Tonic Reflexes/ Behaviors	M	T	W	TH	F	Comments
Placing						
Grasping						
Tonic neck						
Walking						
Startle						
Swimming						
Babinski						
Rooting						

Figure 2.5. Parent observation of reflexes.

Vision Behaviors	M	T	W	TH	F	Comments
Is indifferent to faces						
Prefers bright light						
Shows color preference						
Looks at tops of things						
Turns toward light						
Closes eyelids when light shines into eyes						
Focuses on objects within reach						
Looks at objects in his hand						
Smiles at entire face, but not partial face						

Figure 2.6. Parent observation of child's vision.

Language Behaviors	M	T	W	TH	F	Comments
Moves body in time with speech						
Distinguishes similar speech sounds						
Begins to coo						
Produce noises when feeding						
Begins to laugh						
Links acts to words						
First word						
Can say 10 words						
Responds to limited commands						
Can say 50 words						
Puts two words together						
Anwers routine questions						
Can say 272 words						
Provides yes/no answers						
Puts 3-4 words together						
Can say 446 words						
Answers "what" questions						
Answers "who" questions						
Produces "d'want" questions						
Answers "how" questions						
Can say 896 words						
Understands location words						
Answers "how much" questions						
Can say 1540 words						

Figure 2.7. Parent observation of language behaviors.

Hearing Behaviors	M	T	W	TH	F	Comments
Tightens eyelids when noise is made						
Stops movement when sharp noise is made						
Stops whimpering when hears soothing voice						
Shows alarm						
Smiles when talked to						
Responds to mother's voice						
Turns head toward sound						
Stops what he is doing when hears "no-no"						
Imitates "oh-oh"						
Responds to "bye-bye"						
Differentiates between mother's voice and stranger's voice						
Distinguishes between speech and nonspeech						
Locates sounds from any angle						

Figure 2.8. Parent observation of child's hearing.

Motor Behaviors	M	T	W	TH	F	Comments
Head control						
Rolling over						
Sitting						
Prewalking locomotion						
Standing						
Walking						

Figure 2.9. Parent observation of motor activities.

Cognitive Behavior	M	T	W	TH	F	Comments
Use of reflexes						
Reactions to behaviors						
Repetitions of pleasurable behaviors						
Coordination of various behaviors						
Creative manipulation of behaviors						
Mental representation						

Figure 2.10. Parent observation of cognitive development.

SUMMARY

By more accurately observing the handicapped infants and toddlers, a more precise determination of each child's eligibility can be achieved and more helpful early programs can be implemented for the child and family. No matter what the level of observational skill by parents or professionals, improvements can be made by knowing exactly what to look for with the children. These keen observations, coupled with good clinical information, can provide a basis and guidepost for identifying infants and children who need services and for planning the most appropriate early intervention for each child.

STUDY QUESTIONS

1. Is there infant or preschool screening for handicapped children in your state/community?
2. What are the referral procedures for early intervention programs in your state/community?
3. What assessment materials are used in the local/state early intervention program?
4. What is the eligibility criteria for early intervention services for infants and preschoolers in your state/community?

REFERENCES

Apgar, V. (1953). A proposal for a new method of evaluation of the newborn infant. *Current Researches in Anesthesia and Analgesia, 32,* 260–267.

Bayley, N. (1968). *Bayley Scales of Infant Development.* New York: Psychological Corporation.

Beery, K. E., & Buktenica, N. A. (1967). *Developmental Test of Visual-Motor Integration.* Cleveland, OH: Modern Curriculum Press.

Behrman, R., & Vaughan, V. (1983). *Nelson textbook of pediatrics* (12th ed.). Philadelphia: W. B. Saunders.

Brazelton, B. (1973). *Neonatal behavioral assessment scale.* Philadelphia: J. P. Lippincott.

Bzock, K. R., & League, R. (1971). *Assessing language skills in infancy: A handbook for multidimensional analysis of emergent language.* Gainesville, FL: Tree of Life Press.

Dunn, L., & Dunn, L. (1981). *Peabody Picture Vocabulary Test* (rev. ed.). Circle Pines, MN: American Guidance Service.

Flavell, J. (1977). *Cognitive development.* Englewood Cliffs, NJ: Prentice-Hall.

Golbus, M. (1979). Prenatal genetic diagnosis in 3,000 amniocenteses. *New England Journal of Medicine, 300,* 157–163.

Goldman, R., & Fristoe, M. (1986). *Goldman Fristoe Test of Articulation.* Circle Pines, MN: American Guidance Service.

Mahoney, T. (1984). Large-scale high risk neonatal hearing screening. *Seminars in Hearing, 5,* 25–36.

McCarthy, D. (1972). *Manual for the McCarthy Scale of Children's Abilities.* New York: Psychological Corporation.

Mott, S. E., Fewell, R., Lewis, M., Meisels, S., Shonkoff, J., & Simeonsson, R. (1987). Methods for assessing child and family outcomes in early childhood special education: Some reviews from the field. *Topics in Early Childhood Special Education, 6,* 1–15.

National Institute of Health. (1984). *Osteoporosis: Concensus development conference statement* (Vol. 5[3], 1984-421-132:4652). Washington, DC: U.S. Government Printing Office.

Newborg, J., Stock, J. R., Wnek, L., Guidubaldi, J., & Suinicki, J. (1984). *Battelle developmental inventory.* Allen, TX: DLM Teaching Resources.

Papalia, D., & Olds, S. (1986). *Human development.* New York: McGraw-Hill.

Peterson, N. (1987). *Early intervention for handicapped and at-risk children.* Denver: Love Publishing.

Rittenhouse, R. (1977). *The development of conservation in deaf and normal hearing children.* Unpublished doctoral dissertation, University of Illinois, Champaign.

Serunian, S., & Broman, S. (1975). Relationship of Apgar scores and Bayley mental and motor scores. *Child Development, 46,* 696–700.

Shonkoff, J. (1983). The limitations of normative assessments of high-risk infants. *Topics in Early Childhood Special Education, 3,* 29–43.

Uzgiris, I., & Hunt, J. (1975). *Assessment in infancy: Ordinal scales of psychological development.* Urbana: University of Illinois Press.

White, K. R. (1985). An integrative review of early intervention efficacy studies with at-risk children: Implications for the handicapped. *Analysis and Intervention in Developmental Disabilities, 5,* 7–31.

U.S. Department of Health and Human Services. (1980). *Pre-term babies* (DHHS Publication No. ADM 80-972). Washington, DC: U.S. Government Printing Office.

ADMINISTRATIVE CONCERNS

———————— • ————————

Before any services can be provided to families, efficient and effective administrative structures must be in place. These structures must allow for appropriate communication among serviceproviders. Since focusing on the child's developmental enhancement through the family structure is much more complicated than emphasizing only child needs, professional preparation and role relationships are more significant and staff development is more vital. Ongoing evaluation of the effect of the programming is essential. Planning and coordination is necessary in order to provide specialized services to families in the least restrictive environment.

Chapter **3**

Understanding
Program Costs

W. Steven Barnett and Colette M. Escobar

———————————— • ————————————

Many people recognize that there is an important economic dimension to programs that serve young handicapped children. This is a time when both public and private funding agencies are acutely aware of costs, as well as growing human service needs in many areas (Halpern, 1981). It is also a time when knowledge regarding the economic benefits of early intervention programs is increasing (Barnett, 1986). In this environment, people who operate and advocate for early intervention programs may find it useful to develop a working knowledge of an economic perspective on early intervention. The purpose of this chapter is to introduce the reader to an economic approach to programs for young handicapped children—how to think about economic costs and benefits. The authors hope that this approach will contribute to improvements in developing, planning, and managing early intervention.

COST ANALYSIS

The most obvious and readily measured economic aspect of early intervention is program cost. How much a program costs is a critical consideration for policymakers, program managers, and funding agencies in making decisions about service provision. The economic approach to measuring cost is not the same as the accountant's approach, however. The economic approach is more comprehensive and revealing, and provides better guidelines for making decisions (Barnett, 1986; Thompson, 1981). In this section, the economic approach to cost analysis is illustrated with a simple hypothetical example. In the course of presenting the example, the basic principles of cost analysis are discussed.

An Example: Costs of Clinic- and Home-Based Alternatives

A university program to serve young children with communication disorders is considering the best way to expand its service program. The program currently offers two options. One is a clinic-based program in which children come to the University Speech and Language Center for therapy in individual, small group, and large group settings for a half-day, 5 days a week. A speech clinician, several teachers, and student teachers deliver intervention in the clinic. The other is a home-based program in which parents are taught to incorporate therapy into ordinary interactions with their children and to create a language-stimulating home environment. Parents participating in the home-based program are expected to attend training sessions at the clinic. There are four sessions, each lasting $2^{1}/_{2}$ hours. In order to compare the two options, the University collected data on child progress and conducted cost analyses for one semester of the program.

Economic analysis of costs begins with a definition of the problem (above example) and a complete description of all of the program's resources. Levin (1983) refers to this as the *ingredients* approach. Listing all the ingredients, or resources, that go into providing a service is one of the best ways for a program's administrator, or someone who is contemplating beginning a new program, to develop a clear picture of what a program costs. In this case, the University Speech and Language Center began by listing resources that it uses. These fall into two broad categories: personnel (e.g., teachers, aides, therapists, administrative, support staff); and nonpersonnel (e.g., facilities, equipment, materials and supplies, insurance, utilities, miscellaneous expenses such as the hearing evaluations received by each child entering the program). In addition, the University Speech and Language Center noted that there were some services that the program required that the clinic did not pay for out of their budget. These *donated* services included the amount of time that parents and students provided intervention services, and transportation to and from the clinic.

The basic information about the program ingredients and their costs was organized by the set of data collection forms presented in Figures 3.1 and 3.2, and also in Tables 3.1 and 3.2. Figures 3.1 and 3.2 present a detailed account of personnel resources and their costs. Programs for young children tend to be "people intensive," and this is usually the most important category to attend to in a cost analysis. The remaining information about other program resources and their costs is summarized in Tables 3.1 and 3.2, that are also used to total costs and calculate the average cost per child for each type of program.

Personnel Costs

Figure 3.1 lists all of the paid personnel engaged in providing direct services and calculates their costs. Cost includes all of the benefits paid (e.g., retire-

Program Name *University Speech and Language Center*

A	B	C		D	E	F				G	H
				Period of Employment	Total Salary	Benefits				Total Benefits	Total
Position	FTE	Salary	Per	From — To		FICA	Insurance	Retirement	Other		
Home-based											
Speech Clinician	.25	$25,000	yr.	Semester	$3125	————— 25 % —————				$ 781	$3906
Research Assistant	.25	$ 6.00	hr.	Semester	$ 390	————— none —————					$ 390
Administration											$ 768
Clinic											
Clinic Supervisor	.33	$19,000	yr.	Semester	$3167	————— 25 % —————				$ 792	$3959
Class Teacher	.50	$ 4.40	hr.	Semester	$1144	————— none —————					$1144
Assistant Teacher	.50	$ 4.40	hr.	Semester	$1144	————— none —————					$1144
Student Clinic Super	.50	$ 5.60	hr.	Semester	$1456	————— none —————					$1456
Materials Person	.25	$ 3.35	hr.	Semester	$ 436	————— none —————					$ 436
Student Clinic Super	.50	$ 5.60	hr.	Semester	$1456	————— none —————					$1456
Administration											$1774

Figure 3.1. Paid personnel and their costs.

Program Name *University Speech and Language Center*

A Type of Volunteer	B Activity	C Total Days or Service Hours	D Hourly Rate	E Estimated Value
HOME-BASED				
Parents	Parent-training program	9.5 hours		
	Therapy in the home	7 hours		
	Clinic Observation	1.75 hours		
	TOTAL	18.25 x 20 parents 365 hours	$10.50 / hour	$ 3,833
CLINIC				
Practicum Students	In-class therapy	130 hours x 12 students 1560 hours	$3.35 / hour	$ 5,226

Figure 3.2. Value of volunteer time donated by parents and students.

Table 3.1. University Speech and Language Center resource costs: Home-based program (1986 dollars)

Resources	Total cost	Paid by program	Private contributions (donations)
Personnel			
Salaried staff	$ 5,064	$5,064	
Volunteers	3,833		$3,833
Capital assets			
Facilities	806	806	
Equipment	178	178	
Transportation	2,357		2,357
Materials/supplies	95	95	
Utilities	173	173	
Insurance	115	115	
Miscellaneous	350	350	
TOTAL COST	$12,971	$6,781	$6,190
Cost per child[a]	648	339	310

[a]Number of children = 20.

ment, health insurance, the employers' share of social security tax), as well as the salaries paid. In this case, only two of the staff received benefits. However, in some preschool programs, most of the staff receive benefits, and omitting the cost of benefits could lead to serious underestimation of costs. As can be

Table 3.2. University Speech and Language Center resource costs: Clinic program (1986 dollars)

Resources	Total cost	Paid by program	Private contributions (donations)
Personnel			
Salaried staff	$11,369	$11,369	
Volunteers	5,226		$5,226
Capital assets			
Facilities	1,863	1,863	
Equipment	1,119	1,119	
Transportation	4,089		4,089
Materials/supplies	300	300	
Utilities	399	399	
Insurance	266	266	
Miscellaneous	350	350	
TOTAL COST	$24,981	15,666	$9,315
Cost per child[a]	1,249	783	401

[a]Number of children = 20.

seen, calculating the cost of direct service personnel is a relatively simple matter because it is easy to determine what they are paid and how much of their work time is devoted to each program.

Also included in Figure 3.1 is a cost for the administrative and support personnel required to operate the programs. Unfortunately, it is not as easy to determine the exact contribution of the members of a large organization who do not provide direct service. In this case, there were many people at the University who were required to keep the preschool programs operating, but whose specific efforts for the programs could not be measured (e.g., department heads, secretaries, clerks, bookkeepers, groundskeepers, payroll clerks, vice presidents, maintenance personnel). The total cost of these people to the University, as a whole, could be determined if needed. Thus, their contribution to the program was estimated based on the percentage of the total University budget represented by the clinic's programs. Typically, an approximation like this has to be used to estimate the cost of operating any program within a larger organization. A variety of reasonable rules can be used to estimate a program's share. For example, in a school district, the percentage of teachers or the percentage of students in a program relative to the district total might be used.

Volunteer Costs

Figure 3.2 records the amount of volunteer time that parents and others donate to the program and is used to calculate the costs of people who worked but were not paid. The home-based program required parents to participate in training and then to take time to deliver the service at home. Parent time can be estimated from using mail surveys and program records. In Figure 3.2, parent time represents the average amount of time spent in three intervention-related activities: 1) the parent training program, 2) application of therapy techniques in the home, and 3) in-clinic observations. The clinic program used students to help provide therapy. Both programs required parents to provide transportation. Although the volunteers did not cost the programs anything, they were not "free" from the economist's perspective. To begin with, parents and students were required to participate, making their efforts not entirely voluntary. Both parents and students pass up other productive activities in order to engage in early intervention services. This is called an opportunity cost. The opportunity cost of the volunteer ingredient is calculated as the value of the forgone activities.

Estimating the dollar value of opportunity costs is one of the most difficult tasks of economic analysis. In this case, the simple, but practical, assumption made is that a minimum estimate of opportunity cost for volunteer time would be the earnings that students and parents could make from employment. Knowing that many students were employed on campus at the minimum wage rate of $3.35/hour (U.S. Department of Labor, 1986), an estimate of their opportunity cost was calculated. For parents, the opportunity cost was calculated by using a

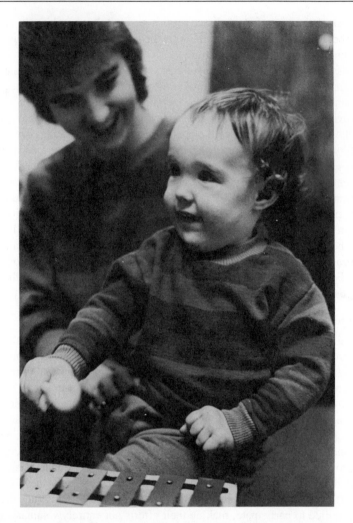

national average rate of total compensation (salary plus benefits: $10.50/hour). For a more in-depth study, the actual compensation rates earned by each parent can be used. In estimating opportunity cost, it is important not to make the mistake of assuming that parents who are not employed outside the home have no time costs. One reason they may not be employed is that they place a value on their time at home that is higher than they could earn in the labor market.

The costs of time for parents of young handicapped children may be quite high. One must be particularly sensitive to the demands on parents' time (that are very high for any infant or preschooler), and the parents' lack of time for recreation and relaxation (Dunlap & Hollingsworth, 1977). A program that places great demands on parent time, assuming that it has a zero cost, can result in parents either not participating as fully as expected, or not implementing program activities at home for the designated amount of time. Consequently, parents who do comply with the program's time demands may experience increased stress or disruption of family function (e.g., other children in the family get less attention). Thus, the program could have unanticipated negative effects on the family.

The home-based program that inspired this hypothetical example was designed to minimize parent costs. Parents were required to attend training sessions, including a visit to the center to observe therapy sessions, and to provide the therapy at home. However, the costs of training were minimized by keeping the training time down as much as possible and making attendance flexible. Make-up classes were provided so that parents weren't restricted to a single time for each session. Parents were also allowed to schedule observation visits any time the clinic was in session. Most significantly, the therapy was designed to be delivered primarily by altering the ways in which parents interact with their children, in their normal daily routine. Only 7 hours of special time were required at home; the rest of the intervention took place in ordinary interactions between parent and child. Thus, little extra time was required, most of the increase was temporary, and there was almost no need to change the amount of time that family members spent with each other or in various activities.

Nonpersonnel Costs

The nonpersonnel costs of the two types of programs are recorded in Tables 3.1 and 3.2. These other costs include materials and supplies, transportation, equipment, facilities, insurance, utilities, and miscellaneous expenses. The importance of these costs varies from program to program. Materials, supplies, and equipment are almost always a very small part of total cost. Transportation and facilities costs can be quite substantial. As can be seen from the tables, nonpersonnel costs are small in relation to personnel costs. In particular, insurance, utilities, materials, supplies, and equipment are not a large part of the costs in the University Speech and Language Center's analysis. Obviously, facilities costs were higher for the clinic-based program than the home-based program. Transportation costs were estimated based on information about mileage and driving time obtained from a parent survey. The time cost of parent drivers is nontrivial, even though parents did carpool.

The costs of materials, supplies, and other operating expenses such as utilities, communications, and insurance are almost always easily determined from a program's operating budget. In this case, the amount that each program spent on materials and supplies was ascertained from the clinic's accounting records. There were no donated materials or supplies so that this represented the entire cost. The amount spent on the other items could be determined for the clinic as a whole, but not for the two programs separately. Each program's share of these costs was estimated based on its share of total personnel costs.

The cost of equipment with a useful life of more than a year is slightly more complicated to determine than cost of materials and supplies. Classroom and office furniture, office equipment, medical equipment, kitchen appliances, and many other capital goods that early intervention programs use are typically not paid for on an annual basis. In other words, the cost of these items does not appear in each year's budget. In order to estimate the cost for the clinic programs, a list was made of the equipment used by each program. To estimate the annual cost of equipment, the replacement value of each item was estimated from current prices, and this value was "annualized" over 10 years. This is only one of several approaches to estimating equipment costs, as is explained below.

The cost of facilities are estimated in much the same way as the costs of equipment. The object is to obtain an estimate of the annual cost, and, again, there are several alternatives. In this case, the University charges the clinic an occupancy fee based on the amount of space that the clinic uses. Thus, the cost of facilities for the clinic as a whole was easily estimated by this fee. However, the total facilities cost was apportioned to the two programs based on the percentage of the space that each occupied over time. For example, the home-based program was charged for 25% of the cost of the speech clinician's office (the remainder of the office space cost is attributed to projects that required the other 75% of the clinician's time) and a small amount for the rooms used for the parent training sessions.

Total Resource Costs and Average Cost Per Child

In summarizing the information about program costs, Tables 3.1 and 3.2 present total cost and also the distribution of costs according to who pays for them. The average cost per child is quite modest for both options, although the home-based program is considerably less expensive. Both of the programs in this example have total social costs that are somewhat higher than the cost to the agency that provides the program. This is because of the costs borne by parents and university students who are not paid for their time. When all costs are taken into account, the home-based program is seen to be less costly by an even greater margin.

In order to be able to choose between the two options, the university clinic also collects data on each child's progress in language development. Given the cost estimates, if the home-based program is at least as effective as the clinic-based program, it makes sense to choose the home-based program for expansion. In fact, the home-based program is found to be more effective. In the case cited, the choice was obvious, the home-based program was better all around.

PROBLEMS IN COST ANALYSIS

Although the example discussed above is a relatively simple one, it illustrates the key concepts and some of the more important practical issues in cost analysis. Perhaps the most important concept is *opportunity cost*. From an economic perspective, the cost of an activity is the value of the resources used to conduct that activity, regardless of what is actually paid for those resources. The value of those resources is best measured by what they would have produced in their best alternative use. In other words, the costs of resources are the opportunities that are foregone in order to use them in the activity under analysis. In many cases, the opportunity cost of a resource can be approximated by what is paid for it. Thus, a teacher's salary and benefits or a building's rent closely reflects the value that those resources produce in their best uses. An individual's opportunity cost varies depending upon background, experience, and how much he or she values his or her leisure time. For example, the opportunity cost of the time that a doctor spends at a soccer match is much higher than that of a laborer, because the doctor earns much more on an hourly basis. Leisure hours typically are even more valuable, which is why employers pay higher rates for overtime hours worked. When a program takes the opportunity cost of its resources into consideration, it is getting a realistic picture of its value.

The importance of the concept of opportunity cost becomes clear when what is paid for a resource is not a good measure of its value. In some cases, what is paid may overestimate the cost of a resource (to society as a whole) because that resource does not have an alternative use, or its best alternative use may not be very productive. For example, if a project hires someone who is unemployed and could not otherwise find work, the opportunity cost may be close to zero. Similarly, if a program uses an empty classroom or vacant building, the opportunity cost is again close to zero, regardless of what is paid. In other cases, what is paid may underestimate the cost of a resource, as when rent or some other expense is subsidized. The most commonly underestimated costs are those of resources that are not paid for at all by a program. The most significant of these resources is probably parent time.

The Value of Parent Time

Most, if not all, early intervention programs require parent time. Parent involvement in program activities is a goal for most programs. At the very least, parent time is required for parents' participation in the development of Individualized Family Service Plans (IFSPs) and Individualized Education Programs (IEPs). In addition, programs may require (or at least pressure) parents to provide transportation for themselves and their children, to take part in home visits, to attend training sessions at a center, to volunteer in the classroom, or to work with their child at home. These activities may require more out-of-pocket costs to parents (e.g., purchasing transportation, buying gas for their own car, or hiring a babysitter for their other children). However, the out-of-pocket costs are likely to be slight in relation to the parents' opportunity costs.

Producing a precise estimate of the opportunity costs to parents is not an easy task. When parents are employed in the labor force, their wages and benefits earned, or compensation rates, reflect the value of their time. However, many mothers are not employed outside the home, and compensation rates cannot be observed for them. This presents a problem because most of early intervention programs' demands for parent time fall on the mother. One solution to the problem is to assume that time costs are the same for women in and out of the labor force. One way for programs to get some idea of the parents' time costs is to ask parents how much the program would have to pay to get parents to work for the program.

The issue of parent time costs is particularly interesting in light of the requirement under Public Law 99-457 that handicapped children ages 3–5 are to be provided with a *free appropriate education*. This has been interpreted as prohibiting programs from requiring parents to provide transportation because it requires out-of-pocket expenses. As yet, it has not been interpreted as prohibiting the imposition of opportunity costs on parents. However, the opportunity costs may be substantially higher than the out-of-pocket costs, as the university center example illustrates. As an illustration of the potential magnitude of these costs, consider a year-long, home-based program that requires parents to participate in a 90-minute home visit once a week and to conduct a program with their child for 15 minutes the other six nights. Using the average hourly compensation rate of American workers, the annual opportunity cost amounts to $1,575 for one parent and $3,150 for two parents (10.50/hr. × 3 hrs. × 50 weeks).

Many may object that parents volunteer because they want to participate even though they are not paid. They get something out of volunteering that offsets the opportunity cost. If they did not, then they would not volunteer. Thus, the net cost to parents can be assumed to be, at most, zero. This objection is valid, if there is no coercion. It is not valid if parents are expected to volunteer by program personnel or if parents believe that their children will not be served or will obtain inferior services if the parents do not volunteer. Also, parents may volunteer because they believe that there will be long-term benefits to the child that make the costs worth it. If parents are incorrect in this belief, then the costs are not offset.

Perhaps the most important issue, with respect to parent costs, is that if program planners assume that the costs to parents are insignificant, then they may find much less parent cooperation and effort than anticipated. This could cause an otherwise good early intervention to be ineffective. All of this is not to say that parent involvement is not highly desirable, just that it should not be assumed to be *free*.

Estimating Capital Costs

Capital costs present special difficulties for estimating and comparing the costs of early intervention alternatives. Capital expenditures may be unevenly distributed over time, as when a new building is constructed or a new classroom is furnished. For an ongoing program, much of the capital may have been purchased long ago and may even be totally paid for by the time of the cost analysis. Because of the difficulties, it is sometimes tempting to simply ignore capital. However, to do so leads to underestimation or uncertainty with respect to costs and a lack of comparability among cost estimates. Thus, cost analyses should estimate the cost of capital per program beneficiary in a way that allows accurate comparisons among programs and that identifies the amounts and types of capital resources needed to start up a program.

To estimate the cost per program beneficiary, the costs of capital (which lasts for many years) must be converted to an annual (or even shorter) basis in order to estimate the costs for the time that the average beneficiary uses it. For example, 4-year-old children who attend a preschool program will only use a classroom for one year. Obviously, the entire cost of the classroom and its furnishings should not be assessed to the children who use the classroom the first year, but to all of the children who will ever use it. This would be simple if the facilities are rented—the cost would be the annual rent. Even if the facilities in question are not rented, it might be possible to see how much rent is being paid for similar facilities in the same area.

Expenses for early intervention facilities and other capital may not be simple matters. They may be donated by a charitable organization or rented from a charitable organization at a special rate that is not available to just anyone. In such cases, the charity is essentially *paying* part of the rent, and the actual rent paid is not a good measure of cost. The capital may be owned by the intervention program or an even larger organization (e.g., a school, hospital, government agency) that does not charge the intervention an occupancy fee (a sort of internal rent that may or may not be subsidized). In such cases, it is necessary to estimate the opportunity cost of capital based upon that capital's replacement cost, its expected useful life, and the available interest rate (a measure of the foregone opportunities). A step-by-step description of this procedure is beyond the scope of this chapter, but can be found in Levin's (1983) lucid introductory text on cost analysis.

Regional Variation in Costs

Perhaps one of the most important things to keep in mind about costs is that they are highly local. It is very difficult to estimate the costs of a program in one place based on its costs in another. One reason is that there are large regional differences in the costs of labor and space. Urban, suburban, and rural costs may be very different even within the same state. Another reason is that when early intervention programs are small and not very widespread, there are plenty of opportunities to make use of slack resources such as school and church space that is underutilized. With such a situation, fairly small increases in the number of children served could produce a big impact on the average cost per child. Up to a certain point, the cost per child decreases as more children enter the program because expenditures on administration, space, and so on, do not need to increase. However, as enrollment continues to grow, the program cost may have to rise sharply to bring in the new resources and facilities required to serve children entering the program as slack resources are no longer available and expenditures rise. Another concern is that in some areas programs may experience constraints that are insurmountable. These constraints will affect the configuration of the program without regard to efficiency of its operation. Examples of such constraints could include: 1) no space for a classroom at any reasonable price, 2) unavailability of some types of staff, or 3) a lack of start-up funds for large purchases.

Variations in costs and constraints often lead to modifications of programs or program choices that make sense in one place, but not another. If everyone used the same model, almost every program would be less efficient than it could be. Cost analyses that are used to make local program decisions should be as local as possible in estimating costs.

METHODS OF ECONOMIC EVALUATION

Completion of the cost analysis of a program is half of the task of an economic evaluation. Generally, two techniques of economic evaluation are appropriate in early intervention: cost-benefit analysis and cost-effectiveness analysis. While these are identical in their analysis of costs, they differ in their treatment of the outcomes, or benefits, of a program. To conduct a cost-benefit or cost-effectiveness analysis, the authors recommend consulting texts by Levin (1983) and Thompson (1980), or Barnett's (1986) article. These contain in-depth discussions of the critical issues that arise in economic analysis, as well as the procedures for conducting such an analysis. The basic techniques are discussed below, as an introduction to familiarize those in early childhood special education with the language and methodology of economic analysis.

Cost-Benefit Analysis

In cost-benefit analysis, monetary values are estimated for costs and for program benefits, or effects. Cost-benefit analysis is a comparative analysis: the state of the world, with the program, is compared to the state of the world without it. The primary criterion for the selection of a particular program is that the benefits exceed costs by a margin wide enough to indicate a sound financial investment. Cost-benefit analysis may be quite complex. Its most significant drawback is that many of the benefits, or effects of early intervention are intangible and very difficult to translate into monetary values. By the same token, once accomplished, the beauty of cost-benefit analysis is that it puts many diverse outcomes of a program into a single, and widely understood, measure—dollars.

Cost-Effectiveness Analysis

Cost-effectiveness analysis seeks to estimate the economic value of all the resources used by a program. However, program effects are not put in monetary terms, making it easier to perform than cost-benefit analysis. Cost-effectiveness analysis is correctly applied when two or more programs, with the same goals, are analyzed and compared. For example, Program A may cost $5,000 and yield an average gain per child of 5 points on some developmental scale. Program B costs $8,000 and children gain an average of 15 points. Taken alone, neither of these results helps a policymaker to make a funding decision. However, a comparison of the results of Program A with Program B provides the basis for making a policy decision.

SUMMARY

Optimal economic evaluations focus on the value of all program ingredients, including those not directly paid for by programs. Program ingredients should be valued according to their opportunity cost to society to portray the true cost of operating the program. Exclusion of the value of contributed or borrowed ingredients, such as parent time, leads to an underestimation of the cost of the program and a misrepresentation on both sides of the cost-effectiveness or cost-benefit equation.

Conducting economic analyses for early intervention programs is a relatively new endeavor. However, such analyses are becoming more widely applied as shrinking funding sources compel programs to demonstrate an efficient and effective service delivery system. Decisionmakers and administrators within the early childhood special education field need to become acquainted with the method of conducting such an analysis, either to apply the techniques to their own programs or to be informed consumers of economic analyses.

STUDY QUESTIONS

1. What are the funding sources for early intervention in your state/community?

2. Do programs in your state/community own or rent the facilities?

3. Are salaries for professional staff comparable to those who may have similar training and who are working locally in other settings?

4. What funds are used to pay for transportation costs?

REFERENCES

Barnett, W. A. (1986). Methodological issues in economic evaluation of early intervention programs. *Early Childhood Research Quarterly, 1,* 249–268.

Dunlap, W. R., & Hollingsworth, J. S. (1977). How does a handicapped child affect the family?: Implications for practitioners. *The Family Coordinator, 26*(3), 286–293.

Halpern, R. (1981). *Economic analysis: A management and fund-raising tool for early childhood programs*. Ypsilanti, MI: Center for the Study of Public Policies for Young Children, High/Scope Education Research Foundation.

Levin, H. M. (1983). *Cost-effectiveness: A primer*. Beverly Hills: Sage Publications.

Thompson, M. S. (1980). *Benefit-cost analysis for program evaluation*. Beverly Hills: Sage Publications.

U.S. Department of Labor, Bureau of Labor Statistics. (1986). *Employment and earnings, 33*(5), 81. Washington, DC: Author.

Chapter 4

Increasing Services through Interagency Agreements, Volunteers, and Donations

Carol Tingey and Fredda Stimell

———————— • ————————

Becoming a "case manager" or contributing to the information to be used by a case manager is a new challenge for early intervention program staff who have been providing educationally oriented services or have been focusing only on the needs of the child (Garland, Woodruff, & Buck, 1988). Since the needs of the entire family are included in early intervention programs, it will be absolutely necessary to call into service the expertise of a variety of different agencies, not only for the ongoing needs during the early intervention years but also to provide smooth transitional services into school-age services for the family.

An almost infinite list of therapies, tutoring, counseling, transportation, medical and respite care, mental health, homemaker, and social services are needed to help promote child and family functions. With even the most generous agency budget, the cost of this variety and intensity of service needs for infants and young children who are experiencing difficulties in development may be excessive. However, it may be possible to literally stretch the typical budget by creative administrative planning that can provide needed services to children and families that cannot be purchased with the available limited or restricted funds. Some services may be within the jurisdiction of other agencies or provided by trained volunteers. Goods and services may also be donated.

INTERAGENCY AGREEMENTS

Agencies begin working together in the same way that people do, by getting to know one another and discovering their common interests. Of course, agencies don't actually meet and talk to each other. It is the people within the agency that must learn to relate to one another. Staff frequently become acquainted at conferences or workshops. LaCour (1982) suggests that one of the first steps is to create beneficial working relationships with the leadership of the agency or organization. Although it is necessary to study the rules and regulations of the other agency, it is also important to know the unwritten procedures for the transaction of day-to-day activities and how they are actually implemented in service delivery. This information can only be provided by someone who has successfully worked within the agency and who is, preferably, still employed there.

For actual discussion of a joint work scope, it will be necessary to deal with someone who can make or direct administrative decisions. In addition, other workers in the agency may become advocates for cooperative action within the system. Professionals, parents, and others who have been living or working in the geographical area for some time will probably have established some of these contacts or relationships. This can be the beginning of the discussion of cooperation that must, of course, be aired through the appropriate administration channels.

Deciding which agencies to approach, and for what services, can almost become a circular proposition. The early intervention project staff may have already identified a certain needed service and begun searching for an agency to provide that service. For other services, staff might go "shopping" in an existing service delivery agency to locate potentially important services that the agency may be providing but of which the staff and families may not be aware. Staff might also discover an existing agency to provide a particular service, but requests may not have come in to the agency (possibly because families did not know that the service could be made available). In some cases, the agency can provide the service by including qualified families of handicapped children in existing services begun for similar target groups. Occasionally, agencies will be seeking agreements with the early intervention project in order to comply with agency policy or mandates to provide services to children and families.

IT PAYS TO ADVERTISE

Rather than discussing program plans for extended services in staff meetings, projects may wish to advertise in various forms of media their need for assistance. For example, programs that have newsletters could run ads to locate an agency or service that might be able to provide 20 hours of respite care, at no charge, to families in the project. Since newsletters often reach more than staff and families, it is possible that someone in that large circle may have a friend or a relative who might be helpful. Such announcements can also be made in the local public media. A human interest story, highlighting needs and information, and placed in the public media, could be quite beneficial to an agency. If radio and television public service spots or personal appearances are used, it is important that they be aired at different times of the day to reach a variety of audiences.

Another way of announcing specific project interests is to become active in local professional associations, to attend public hearings for related issues, and to travel to other places where staff from other agencies may interface in service planning meetings concerning similar issues. Serving on committees in community and professional organizations can also be helpful. Although actual attendance may be low, just announcing an open house can help spread the word that the project is interested in the needs of families with handicapped children. Displays in public places such as libraries and shopping centers, and talks to service organizations, should include not only the good things that the project is doing, but the unmet needs that still exist.

It usually helps to create a brochure that describes the project and present it to interested parties. In order to attract sophisticated agencies, it is important that the brochure be dignified and attractive. Professional quality is possible, with little cost, if a clear original is taken to a good copy shop and produced on paper that is a bit heavier than letter paper. A typed list of needs could also be prepared.

FIRST THINGS FIRST

It is easier for each early intervention program to make a list of the services needed, then proceed immediately to secure all of them. Each program needs to determine which agencies to contact first, and what amount of effort to put into each contact. Sometimes this determination is made by the strength of the need; other times it is made by the strength of the existing relationship with the other agency. A currently available service may increase program effectiveness more than a grandiose service that takes years to negotiate. Cooperation on a simple project can help pave the way for a more intense cooperative agreement later.

Interagency agreements must be beneficial to each agency involved. Something should be provided to the other agency in order to secure the service needed. In negotiating these agreements, the following should be included in the calculations: the cost in time of providing the record keeping, exchange of documents, staff meetings, and other activities necessary to secure the service.

Sometimes after one agency agreement is made, it is easier to make agreements with others and to join a "network" of agencies that work together. It appears that at least facilitative agreements are necessary in order to assist families in securing services that promote family function, as required by Public

Law 99-457. This is particularly true for those families who are experiencing life stress unrelated to the handicapped child. In discussing the difficulty of protecting children's rights in complex organizational systems, Julius and Handal (1980) suggest that there be professional training for *systems negotiation*. This training might include procedures and processes to protect existing structures, mandates, and regulations, while allowing for adequate services to be provided with minimal red tape. It is necessary to clarify exactly who will perform the service, and whether it is provided directly to the child or family, or to the early intervention project. Only through such coordinated service delivery can services be provided to the whole person (Goldman, 1982; Ozarin, Shartstein, & Albert, 1981).

CONFIDENTIALITY

Whenever personal information concerning the child and the family is transmitted from one agency to another, it is necessary to have specific permission from the family to share that information with another agency (LaCour, 1982). This can be a particular problem if the information is in automated data systems (Lipscomb, 1980). It may be beneficial in the intial intake procedures to discuss confidentiality issues with the family, and to receive general permission to share some information, at least for the negotiation of services. It would be beneficial to the family if certain kinds of information such as birth history could be standardized so that it might be transmitted without repeated intake procedures. As interagency relationships become more secure, it may be possible to have one intake procedure or a central point of entry that would make early intervention and other agency services available through the same procedure. This, of course, would save time for the family as well as both agencies (LaCour, 1982).

GENERAL PROBLEMS IN INITIATING AGREEMENTS

Agencies may be reluctant to initiate agreements when: the services that the agency is providing must be clearly documented, and the diversity or the unique perspective of the agency must be preserved (Goldman, 1982). Other problems may arise from differences in the quality of service (LaCour, 1982), from difficulties in implementing third-party payment for services provided (Shartstein, 1982; Cummings, 1979), or from determining which agency pays a particular part of the costs (Gilman & Diamond, 1985; LaCour, 1982).

Steps in initiating an interagency agreement include:

1. Conducting a needs assessment to clearly identify essential, supplementary, or complementary services needed

2. Reviewing laws and regulations of your own organization and prospective cooperating organizations
3. Getting to know the leadership of the prospective organizations
4. Learning how the other organizations function both formally and informally
5. Explaining your mandates and needs to the other organization by both written documents and verbal discussion
6. Identifying the resources, services, and information to be exchanged
7. Examining the benefits to both agencies
8. Developing a draft of a written agreement that is acceptable to the leadership in both orgnizations

(Adapted from LaCour [1982] and Newman [1982].)

Although a written agreement appears to take more time than necessary, it is essential to the implementation of the details of the agreement, especially when there are large numbers of staff involved. The written agreement does not need to be long, and should be written in simple, clear language. It should include: 1) the reason for the agreement; 2) the responsibilities for each agency; 3) the standards for each activity to be performed; 4) the process for the exchange of information, including any forms that might be created for the process; and 5) methods and procedures to modify the agreement (LaCour, 1982). Figure 4.1 is a sample agreement between an early intervention program providing services to infants and children with Down syndrome and a hospital that provides assessment in hearing for the children. The actual agreement was an outgrowth of a more general agreement with a child development center at the same hospital. The agreement took a year to negotiate, and revisions are continually made.

VOLUNTEERISM

Providing service to others as a volunteer is just as much a part of modern America as it was when the early settlers grouped together to protect one another from dangers and to share in the care of the sick or aged. One out of two Americans volunteer for some worthy cause (Henderson, 1985). Volunteers provide services to the aged (Nettings & Hinds, 1984), abused (Wert, Fein, & Haller, 1986), and handicapped (Marrs, 1984), as well as others in need. Sometimes, volunteers are needed because of the lack of comprehensive services provided in rural locations (Marrs, 1984), because advocacy is needed for those unable to be responsible for themselves (Nettings & Hinds, 1984; Zischka & Jones, 1984), or because the person volunteering has a need to do something that is seen as worthwhile or contributing to a cause (Henderson, 1985; Marrs, 1984). In general, volunteers can provide more personalized service, and are frequently seen as creative and enthusiastic. They see their work as an oppor-

TO: Speech and Hearing Staff at Children's Hospital
FROM: Head Speech Therapist
         Early Beginnings Program

In the consultative arrangement between Children's Hospital Speech and Hearing Center and the Early Beginnings Speech Department for the Sept. ____–June ____ school year, the following points are agreed upon:

1. Staff from both programs will meet a minimum of two times during the calendar year.

2. The content of the meetings will be flexible, the goal being to better the existing speech and language programs at the Early Beginnings Program. Meetings will be either observational or discussion oriented and will stress:
a. Innovative speech and language programs
b. Therapy models
c. Sharing of material (both therapeutic and diagnostic)
d. Specific caseload concerns
e. New research in the field of speech, hearing, and language as particularly relevant to Down syndrome

3. At least one of the meetings will be at the Early Beginnings Program.

4. The Children's Hospital Speech and Hearing staff will remain available as a phone contact throughout the school year. These contacts will be on a regular basis.

5. Children's Hospital Speech and Hearing Center will remain a referral source for children of the Early Beginnings Program seeking additional private speech and/or hearing consultations.

6. The Children's Hospital Speech and Hearing staff will be available for any Early Beginnings staff members seeking input. The above has been read and agreed upon.

Signed:
_____   Date _____
_____   Date _____
_____   Date _____
_____   Date _____

Figure 4.1. Sample agreement between an early intervention program for Down syndrome children and a hospital.

tunity to provide something to others rather than an obligation (Henderson, 1985). Volunteers are doing the work because they place value on personal expression and growth rather than on social and economic success (Williams, 1986, 1987).

As more women (the traditional volunteer force) become employed and have less time for volunteer activity, a new source has become increasingly available—the older citizen (Henderson, 1985; Salmon, 1985; Tierce & Seelback, 1987). Today's volunteer is typically more experienced and therefore has the potential for providing more sophisticated service to the organization than past volunteers (Henderson, 1985; Salmon, 1985). Along with this trend for sophistication comes a need for the potential agency to become more professional about volunteers.

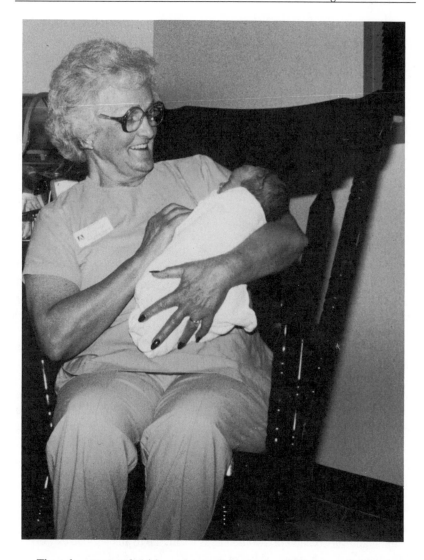

The advantages of paid employees include the ability to maintain closer organizational control over the work activities and to make sure that there is not a conflict of interest between the worker, agency, and/or client (Zischka & Jones, 1984). It is likely that these issues have been partly responsible for the growth of the attitude that only professional staff could provide services to those in need (Salmon, 1985). However, there are also some distinct advantages to the work that a volunteer might provide. The volunteer is likely to have more knowledge about the community and community resources and can function as a true advocate for the client. It is through this personal interest that the volunteer enhances the client's sense of competence and worth (Zischka & Jones, 1984).

Tasks Performed by Volunteers

Although there are certain activities within each agency that must be performed by paid staff, for wise leaders the list of jobs that volunteers might be "given" is extremely broad and includes such things as: 1) yard work, 2) personal care, 3) home care, 4) construction of special equipment, 5) teaching homemaking skills, and 6) assistance to secure other services (Marrs, 1984), as well as the more traditional assistant teachers or clerical work. A more mature volunteer or well-trained younger volunteer makes it possible to provide services in the home, such as collating papers or creating teaching materials (Salmon, 1985). Marrs (1984) suggests that nearly everyone can do *something* that can be beneficial to the agency. Mature volunteers have been most helpful in providing expertise at the level of organization and management of programs such as serving on a voluntary board of directors (Conrad & Glenn, 1983). Many volunteers have a significant effect on programs such as Herbert Stimell (1933–1986), who was a volunteer board member for 13 years and who generously assisted with conceptualization, development, and implementation of a comprehensive early intervention program in New York.

It may be an advantage, especially to older volunteers, to provide transportation and lunch so that the effort expended would not cost the volunteer any money (Salmon, 1985). Of course, it is important to make sure that the early intervention project is not using funds for volunteers without receiving adequate service in return. However, it is likely that even if the volunteer is provided lunch and transportation, the cost for the work that is done for the agency is minimal compared to what that service costs if purchased in the labor market (Salmon, 1985). Sometimes retired senior citizens' agencies provide in-service or mileage reimbursement for volunteer workers.

Reactions of Professional Staff

Although most staff would like to have their work load reduced, few see the training and supervision of a volunteer as a solution to an overload of work. In fact, many see such supervision not as an asset, but as an addition to the work load (Salmon, 1985) and "subversive" to professionalism (Henderson, 1985; Marrs, 1984). In order to have the professional staff comfortable with the volunteers in the project, it is necessary to include staff in the planning for use of the volunteers and in the ongoing plans for supervision. Some of the issues that might need to be aired include the following:

1. What additional work needs to be done and which tasks can be performed by volunteers?
2. How can confidentiality be ensured?

3. How will medication be dispensed and specific therapies implemented?
4. What are the supervision and liability responsibilities?
5. What is the content and organization of initial and continued training?
6. What methods are used to enhance dependability and regular attendance of volunteers?
7. What are some of the issues concerning loyalty to the organization and staff?

Implementation Procedures

In order to have a successful volunteer/agency relationship, it is important that job roles, recruitment, and training for volunteers be given the same serious attention as would be given for paid staff (Firth & Mims, 1985). Responsibilities of the agency include:

1. Recruitment and individual interview of applicants
2. Formal orientation to agency and inservice training
3. Written job description
4. Mutually agreed upon time schedule
5. Procedures for ongoing evaluation of work and feedback given to the volunteer
6. Procedures to maintain records of volunteer's work
7. Providing regular informal and formal thank you for the work
(Adapted from Tierce & Seelback [1987].)

After some staff consensus is reached, it is possible to begin to plan for the organized inclusion of volunteers into the project. From the agency point of view, the plans for training come before the actual recruitment. The training is a significant part of the success of the volunteer experience, not only for the volunteer, but also for the organization. For this reason, it is particularly important that staff members have input into the plans for training (Marrs, 1984).

Some projects find it advantageous to create a certification procedure in which the prospective volunteer completes a series of training sessions and hands-on work before the commitment to being a volunteer is made (Nettings & Hinds, 1984), just as one might train and evaluate a paraprofessional employee (Michaelis & Williams, 1978). Although some of this type of generic training could be handled as generalized training for the role of the volunteer, shared by volunteers in various organizations and done in connection with other agencies, specific training will still be needed before working in any individual site. Along with the cognitive material to be covered in the training, some time should be set aside for the trainee to talk about his or her feelings, insecurity, discomfort, pity, and anxiety that might surround the possibility of working with the handicapped and their families (Marrs, 1984). A typical training sequence might include:

1. Orientation to the facility
2. Discussion of handicapping conditions in infancy and early childhood, with special emphasis on problems of infants and children served by the project
3. Description of exact duties to be performed
4. Designation of whom to report to each day
5. Designation of who will supervise and evaluate, including what the criteria will be and when the evaluation will take place
6. Procedures and equipment necessary to report that work has been completed and how much time was spent on the activity
7. Procedures for reporting problems and concerns, including appropriate contact person

It might help to create a flow chart of authority for volunteers, just as one might be done for other personnel. A checklist such as the one shown in Figure 4.2 might also be used for training and supervision. This particular chart was used every 2 weeks by the supervisor, and served as a combination evaluation and in-service training tool. In some cases, volunteers may be recruited one at a time. However, it can be more beneficial, if possible, to recruit and train them in groups so that volunteers might enjoy one another's companionship and have

Name: _____

Evaluator: _____

	Always 100%	Usually 75%	Sometimes 50%	Occasionally 25%	Never 0%	Not apply
1. Arrives at work promptly						
2. Calls children by name						
3. Handles children as directed						
4. Interacts courteously with others						
5. Handles equipment carefully						
6. Follows instructions						
7. Dresses appropriately						

Figure 4.2. Volunteer evaluation form.

someone with who to share experiences (Marrs, 1984; Salmon, 1985), thus using staff time more efficiently.

Recruiting Volunteers

Although recruitment can be initiated through media campaigns (as described earlier in this chapter for agency agreements), recruitment of volunteers through direct person-to-person contact is more successful (Marrs, 1984). Although volunteers could come from almost anywhere, several key possibilities are: 1) friends and relatives of parents and staff, 2) members of civic and business groups, 3) high school students as part of a class or in the summer, and 4) retired persons.

Some service organizations promote the concept of volunteering for a cause as part of a community or religious mission (Marrs, 1984) or to become a "better person" (Henderson, 1985). Perhaps the most effective method of recruitment is for those who are already volunteering to invite their friends to come. One of the benefits to the volunteer is companionship (Marrs, 1984), and volunteers can help to fill a void stemming from the loss of a loved one or the memory of a child who has passed away. It would be appropriate to ask for a personal recommendation from a volunteer who does not know anyone in the agency. The simplest way to obtain a reference would be to prepare a form that, in addition to providing volunteer data, asks for the name of a reference to contact (see Figure 4.3).

Making It Rewarding for the Volunteer

Usually, agencies consider only one side of the volunteer situation, that is, how the agency can benefit. In order to keep the volunteer coming back, there should also be concern for how it feels on the other side of the fence. Since there is no paycheck to say thank you, the thought must be expressed frequently by the teacher, administrator, or whoever is in day-to-day contact with the volunteer. Another important way to show appreciation is to make sure that equipment needed to perform the task is available and that the task is one that has some obvious value to the program. No one wants to volunteer for a task that does not appear to be important to the purpose of the project. Likewise, no one wants to volunteer for a service only to find that it is not needed today, or to find that someone else has already completed the task, or to realize that several people are expected to help with a task that could be completed by one person in a rather short time. A volunteer wants to be kept busy with something that appears to be worthwhile (Marrs, 1984).

Many people who volunteer in early intervention projects are anxious to work directly with the children, but there may be others who would prefer to make telephone calls, create toys, or even keep the playground in shape. For those working directly with children, it is important that they have a complete physical before beginning their volunteer work, just as paid staff (see Chapter

Name _____

Address _____

Phone ( ) _____

Sex _____ Date of birth _____

EXPERIENCE

Schooling _____
_____

Work _____
_____

With children _____
_____

Hobbies _____
_____

Special interests _____
_____

TIME AVAILABLE FOR VOLUNTEER WORK

Day of week	Time of day
_____	_____
_____	_____
_____	_____

VOLUNTEER ACTIVITY PREFERRED

☐ With children   ☐ Clerical work   ☐ Toy repair

☐ Therapy   ☐ Other (specify) _____

FRIENDS, RELATIVES, SUPERVISORS

We may contact as a reference:

1. Name _____ Title _____

   Address _____

   Phone ( ) _____

2. Name _____ Title _____

   Address _____

   Phone ( ) _____

3. Name _____ Title _____

   Address _____

   Phone ( ) _____

Figure 4.3. Volunteer data sheet.

14). The important thing is not so much what the person does, but making sure that whatever the activity is, that it is seen as valuable both to the staff and to the volunteer. It is also important to ensure that the volunteer is not expected to wait around to be told what to do next. Perhaps the most effective way to accomplish this is to be sure that there is something that always needs to be done, even in slack times. Such activities as organizing the toys, dressing the dolls, cleaning the toys that have been mouthed, cleaning potties, setting up the water color easels, or working with a child on his standing balance could be done at almost any time.

Providing a regular schedule for the volunteer helps prevent him or her from wasting time. One of the most efficient ways to do this is to set up an agreement that stipulates exactly what times the person should come in and what the usual activities that should be performed at that time will be. This could vary for individual volunteers and for the same volunteer on different occasions (Sharow & Levine, 1984). For those who may be preparing things at home rather than coming in regularly, it is important to let them know just exactly how many bibs, dolls, or tote bags are needed and how often they are needed. Sometimes it helps to draw up a written agreement that states something like, "Jane Doe will come in on Tuesday and Thursday from 9:30 a.m. to 11:30 a.m. to assist the physical therapist in providing therapy to the children in Room 3" or perhaps, "Dick Anderson will come to the school between 8:00 a.m. and 8:30 a.m. each weekday morning to assist the children from the family car into the building safely." If the volunteer is not able to provide the service, it is important to ask him or her to notify the agency as early as possible. Absentees should be followed up, just as they would be for paid staff. Comparing the volunteer to the paid worker has shown that the attendance of the volunteer worker is just as dependable as that of the paid worker, even when the health problems of older volunteers has been taken into consideration (Salmon, 1985).

In addition to evaluation and feedback given to the volunteer, it is important that the project also provide him or her with an opportunity to give input to the organization. Volunteers who have worked professionally in other organizations may have some specific suggestions. Others may have contacts with people and agencies in the community that might be able to provide additional resources or suggestions for more efficient use of present resources. It is important that specific times for feedback be arranged so that reporting each day does not interrupt programming for children or other ongoing activities because of discussion between the volunteer and teacher or other staff supervisor.

Formal Recognition of the Volunteer

It is helpful for both paid staff and volunteers to have a formal recognition of the volunteer service. There are a variety of ways that this can be done. Luncheons, dinners, or in-house potluck parties can celebrate the pleasure of working together. Volunteers could be honored at public award ceremonies connected with civic organizations, or the local newspaper might join with the agency to honor the volunteers in the program. There may also be a time when the community as a whole honors those who volunteer in a variety of activities within the community (Hinds, 1987).

DONATIONS

It is possible for early intervention projects to attract the donation of goods as well as services. The *donations* could be anything from toys to assist with motor development, to taxi service for door-to-door transportation, to an unused portable classroom for center-based programming, and almost everything in between. Advertisement of the needs for agency coordination and volunteer services could also include the need for large and small items and for donated services.

Generally speaking, methods to attract donations are similar to methods for attracting agency agreements or volunteers: Know exactly what is needed and let those needs be known to those who may be in a position to donate them or who may be in contact with someone who might be able to donate. Even people with modest means may be interested in making a donation on behalf of a family member who is handicapped or someone close to them. It is important to ascertain whether the individual or agency wishes to be publicly recognized or if they wish to remain anonymous. For those who would like public recognition, anything from a ceremony of acceptance to renaming the school could be appropriate. Written appreciation should be sent to those who wish to be publicly recognized and those who do not. For tax purposes, some who donate may appreciate a receipt for their records.

SUMMARY

Early intervention personnel can significantly increase the quality and intensity of services provided to infants and children with handicaps and their families by productively tapping the natural interest and feeling that people in the general public have for all children, and the depth that accompanies those interests and feelings when the child is handicapped. Mature members of society, of all ages, are interested in making their own lives richer by providing something of worth to society or to individual members of society. Wise early intervention personnel can orchestrate ways for this interest to fill gaps in services and to add enrichment to programs. Without the volunteer program, agreements with other agencies, and public donations, such improvements would probably not be possible with ever present budget constraints.

STUDY QUESTIONS

1. What agencies provide services to infants and young children who are handicapped? Which agency is the primary agency?

2. How do these agencies work together?

3. Is there a cooperative transition program for the state/community early intervention programs?

4. Are volunteers used in state/community early intervention programs? In what way?

REFERENCES

Conrad, W. R., & Glenn, W. E. (1983). *The effective voluntary board of directors.* Athens, OH: Swallow Press.

Cummings, N. A. (1979). Mental health and national health insurance: A case history of the struggle for professional autonomy. In C. A. Kiesler, N. A. Cummings, & G. R. VanderBos (Eds.), *Psychology and national health insurance: A source book* (pp. 5–16). Washington, DC: American Psychological Association.

Firth, G. H., & Mims, A. (1985). Burnout among special education paraprofessionals. *Teaching Exceptional Children, 17*(3), 225–227.

Garland, C., Woodruff, G., & Buck, D. M. (1988). *Case Management.* Reston, VA: Council for Exceptional Children.

Gilman, S. R., & Diamond, R. J. (1985). Economic analysis in community treatment of the chronically mentally ill. *New Directions for Mental Health Services, 26,* 77–84.

Goldman, H. H. (1982). Integrating health and mental health services: Historical obstacles and opportunities. *American Journal of Psychiatry, 139*(3), 616–620.

Henderson, K. A. (1985). Issues and trends in volunteerism. *Journal of Physical Education, Recreation, and Dance, 56,* 30–32.

Hinds, H. N. (1987). Volunteer advocates. *People Today.* Knoxville: East Tennessee Area On Aging.

Julius, S. M., & Handal, P. J. (1980). Third party payment and national health insurance: An update on psychology's efforts toward inclusion. *Professional Psychology, 11*(6), 955–964.

LaCour, J. A. (1982). Interagency agreement: A rational response to an irrational system. *Exceptional Children, 49*(3), 265–267.

Lipscomb, C. F. (1980). Confidentiality and automated health data systems: The position of the Canadian Psychiatric Association. *Canadian Journal of Psychiatry, 25*(7), 595–597.

Marrs, L. W. (1984). Should a special educator entertain volunteers? Interdependence in rural America. *Exceptional Children, 50,* 361–366.

Michaelis, C. T., & Williams, L. (1978). Checklist for teacher use to train and evaluate aides in the severely and profoundly handicapped classroom. *The Journal for Special Education, VXV*(1), 26–58.

Nettings, F. E., & Hinds, H. N. (1984). Volunteer advocates in long-term care: Local implementation of a federal mandate. *Gerontologist, 24*(1), 13–15.

Newman, I. M. (1982). Integrating health services and health education: Seeking a balance. *Journal of School Health, 52*(8), 498–501.

Ozarin, L. D., Shartstein, S. S., & Albert, M. (1981). Integrating mental health and general health care. *Hillside Journal of Clinical Psychiatry, 3*(1), 97–105.

Salmon, R. (1985). The use of aged volunteers: Individual and organizational concern (Special issue: Gerontological social work practices in the community). *Journal of Gerontology Social Work, 8*(3–4), 211–223.

Sharow, N., & Levine, S. (1984). *Training babysitters and volunteers for children with disabilities*. Springfield, IL: Charles C Thomas.

Shartstein, S. S. (1982). Competition or catastrophe: Insurance for psychiatric care. *Comprehensive Psychiatry, 23*(5), 430–435.

Tierce, J. W., & Seelback, W. C. (1987). Elders as school volunteers: An untapped resource. *Educational Gerontology, 13*(1), 33–41.

Wert, E. S., Fein, E., & Haller, W. (1986). Children in placement: A model for citizen-judicial review. *Child Welfare, 65*(2), 199–201.

Williams, R. F. (1986). The values of volunteer benefactors. *Mental Retardation, 24*(3), 163–168.

Williams, R. F. (1987). Receptivity to persons with mental retardation: A study of volunteer interest. *American Journal of Mental Retardation, 92*(3), 299–303.

Zischka, P. C., & Jones, I. (1984). Volunteer community representatives as ombudsmen for the elderly in long-term care facilities. *Gerontologist, 24*(1), 9–12.

Chapter 5

Staff Development in Early Intervention

Strategies for Quality Service

John Killoran and Carol Tingey

———————————— • ————————————

Administrative commitment and educational innovation are increasingly recognized as important characteristics of effective schools (Bickel & Bickel, 1986; Gersten & Guskey, 1985; Striefel & Killoran, 1987). Administrative commitment has been cited as a key variable in the development of innovative early intervention programs (Striefel & Killoran, 1987). This commitment to innovation, combined with the ability to remain flexible in the attainment of established goals (Bickel & Bickel, 1986), provides leadership and guidance that enhance program quality and services to children and families.

Even though administrative commitment to early intervention is vital, teachers and therapists are the primary ingredient in a child's program (Gersten & Guskey, 1985) and in services provided to families. For the most part, teachers and therapists take this role seriously and interact with the child and family with ongoing enthusiasm and steady purpose. However, teachers and therapists are sometimes prone to repeat the same procedures and activities, even when those interventions do not seem to be working because of the continued need to attend to the child. Occasionally, they also seem to hesitate to implement innovation (Gersten & Guskey, 1985). Often this hesitation is not due to a reluctance to change, but is a result of an individual's lack of knowledge or skills to determine what changes may improve the situation. Using current and innovative therapeutic strategies benefits both children and staff, and even the community at large. Children benefit from more effective intervention and increased family involvement. Staff benefit through increased skills, knowledge, and satisfaction from the work as well as through enjoyment of the varied daily routine. Administrators benefit because less energy is expended due to staff turnover. Communities may benefit through increased cost-effectiveness in early intervention programs that result in the eventual increased self-sufficiency of the citizens who receive services.

One of the major tasks of administrators in early intervention programs must be to stimulate staff implementation of current best practices. Since teachers and therapists are usually unable to attend national, regional, and state conferences because of the need to remain with children during programming, they must depend on local administrators to transfer that information to them. This taks can only be accomplished through the use of well-designed, comprehensive staff development programs. In order to be effective, in-service cannot be thought of as the traditional opening in-service that is required to meet regulatory guidelines. Such in-service is often attended and forgotten. In contrast, in-service should be thought of as an ongoing process allowing for practice, feedback, and opportunity to see that the information or new procedures actually improve the intervention (Gersten & Guskey, 1985). The importance of staff development is obvious; as job responsibilities increase, performance demands change. With this change comes the need for training to understand and perform the new role.

There are currently thousands of practicing teachers struggling to work with students they were never trained to teach (American Association of Colleges of Teacher Education, 1980). These teachers urgently need, and in many cases are requesting, in-service training. The amount and form of training needed for early intervention personnel are not known (Tingey-Michaelis, 1985); few people have had specific interdisciplinary training as early intervention specialists. The need for in-service training for early intervention personnel is obvious.

Early intervention practitioners represent a variety of disciplines. Special educators; physical, occupational, and speech/language therapists; psychologists; health care providers; and paraprofessionals are all part of the early intervention program and must be recruited by administrators. Staff development for these individuals begins with the hiring procedure and remains an ongoing process throughout the professional relationship. Responsibilities and qualifications vary for each team member, yet revolve around the following basic competencies (Bailey & Wolery, 1984):

1. Understanding of normal child development
2. Skill in early childhood assessment strategies
3. Understanding of instructional theory and research
4. Ability to use principles of behavior

5. Knowledge of how to plan for skill acquisition and generalization
6. Ability to interact effectively with parents

It is important to keep these basic competencies in mind during the staff hiring and development process.

STAFF HIRING

Hiring new staff as early intervention practitioners is a five-step process. These steps include:

1. Developing job descriptions and announcements
2. Making these announcements public
3. Screening applicants
4. Interviewing finalists
5. Selecting applicants and providing orientation

Developing Job Descriptions and Announcements

The first step in hiring a new staff member is the development of the specific job description and announcement. This description delineates the tasks and skills required to satisfactorily perform the job, as well as the minimum qualifications that applicants must demonstrate. Program planning (see Chapters 3, 4, and 6) decisions, concerning the variety and intensity of services, guides administrators to identify the type of staff and the qualifications necessary to perform the services as planned. For example, a home-based parent-training model may need staff with training different from that required for personnel in a center-based program to implement transdisciplinary services (see Chapter 8). Job descriptions should be based on a task analysis of the position's general and specific responsibilities and include any unusual skills required.

As job descriptions are completed, they are converted into job announcements. Job announcements should include a brief description of the program and the unfilled position, minimum qualifications and experience required, salary ranges, application procedures and contacts, and a closing date. The application process for professional staff usually entails the submission of a letter of intent, current vita, academic transcripts and certifications, and three to five letters of reference.

Making the Announcement Public

Active recruitment of new staff begins with the dissemination of the job announcement. Notice of vacancies may be made through newspaper and radio advertising; professional organizations; journals and newsletters; and public, private, and university employment agencies and placements offices. Obviously it is important to let current staff assist with the plans and be aware of job openings. Contacts they have through professional friends and organizations can be almost helpful in getting the information to appropriate potential applicants. Funding for recruitment, availability or shortages of desired personnel, and compliance with affirmative action regulations must all be considered when recruiting new staff.

Screening Applicants

Screening applicants is usually conducted through a committee process. The committee, commonly known as a search committee, serves the dual function of screening and interviewing potential staff. Committee members should include the program administrator, representatives from the program's advisory board, a parent of a child in the program, and professionals who will be working with the applicant.

It is the responsibility of the search committee is to identify the best qualified applicants for whom interviews are appropriate. This is accomplished by reviewing the materials submitted by the candidates and by personally contacting and verifying references. In early intervention programs, it is imperative to ensure there is no history of child abuse or neglect before considering an applicant for a position (Striefel & Cole, 1987). This may be accomplished through requests to local and state social service agencies.

Written criteria should be developed in order to rank applicants. In most situations, the search committee recommends three to five applicants to be interviewed. Due to the shortage of some professionals, especially therapists trained to work with young children, there may be few qualified candidates, particularly in rural areas. If inexperienced people must be hired, in-service training either on-site or in university training settings is even more vital (see later section of this chapter). Hiring in these cases may be with stipulation of additional training within a specified time as part of the job responsibility.

Interviewing Finalists

Based on the search committee's recommendations, the program administrator schedules interviews for the finalists. Reasonable advance notice should be provided to the applicant and search committee members. This allows the applicant to prepare for the interview as well as ensures that all search committee members may be present. Prior to the interview, a standard list of questions to be asked of all applicants should be developed by the search committee. Questions must specifically address the applicant's skills, knowledge, and qualifications to perform the tasks required as pointed out in the job description. Responses to questions must be kept confidential at all times. In some settings, it is helpful to have the candidate make a presentation to a group of staff, parents, advisory board, or other interested people.

During the interview, the search committee should show interest in the applicant and attempt to make him or her feel comfortable and at ease. Applicant questions and clarification of job responsibilities should be encouraged and factually answered. Tours of the facility should be conducted and timeliness for selection should be discussed.

Selecting Applicants and Providing Orientation

When all interviews are completed, the search committee ranks the applicants and recommends a finalist to be offered the position. The administrator then schedules a second interview with the finalist to: 1) offer him or her the position; 2) negotiate salary, benefits, and start date; and 3) answer any questions that may remain. Position offers should be made in writing and include the job title, salary range, and start date. Follow-up letters to notify and thank nonselected finalists should be mailed as soon as a candidate accepts the position.

Orientation activities should include an overview of the program's philosophy, goals, policies, and procedures. Orientation should be planned and systematic rather than delivered "on the go." Expectations should be elaborated and clarified since role clarity is essential to staff performance, interaction, and significantly reduced staff stress (Striefel & Cole, 1987). Many programs have found that preparing a simple slide presentation that shows people working with the children, and that gives a brief description of the program, is helpful during orientation and in other situations as well (including recruiting volunteers, see Chapter 4). Although a commercially prepared slide/tape package is easy to use, it is not necessary to stretch the budget to pay for one. Slides and a personal narrative by a staff member are just as effective. Orientation is the starting point for systematic staff development.

ORGANIZING STAFF DEVELOPMENT

Brookfield (1981) defines staff development and in-service training interchangeably as: "A systematic process for planning and implementing directed change to improve behaviors and performances in order to meet the needs of individual staff members in concert with the philosophy and goals of the organization" (p. 1). This definition implies that the agency has in writing a current philosophical framework by which it is guided and has identified the goals it wishes to achieve.

Program Philosophy

A philosophical statement serves as a purpose and mission of the agency. By having this guiding philosophy, staff members are consistently reminded of the purpose of their agency, as well as the theoretical framework that guides the program.

Agency Goals

The first task in implementing a systematic staff development program is the development of agency goals. An agency's goals should guide its activities on a daily basis. In early intervention programs, goals reflect the agency's commitment to providing service to children and their families. However, communities, agencies, and funding patterns change over time, and established goals may become obsolete or moot, or methods for reaching ongoing goals may change. Goals should be established and reviewed annually by both administrators and staff (staff should be seen as critical members in the development and revision of agency goals). Staff members' clinical and classroom experience provides valuable information and adds to the knowledge base of successful decisionmaking. When individuals are part of the decisionmaking process, more cooperation is assured and the likelihood of successful change increases.

Goals should reflect any changes desired and the direction in which the program wishes to move. For example, agency staff may wish to modify their service delivery to include servicing nonhandicapped children, in order to provide integrated settings within a previously self-contained setting. There should also be an outline for strategically planning implementation. The strategic plan for implementing each goal should include:

1. A task analysis of the goal
2. Activities to accomplish for each step of the task analysis
3. Funding needed to implement the activities
4. Timeliness and identification of persons responsible for accomplishing each activity
5. Identification of obstacles to overcome
6. Staff training needs to ensure success

Using Task Analysis   Many early intervention practitioners employ task analysis strategies when changing the behavior and skill levels of their students. However, this familiar strategy is often overlooked when professionals are either assessing their own work or desiring to implement systems change. As a result, the activities necessary to achieve a goal often seem overwhelming. By task analyzing goals, staff can set systematic steps that are realistic, organized, and, most important from staff perspective, achievable. Although this might be seen as an administrative task, it may also be beneficial to have all or part of the staff assist in this procedure.

Designing Activities   To accomplish each step in the goal, activities must also be identified. This provides staff with concrete tasks to perform and allows for feedback and direction. For example, an early intervention agency may identify the need for increased coordination of agency "child find activities" as a critical need. Activities to accomplish this goal may include:

Goal: To develop procedures to increase the effectiveness and coordination of agency and community child find procedures.

Activities: The following are a list of activities used to increase the effectiveness and coordination of agency and community child find procedures. They include:

1. Coordinating agency and community child find through interagency planning
2. Developing interagency child find activities through written memos of agreement
3. Operationalizing implementation procedures for joint child find activities
4. Developing a procedural manual and guidelines for child find activities
5. Incorporating coordinated child find activities into appropriate regulations, plans, and monitoring and compliance procedures
6. Disseminating revised activities to all participating agencies
7. Providing joint in-service to participating agencies
8. Providing technical assistance and support to participating agencies
9. Monitoring compliance

Administrators must keep in mind that the primary function of most of the staff is direct service delivery to children and their families. As such, staff activities must be achievable in daily routines or released time from assigned responsibilities must be provided.

Locating Funding   The hidden saboteur in program development is most often funding. All to often, goals are set, activities planned, then change stops due to the lack of funding. This cycle quickly becomes self-defeating since staff hesitate to invest their own time and resources on a project that never gets off the ground. Whether by shifting present funding priorities or by generating extramural funds, a program administrator must commit the resources needed to enhance success (see Chapters 3 and 4). Funding for in-service activities may be obtained from federally funded projects, state systems of comprehensive personnel development, and state and federally funded discretionary grants.

Establishing Timeliness   A timeline should consider staff workloads and commitments, and must be established for each step of the goal. Activities should be sequenced and combined where feasible. One staff member should be assigned as the primary person responsible for achieving each task. Specific times should be allocated and devoted to goal achievement. Again, the administrator must ensure that the time is part of, not in addition to, regular staff assignments and expectations.

Identifying Obstacles   Obstacles that must be overcome during the planning process should be identified to save both time and energy. Addressing difficult issues, such as a lack of funding, at the onset of planning provides an opportunity for solutions and strategies to be built into each step. Involving all staff in the planning and implementation process brings problems to the surface and can turn opposition into support. Confronting obstacles at the outset increases the likelihood of successful change.

Providing Staff Development and Training   Providing staff development and training throughout the year ensures that the knowledge and skills needed to implement best practices and education change are in place and continually reinforced. Staff development must encompass both acquisition of basic skills and instruction in new practices. Training should not only target knowledge level, but should also give staff opportunities to try out new ideas and techniques while receiving feedback on their performance.

STRUCTURES FOR STAFF DEVELOPMENT

Three management structures for designing staff development programs have been described by Brookfield (1981): 1) agency administrator, 2) staff development specialist, and 3) staff development committee.

In an *agency administrator* structure, the administrator designs and implements the staff development program. Programs may be based on needs assessments or the administrator's impression of staff in-service needs. Unfortunately, administrative time constraints often mean that staff development becomes a low or last priority. With time limited, staff involvement and input decrease or become nonexistent.

A *staff development specialist* usually has in-service training as his or her primary job responsibility. Although this allows the time and expertise of a staff member to be concentrated solely on staff development (Brookfield, 1981), its cost usually makes it a prohibitive option in early intervention settings.

The use of a *staff development committee* continues the team involvement that is fostered in the goal-setting process. This continually shared ownership increases staff motivation and morale since they identify their own needs and establish their own commitment to growth. The staff development committee membership should be representative of all disciplines in the agency. This structure has the advantage of sharing this responsibility of needs assessment, planning, and implementation of training across many rather than one staff member. As such, the staff development committee is recommended for use in agencies where budgetary restraints prohibit the hiring of a single staff development specialist.

Staff Development Process

The four steps of systematic staff development are:

1. Needs assessment
2. Planning
3. Implementation of in-service activities
4. Evaluation of staff development

Needs Assessment The gathering of information to identify needs as seen by the staff and to expose discrepancies between program standards and demonstrated skill levels is referred to as needs assessment (Kaufman, 1972). Needs assessment for staff development includes formal and informal measurement by staff and consumers. By restating the identified needs and discrepancies as behavioral objectives, activities and training can be planned to master the goals of staff training (Brookfield, 1981).

Needs assessments are conducted using various formats including questionnaires, direct observation, performance evaluations, and consumer satisfaction surveys. There are numerous needs assessment instruments commercially available. As with most commercially available products, however, their lack of specificity to program goals can be a major drawback to their use. Consequently, most needs assessments are developed as "in house" projects reflecting an agency's goals and the specific needs of its geographic area (e.g., rural or urban interests).

In addition to these specific needs, an agency will also find that its assessment identifies some generic staff development needs, vital to any early intervention program. Examples of two such needs are cardiopulmonary resuscitation (CPR) training for safety of children and sanitation precautions (see Chapter 14).

Planning The second phase of the staff development process is the planning of in-service training based on staff needs. Identified needs are converted into behavioral competency statements and training objectives that provide the framework for the training activities to follow. Individual and group training sessions can then be identified or developed for single or combined objectives.

Competencies can be grouped into two broad categories: knowledge competencies and performance competencies (Adams, Quintero, Killoran, Striefel, & Frede, 1987; Horner, 1977; Wilcox, 1977). *Knowledge competencies* encompass the academic and intellectual components. In a sense, the knowledge competencies are prerequisite to, and underlie the acquisition of, *performance competencies*. These latter include the skills and behaviors. Mastery of knowledge competencies can be evaluated with written tests. Performance competencies, however, must be demonstrated in work with children, their parents, or other service components. Both types of competencies are needed for effective intervention.

Priorities for in-service activities are established based on project goals, program resources, individual preferences, and logical sequence (Brookfield, 1981). Training activities must be planned to meet individual and group needs. Activities range from formal course work and training seminars to informal observation of colleagues and professional readings.

After activities are delineated and assigned priorities, trainers must be identified. Adams et al. (1987) suggest the development of a directory of local training resources. This directory is intended to provide practitioners with an organized list of local personnel and resources available to assist in staff development. A complete, up-to-date directory should help increase the cost-effective use of training time and dollars. Developing a directory of local trainers is accomplished by:

1. Listing competencies identified as priorities and identifying the appropriate activity to train each competency
2. Listing the name of one or more individuals who could, and would, be willing to train each competency
3. Identifying resource organizations that could provide training, technical assistance, and/or materials. (Organizations include universities, regional resource centers, model programs that may exist in the local area, and state comprehensive systems of personnel development. With the new emphasis on implementation of PL 99-457, such institutions are likely to be interested in some form of field-based training and may have specialized funding. Names and telephone numbers of organization contact persons should be included.)

Chapter 1 provides a list of Joint Dissemination Review Panel (JDRP)-approved early intervention programs that will contract with an agency for a specific in-service training.

It may also be possible to provide some of this service through interagency agreement or by volunteers (see Chapter 4). CPR training, for example, is frequently provided free of charge by volunteers from the Heart Association or the local hospital.

Another alternative may be to look within an agency's own staff. The following questions may help identify appropriate trainers:

1. Which people within the agency have the most knowledge and practical experience in this competency area?
2. Of those people, who would be best able to train others? ("Best" in terms of relevant expertise, training ability, and perceived credibility by their peers.)
3. Does the person (or persons) identified have the time to do training; or could time be made available by changing that person's responsibilities and schedule; or could compensatory pay or time-off be arranged?
4. Is the person (or persons) identified willing to do the training?

Implementation of In-Service Activities

When needs have been identified and converted to competencies, activities sequenced in order of priority, and trainers contacted, in-service training can be implemented. There appear to be three types of in-service training needed by practitioners. These are: *general skills training, student-specific training,* and *problem-focused training.* All three types are need to help acquire the increasingly broad range of competencies required for innovative leadership in early intervention. Unfortunately, it appears that most current in-service is limited to problem-focused training.

A few 1- or 2-hour training sessions at the end of a programming day to discuss problems are simply not sufficient. Such training yields an isolated acquaintance with knowledge competencies and on incomplete grasp of the vital performance competencies. Individual reading of journal articles or books may suffice for certain knowledge components, but this barely begins to address the performance aspects of the competencies. The results of teaching many of the performance components exclusively by lecture, reading, or discussion would be equivalent to the success one could expect from teaching piano or swimming by such methods. When 1- or 2-hour-a-day training sessions are continued for extended periods of time, however, and focus on general skills and student-specific training as well as specific problem-solving, a full complement of early intervention skills can be acquired.

Required to meet the needs of practicing professionals more adequately is an in-service training program that is *comprehensive* and *sequential* (Fredericks et al., 1977). A comprehensive plan should include: 1) guided reading, 2) brief (1–2 hour) didactic training, 3) short workshops or mini-classes, 4) specially designed summer quarter college classes, 5) supervised practica, 6) in-classroom demonstrations and shaping of teacher behaviors, 7) in-classroom consultation with specialists, and 8) consistent, long-term follow-up by trainers. Such a staff development program could be designed and jointly sponsored by university faculty from special education and regular education departments, as well as personnel in other early intervention programs. In necessitates closer interaction between university staff and practitioners in the field and should include built-in assessment procedures to evaluate efficacy. Trainers should be able to demonstrate competencies identified in the needs assessment. The training should be designed to focus on those major areas that have not typically been a part of the training experience of most regular staff (e.g., attitudes, behavior modification skills, adaptive equipment, exceptional conditions, and working closely with parents).

Evaluation of Staff Development   Evaluation of training activities is the final step in the staff development process. Evaluation should address both staff development activities and individual performance.

Training Activity Evaluation   Evaluation of training activities provides feedback needed to verify program effectiveness or to modify training. Jessien and Wolfe (1984) have identified a three-step process, which includes:

1. Self-evaluation
2. Participant evaluation
3. Knowledge and performance testing

Self-evaluation refers to the trainers critiquing themselves to decide the effectiveness and success of the training activity. Organization, presentation style, and accomplishment of objectives are addressed in self-evaluation.

In *participant evaluation,* trainees are the source of feedback. Participant evaluation determines pre/post knowledge levels of material presented, assesses organization of the activity, lists strengths and weaknesses of the activity, and offers suggestions for improvement. Overall quality and usefulness of the activity are also usually measured by the participant rating the training on a scale that allows for a degree of satisfaction to be specified.

Knowledge and performance testing is the ultimate measure of the effectiveness of the training. This may include formal testing on the training content, but is usually measured by direct observation when the participant is working with children or parents. Formal knowledge testing should objectively measure the participant's mastery of learning objectives (Jessien & Wolfe, 1984).

The primary purpose for evaluating individual performance is to improve effectiveness (Kukic, Ryberg, Link, & Freston, 1986). Evaluation must result in improved performance and be based on objective strategies rather than personal opinion. Individual performance evaluations are created by converting goals of the in-service training into performance objectives. The observed behavior is then rated on a scale that allows for performance to be measured as outstanding, good, fair, adquate, or inadequate.

Individual Staff Performance Evaluation In order to maintain a consistent level of service and to ensure that each staff member is continually performing satisfactorily, an individual evaluation of work performance is necessary at least yearly. Components of a good performance evaluation are (Striefel & Cole, 1987):

1. Development of accurate measurable job descriptions
2. Identification of evaluators
3. Development of ongoing feedback systems
4. Use of corrective actions plans; these plans specify:
   a. Behaviors to be changed
   b. Target behaviors to be developed
   c. Remediation strategies to be employed
   d. Methods for measuring progress
   e. Timeliness for change to occur

In addition to competencies based on individual job descriptions, Kukic et al. (1986, p. 7) define 14 areas of teaching that should be included in performance evaluations for teachers:

1. Identification of learning outcomes
2. Utilization of instructional materials

3. Instructional techniques
4. Academic learning time
5. Use of positive reinforcement
6. Systematic correction of errors
7. Classroom discipline
8. Instructional style
9. Instructional efficiency
10. Progress monitoring
11. Communication
12. Transdisciplinary teaming
13. Organizational commitment
14. Professional development

Despite the procedures used in evaluating teacher performance, evaluation techniques must be behaviorally oriented and objective, include constructive feedback, and result in increased teacher effectiveness.

Staff who work with children or families toward therapeutic goals also need to be evaluated individually on performance goals suitable for the professional goals. Such performance goals include testing and report writing skills for psychologists, and methods of facilitating sensory integration for therapists. In this respect, administrators in early intervention programs are responsible for creation of job descriptions and performance evaluations for support, clerical, and custodial, as well as, in many settings, bus drivers and food service personnel. Obviously each of these jobs would require different competencies and methods of evaluation.

Preventing Burnout

No matter how well an administrator attempts to meet staff needs, there are times when everyone experiences strain. It is often said that being a parent is the hardest job one will ever have. If this is so, working with or around children may just be the next hardest job. Staff are expected to be nurturing, yet disciplined; structured, yet flexible; child-centered, yet adhere to administrative consent. The energy expended while working with 3-year-olds is enormous, yet must be replaced the next day. Often child progress is slow and staff become discouraged and tired. Coupled with the need to attend meetings, complete paperwork, and undergo repeated assessments, early intervention personnel are faced not with a question of will stress and potential burnout be a problem, but what to do to prevent them from occurring. One of the biggest challenges administrators face is to maintain the morale and motivation of staff.

STAFF ENVIRONMENT

Emotional Climate

Although each staff member is personally responsible for interacting with others in a pleasant and cooperative way, the administrator is responsible for setting the emotional climate of the project. The formal and/or informal ways in which the director/principal (or other title of a chief administrator) interacts with staff sets the official climate. This environment may be nurturing and supportive, or fraught with jealousy, distrust, and competition. Although staff members in a cold atmosphere may stick together and even become close friends, enthusiasm for and dedication to their work suffer when emotional energy must be used to find ways of working in spite of a lack of respect for their work.

A healthy emotional climate also acknowledges that, in any organization, there are employees with advanced training and experience and others who perform what might be considered more mundane work. In a well-organized program, all job roles are recognized as essential for the successful implementation of the program. Custodial services are just as pertinent as developmental therapy.

An administrator who respects each staff person's skills helps others to do the same. It is also important to respond to the personal needs of staff members. Since many of the direct service staff are likely to be young, they may also have young children. These staff members may need to go to their child's school for a conference or take their child to the pediatrician during regular working hours. The ACDS project discussed in Chapter 8 has, in its center-based program, a preschool class for the children of the staff. Other staff members may have to assist aging parents or cope with problems in the lives of their teenage children. Although it is important that implementation of the program not suffer due to the personal needs of the staff, it is important that staff members be recognized as individuals whose personal needs will sometimes require administrative time and support. The key to having a nurturing intervention program for children and families is to have an atmosphere of nurturing for staff as well.

Motivation

Striefel and Cadez (1983) have identified administrative support, performance feedback, and task diversity as critical to staff morale, ranking higher in importance than salaries. In a field in which salaries are likely to be low, wise administrators capitalize on this fact and provide individual feedback on performance and skills to increase performance (Striefel & Cole, 1987).

The intensity and routine climate of the work environment also critically influence staff morale. No job is all fun, but productivity increases when the emotional climate is pleasant. Social activities such as birthday breakfasts and happy hours often increase staff social interaction, diffuse stress levels, and provide a vehicle for enhancing staff satisfaction. In most settings, staff are willing to rotate responsibility for planning simple, inexpensive socials. Some programs have enjoyed including families served by the program in their socials (see Chapter 16).

SUMMARY

If early intervention programs are to become increasingly more effective, it is essential that excellence is approached systematically rather than haphazardly. The key to success, although highly dependent upon the commitment of program administrators, is in the hands of the program's direct service providers. Through the cooperative decisionmaking of staff and administrators, staff development programs can be designed that result in increased skills, motivation, and morale, and as a result, produce high-quality services to children and families.

STUDY QUESTIONS

1. What is the training/experience of staff who are working in the state/community early intervention programs?

2. What in-service is provided for staff of early intervention programs in your state/community?

3. Interview an early intervention staff person to discuss the rewards and stresses of the work.

4. Interview an early intervention administrator to discuss the rewards and stresses of managing programs/staff.

REFERENCES

Adams, P., Quintero, M., Killoran, J., Striefel, S., & Frede, E. (1987). A review and synthesis of teacher competencies for effective mainstreaming. *FMS Final Report Project Review Papers*, Logan, UT.

American Association of Colleges of Teacher Education. (1980). *A common body of practice for teachers: The challenge of Public Law 94-142 to teacher education.* Washington, DC: Author.

Bailey, D. B., & Wolery, M. (1984). *Fundamentals of early intervention: Teaching infants and preschoolers with handicaps.* Columbus, OH: Charles E. Merrill.

Bickel, W. E., & Bickel, D. P. (1986). Effective schools, classrooms, and instruction: Implications for special education. *Exceptional Children, 52,* 489–500.

Brookfield, J. (1981). *Staff development: A systematic process.* Seattle: WESTAR.

Fredericks, H. D. B., Anderson, R. B., Baldwin, V. L., Grave, D., Moore, W. C., Moore, M., & Baird, J. H. (1977). *The identification of competencies of teachers of the severely handicapped* (Grant No. OEC–0–74–2775). Washington, DC: Bureau of Education for the Handicapped, Department of Education.

Gersten, R., & Guskey, T. R. (1985). Transforming teacher reluctance into a commitment to innovation. *Direct Instruction News,* Fall.

Horner, R. D. (1977). A competency based approach to preparing teachers of the severely and profoundly handicapped: Perspective II. In E. Sontag (Ed.), *Educational programming for the severely and profoundly handicapped* (pp. 430–444). Reston, VA: Division on Mental Retardation, Council for Exceptional Children.

Jessien, G., & Wolfe, B. (1984). *How to conduct a training workshop*. Chapel Hill, NC: TADS.

Kaufman, R. (1972). *Educational systems planning*. Englewood Cliffs, NJ: Prentice-Hall.

Kukic, S. J., Ryberg, S. L., Link, D., & Freston, J. (1986). *SET: The scales for effective teaching*. Alpine, UT: The Change Agency.

Striefel, S., & Cadez, M. J. (1983). *Serving children and adolescents with developmental disabilities in the special education classroom: Proven methods*. Baltimore: Paul H. Brookes Publishing Co.

Striefel, S., & Cole, P. (1987). *Providing psychological and related services to children and adolescents: A comprehensive guidebook*. Baltimore: Paul H. Brookes Publishing Co.

Striefel, S., & Killoran, J. (1987). *Functional mainstreaming for success: Final report* (Grant No. G008–401757). Logan, UT: Developmental Center for Handicapped Persons.

Tingey-Michaelis, C. (1985). Early intervention: Is certification necessary? *Teacher Education in Special Education, 8*(2), 91–97.

Wilcox, B. (1977). A competency based approach to preparing teachers of the severely and profoundly handicapped: Perspective I. In E. Sontag (Ed.), *Educational programming for the severely and profoundly handicapped* (pp. 418–429). Reston, VA: Division on Mental Retardation, Council for Exceptional Children.

Chapter **6**

Evaluation of Effectiveness

Carol Tingey

———————————— ● ————————————

Time, money, distance, length, weight, and volume can, using the appropriate equipment, be measured with precision; for a variety of reasons, however, human characteristics and values cannot. These reasons may be grouped into four complicated clusters of unknowns that create difficulty in determining: 1) exactly *what* is being measured, 2) the exact *unit* of measurement, 3) how the characteristics to be measured are to be *valued* in relation to other characteristics, and 4) a *standard* that can be used to measure the entity for a variety of purposes and circumstances. Human behavior and values are both complicated and interrelated; neither has discrete or consistent units (Lamping, 1985). Therefore, even when circumstances are similar, nuances of an event can cause the evaluation to change. The whole question of evaluating the effectiveness of early intervention programs or segments of programs can change, depending on who is interested and for what reason.

To date, early intervention programs have usually rated the effectiveness of their programming by measuring a child's developmental attainment (usually on an intelligence or developmental scale) (Weatherford, 1986). This is frequently done as soon as the child finishes the program (see Chapter 1 for description of the integrated analysis of early programs). Since many of these programs were enacted as pilot or demonstration programs, they were not mandated or funded to collect data concerning the long-term effect on the family or the child. Therefore, these programs should not be faulted for not expending the resources necessary to collect such information. Current interest in the quality of education for all children (Goodlad, 1984), however, and in the practical need to document effectiveness of early intervention programs for fiscal purposes (Bickman & Weatherford, 1986), dictates that broader evaluations must be performed. These evaluations will have to assess difficult-to-measure characteristics by using imprecise instruments to answer a variety of questions still being specified. It will be necessary to determine such issues as: 1) what child and/or family characteristics are to be selected for measurement; 2) what procedures or instruments can be used to describe current and future status; 3) if the variables chosen for examination are the same as family goals, program goals, and actual practice; and 4) if the measures produce consistant results in meaningful life settings outside the program, and can be used as a tool for future reference.

WHO IS INTERESTED AND WHY?

Although it is not possible to create one evaluation that addresses all of the possible areas of assessment (Glenwick, Stephens, & Maher, 1985; Rosenberg, Robinson, Finkler, & Rose, 1987), it is possible to create evaluations that meet specific needs of specific audiences (Smith, 1986). First, the focus and scope of the desired evaluation must be determined (Shadish, 1986). Figure 6.1 lists seven core questions to determine the evaluation emphasis. Professionals, parents, the children themselves, and the community at large are all potential evaluators of the early intervention services and may see each of the elements that are chosen for emphasis in a different light. For example, parents might see the ability to recite the alphabet as an appropriate measure of child progress while

---

Questions to Determine Focus and Scope of Evaluation

1. Why is the evaluation needed? (e.g., program planning, funding concerns, student progress, family satisfaction, community interest, combinations of concerns)
2. What resources are available for evaluation? (e.g., time of current staff, funds for additional staff or consultants, testing, other information from various agencies)
3. How soon is the information needed? (e.g., for immediate funding use, at end of school year, when the children reach school age)
4. What kind of information is needed? (e.g., data on child progress, effective use of funds or space, number of children served compared to number identified who need service)
5. Who will be responsible for gathering what information and when? (e.g., teachers, physicians, nurses, therapists, administrators, parents; to be gathered immediately, throughout the year, as the children leave the program)
6. How will the information be reported and who will organize the information for the report? (e.g., budget sheets, program description, test results; in a printed format, by oral presentation, or combination)
7. How will the value/significance of the evaluation be determined? (e.g., regular administration/staff, committee of professionals organized for this purpose, representatives of community, legislative committee)

Figure 6.1. Pertinent evaluation questions. (Adapted from Glenwick, Stephens, & Maher, 1985.)

program personnel may be more concerned about developmentally appropriate play skills and independence in self-care skills as measured on a standardized test.

Professionals as Evaluators

The questions and answers can further be delineated by considering the methods of determining what information would be considered valid, from which perspective or for which audience (Lamping, 1985; Wykes, Sturt, & Creer, 1985). For example, the questions and answers could be used to examine what might be pertinent to early intervention professionals from various disciplines. Table 6.1 is a listing of evaluation emphasis and outcome criteria used by professionals in a variety of fields. To minimize the possibility that important criteria will be overlooked in the evaluation, it is important that the process be implemented by a team, representing a variety of professions, perhaps one with rotating membership.

Parents as Evaluators

Another significant group that may have different criteria for evaluation of effectiveness are parents. Parents may see the program as effective for any of the reasons stated in Table 6.1. Or, they may rate the program on its provision of

Table 6.1.   Evaluation emphasis and criteria for various professions

Profession	Emphasis	Criteria
Medicine	Physical health	Height and weight gain, absence of disease
Psychology	Development	Standardized assessment of developmental milestones
Physical and occupational therapy	Motor function	Clinical assessment of reflex control, quality of movement in mobility and self-care
Speech/language therapy	Communication	Standardized and clinical assessment of functional speech and language skills
Social work	Social environment	Family function and family relationships examined by interview, visit, and case management format
Mental health	Coping and daily function	Ability to handle stress and deal effectively with each new life challenge
Teaching	Child progress	Child attainment of teaching goals
Administration	Program plans	Implementation of services as planned and resources distributed most efficiently

safe or acceptable care for their child for a few hours a day so that they can turn to other chores or relax from the intensity of providing care for a child who is experiencing difficulties in development. The parents may also view the program as effective because it helps them by providing a much needed supportive atmosphere (Tardy, 1985). Parents rate the importance of the early intervention program by indicating its value to them. Parents are, quite naturally, only interested in the program which serves their child. Evaluation questions for parents are more personal and may differ from those for professionals. The following are questions that parents might ask (Tingey-Michaelis, 1986):

1. Who will be working with my child?
2. What kind of training/experience does this person have with children who have problems like my child?
3. How much of my child's time will it take?
4. How much of *my time* will it take?
5. How much of the time of other family members will it take?
6. Is transportation available?
7. Is there a fee for the program?
8. Will my child have individual attention and individual goals?
9. If I did not have to rush off to the program, would I have more time and energy to give to my child?
10. Exactly what can my child get from the program that he or she is not already getting?
11. Exactly what can *I* get from the program that I am not already getting?

Children as Evaluators

Although considering a young child's response to be an evaluation per se would be inappropriate, a child may be observed for his or her reactions to a program. If the child begins to cry when mother leaves or screams during therapy, he or she may not feel comfortable at the program. However, if the child does not want to be taken from the program at the end of a session, it could be assumed that he or she enjoys the surroundings.

Although it would generally be assumed that a child "doesn't know what is good for him or her" and that adults should be deciding the value of a program for a child, few adults would want intervention to continue unchanged if a child were screaming throughout treatment. Disruptive child responses or reluctance to attend on the child's part would surely affect a parent's attitude about the effectiveness of a program.

Community as Evaluator

Community pride and a willingness to participate in community life vary from person to person. For some, an interest in the condition of the roads, parks, and schools leads to involvement in "clean-up" campaigns and volunteer programs;

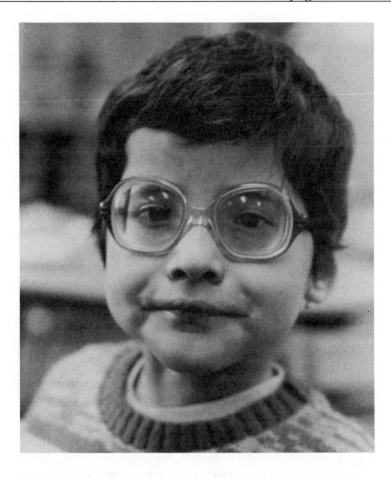

others remain apathetic. Interest in providing services to the more needy of a community also fluctuates. For some citizens, taking care of everyone in the area is a priority (Marrs, 1984), while for others concern extends only to ensuring an adequate police force to protect taxpayers from the vagrants who may be dangerous. United Way and other civic groups are interested in how volunteers and donated services are utilized.

Real estate agents and long-term residents usually tout the benefits of their community by describing the quality of the schools. This interest in the educational system may intensify and be taken up by more residents when the schools are crowded or need to be replaced, or when there is a bond issue on an election ballot. From this perspective, the adequacy of the services designed to meet the needs of children who have developmental difficulties is part of the wealth of a community and is one of the concerns of a city's elected officials and other community leaders (Swift, Fine, & Beck, 1985). Although a community's leaders may not be conversant with the details of their area's early intervention programming, they will have some knowledge of the services for "these special children" and will be interested in the results of those services.

USING THE EVALUATION

Another way of identifying the purpose of an evaluation, besides looking at who is doing the evaluating, is to clearly define all of the parties who will be using the data gathered. Professionals may be concerned foremost with how the data collected answer specific questions pertinent to that discipline. Yet, ultimately, the data may be for another purpose. Data may be needed to defend the budget to the United Way, to a local legislature, to a school board, or at a community hearing. For these purposes, a parent's description of his or her child's improvements, a parent's testimonial on the supportiveness of the program, or the personal comments from the president of the Junior League concerning a visit to the center may be more effective than any statistical analysis of carefully gathered numerical data. Although statistics are helpful, it is possible to describe the impact of an early intervention program from a variety of perspectives, and the ultimate use of the information should always be considered when an evaluation is planned.

Another consideration is the timeframe of the evaluation. Just when should an evaluation be conducted? Obviously, it is easier to complete an evaluation of a recent event, but for early intervention (as for all training services), the important thing is not the immediate result but the long-term effect of the service (Glenwick et al., 1985).

No matter how the evaluation is conducted, there are three general sources of data: 1) child progress, 2) family measures, and 3) community measures. These three areas are discussed in the following subsections of this chapter. (A fourth area, satisfaction of employees, could also be listed as a source of data but because it is an administrative concern rather than a program effectiveness concern, and, is thus, not discussed here; refer instead to Chapter 2.)

Child Progress

Although parents and other careproviders sometimes become bored with day-after-day care routines and may not notice a child's changes from week to week, even the most preoccupied adult notices that over the summer children not only outgrow their clothes but also their favorite foods, toys, and games.

For children with developmental delays; it is particularly important to monitor these changes and the new skills they are acquiring. For professionals, there are a number of carefully constructed lists of behaviors and performance criteria that can help plot a child's attainment of skills in rather precise increments. These tests can be standardized or criterion-referenced, as described below. It is important to note, however, that since many of the same items appear in each type of test, it is sometimes difficult to distinguish between the types.

Standardized Assessment Standardized measures are created by carefully noting observable behavior, and then designing interactions with the child to elicit those behaviors or interviewing the careprovider to determine whether the child does indeed produce these behaviors.

Standardized tests are created only after many children of different capabilities and backgrounds have been observed. The average age at which these children were able to perform each task is calculated. The tasks are then listed in the order in which children learned them (a developmental sequence) and an age range for the acquisition of each behavior is identified. This makes it possible to compare any child's behavior to the average behavior of the larger group of infants and to calculate a *developmental age* for that child. Since long lists can become awkward, the items are usually grouped into *domains* or types of behavior. The most common are: motor, language, social, and self-care. The motor domain is frequently divided into gross and fine, and the language domain into receptive and expressive. The domains in most scales are similar, but some test developers have divided these skills into other groups. For example, the Battelle Developmental Inventory (BDI) uses five domains: 1) personal-social, 2) adaptive, 3) motor, 4) communication, and 5) cognitive (Newborg, Stock, Wnek, Guidubaldi, & Svinicki, 1984).

Standard Procedures Typically, standardized tests describe how the instrument was developed. This information is given in the examiner's manual, which also typically includes tables to calculate various standard score measurements from the child's chronological age and developmental age. The information about standardization also usually describes the number of children who were tested and gives a geographic and socioeconomic description of them. When a standardized test is used, the child tested is compared to the children who were tested in the original group.

The examiner's manual also includes data that describe how *reliability* was determined (by the use of the same test a second time with the same child at a later date, and by comparing different examiners' scores for the same child). Likewise, the manual describes the *validity* of the test. This is done by examining both the content of the items and the way they are worded, and by then studying how infants of both sexes and from different ethnic backgrounds responded to the items.

Some standardized tests also provide information concerning how handicapped infants and children have responded to various parts or a test of specify adaptations that can be made for various handicapping conditions (e.g., BDI). Typically, however, standardized tests do not provide such accommodations. Although not having this may seem like a serious problem (Fuchs, Fuchs, Benowitz, & Barringer, 1987), having handicapped children in the standardized sample (frequently called the norming group, since averages are computed for this group and a "normal" score is determined) may actually compromise the procedure. This is possible because the objective of the standardization is to identify what skills most children of each age can perform successfully so that children who are having problems can be compared to this standard.

The examiner's manual also includes a description of how the items should be administered to the child and the kinds of materials that should be used to help elicit the child's performance. In some of the tests, the exact words are given. In others, a description of probes to refine responses that pinpoint the behavior to be assessed are given. In order to make sure that the results are standard, these measures must be performed exactly as written. Performance adaptations for children with disabilities, such as having objects rather than pictures for a blind child to describe or allowing more time to respond (Van Hof-Van Duin, Mohn, & Batenburg, 1982), must be noted by the assessor on the scoring form or in a written report.

The examiner's manual also specifies answers that are both acceptable and unacceptable for scoring purposes. Some tests allow partial scores, while others do not. In some instances, standardized tests are protected tests that can only be administered by someone who has been trained as a psychologist. In other cases, the person to administer the test is expected to study the procedures and practice. Obviously, some people are better than others at standardized test administration because they are more familiar with the test's procedures or because they are more relaxed when working with children.

Norm Samples   All standardized measures of child progress are in some way comparing that child to other children. The number of and manner in which these other children are selected are of extreme importance. If the norm sample is small or if all the children come from only one region, ethnic group, socioeconomic status, or religion, the comparison may not be a significant one. If children in the rural midwest are compared to children living in apartments in New York City, there will likely be general differences in language and motor abilities for the two groups.

Since there are so many different characteristics of children and families to compare, creating a norm sample usually takes a number of years. This is a problem because it is never possible to compare a child to today's children (Hoko, 1986). Comparing today's child to a child of the 1920s would be interesting, but obviously not a good measure of the effectiveness of the early intervention program. When effectiveness of the program is to be measured in some way by the progress of the child, it is necessary to select a measure that has been generated from a large population sample and has been completed recently.

Criterion-Referenced Tests   Criterion-referenced tests usually consist of items that represent developmental milestones from standardized tests. The difference is that only attainment of the skill is observed; the age at which the child masters the skill is not significant. Therefore, a developmental age is not calculated. The items on a criterion-referenced test could also encompass skills not usually considered to be directly related to developmental milestones, but instead are related to a specific task or skill that adults may see as important to the child (Hoko, 1986). Sometimes these skills are the emphasis or goals of a specific curriculum.

Criterion-referenced measures many also focus on skills related to difficulties that the child may have due to his or her handicapping condition. A criterion-referenced instrument may also specify the skill in finer detail than items that cover similar skills on a developmental scale. For example, a child who has motor problems may be evaluated on a criterion-referenced test on the following: 1) able to reach out to touch the spoon, 2) able to grasp the spoon with adult assistance, 3) able to grip the spoon when placed in his or her hand with fingers placed around the handle, 4) able to pick up a spoon from the table, 5) able to pick up the spoon from the table and grasp around the handle, 6) able to put spoon to mouth without assistance, and 7) able to scoop food with the spoon from a plate with a lip. The comparable skill on a standardized test might read as follows: able to use spoon to eat.

An evaluator may use a list of skills from a general list in an already published criterion-referenced scale, or generate an individualized list for a specific child in order to more finely describe the behaviors that must be learned or maladaptive behaviors that must be "unlearned" (Aman, Singh, Stewart, & Field, 1985). (See Chapter 13 for criterion-referenced skill lists for attainment of self-care skills.)

The major benefits of criterion-referenced tests include their ability to: 1) show a child's progress by comparing the child's present performance to the same child's past performance, 2) avoid comparing a child's progress to the status of other children, and 3) offer goals detailed enough to be used for teaching objectives. Criterion-referenced tests are valuable for identification and attainment of child goals (Anderson, Hodson, & Jones, 1975; Marston & Magnusson, 1985). However, since criterion-referenced tests do not allow for comparison with other children, they cannot be used to identify or classify a child as handicapped.

Limitations of Testing In evaluating a child's progress, whether by standardized or criterion-referenced measurement, the limitations of testing must be kept in mind. Three cautions may bear particular mention.

First, many full-length tests have shorter versions that are useful for screening and may seem to offer time savings to the evaluator. Although these abbreviated versions are very valuable in the beginning process of identification, they have little value in the measurement of effectiveness. In screening instruments, only a few representative behaviors are sampled; therefore, they cannot show fine increments in child skill or change of skill. (See Chapter 2 for more discussion of procedures for initial assessment and assessment measures.)

The second caution focuses on the possible inaccuracy of measurement of the progress of infants and young children. Since these children have had less time for learning than older students, there are fewer skills or behaviors to examine to determine their progress. With so few items to examine, there is little confidence that early measures of child function will relate to later function of that child, especially for more mildly handicapped children (Valus, 1986). This limitation is frequently cited as a problem if these instruments are used to document effectiveness (Weatherford, 1986).

A third area of concern in early intervention evaluation is the experience and familiarity of the individual administering the test. Few assessors have had enough experience to have developed clinical expertise with infants and very young children. This problem is encountered frequently, since most people trained in assessment have been taught how to measure the function of school children, and are sometimes uncomfortable or at least unfamiliar with the skills of infancy and early childhood. Consequently, they do not always detect fine differences in the quality of the behavior and how it relates to the child's immediate physical state or mood. The situation may be further complicated by the relationship of the assessor to the child. Rapport is necessary between assessor and child for accurate results, and yet to be assured that a child has attained the skill in question, it must be performed in the presence of an unfamiliar person in order to obtain an accurate assessment for the purpose of evaluating the program.

Family Measures

If measurement of child progress seems difficult, measurement of change in the family unit is even more problematical (Fewell, 1986). Each family member, adult or sibling, introduces a new set a characteristics that grows broader as the individual ages. As those characteristics expand, the range of interactions among those characteristics likewise increases. As interactions between people and among characteristics unfold, secondary reactions occur. Indeed, the family unit becomes an everchanging system. Yet, it is not possible to make an accurate evaluation of a child's skills or progress if the characteristics of the family are not known. Describing those characteristics is an intricate task.

To begin, there are a variety of areas that may be categorized as family descriptors. These include:

Number of parents in family
Number of children in family
Education of parents
Occupation of parents

Income of parents
Physical health of family members
Mental health of family members
Total funds available for family use
Size of dwelling

Although such demographic data may be the easiest measures to collect on a family, they will perhaps be of the least value in documenting effectiveness of the early intervention program. It is highly unlikely that working with the child will change any of these family variables. Take, for instance, the second characteristic listed, "number of children in family." There is a slight possibility that if services are provided that help the family with the handicapped child, the family will feel more confident in having another child and therefore increase the number of children in the family. Decisions concerning the number of children in a family, however, are made in some families by careful calculation of resources and circumstances and in others by chance. Other family variables such as the availability of child care assistance and emotional attachment of family members are related more to family function and may possibly change due to the results of the early intervention program, but they, too are likely to be influenced by other events or activities. For example, a change of employment, the death of a grandparent, or moving into a new neighborhood has the potential of affecting a family as much as (or even more than) the early intervention program.

Table 6.2 lists some of the instruments frequently used to take family measures and the focus of the instrument. These instruments can identify areas that may be creating problems for the family. In some incidences, the instruments can provide a clearer picture of possible problem situations or highlight potential problem areas for families. The data gathered from these instruments can be used to design services for families (see Chapter 16 for a description of services to families). After services are delivered, data can be gathered again with the use of these instruments and parent interviews.

The parent interviews can be used to document any change in the emotional status of the family. The following are examples of interview questions used in the evaluation:

Do you feel comfortable with your understanding of how a child develops?
Do you know how to help your child relate to other children?
Do you feel that you have all the information about your child's special needs?
Do you have someone to talk to about your child's problems?
Do you have someone to call when you need assistance with your child?

Parents are asked to respond to each question during the interview with one of the following answers: always, usually, sometimes, and never. These responses could be incorporated into a numbering system, where as each response is

Table 6.2. Summary of selected family measures used in cooperation with early intervention programs

Measure	Description

Family Inventory of Life Changes and Family Adaptability and Cohesion Evaluation Scale (FACES 111)
   Family Stress & Coping Project
   290 McNeal Hall
   University of Minnesota
   St. Paul, MN 55108
	Family Inventory—seventy-one item list in areas of potential stress, including: finance, work, child bearing, illness, legal, loss of family member, marital, and transition issues. Parent's check-list for events in last year and before that time. (Approximately 20 minutes to complete.)
	
	 Family Adaptability—forty items used for data on communication, organization, child rearing attitudes and closeness of family members. Parents respond once for ideal family function and once for actual function of own family. (Approximately 15 minutes to complete.)

Family Resource Scale and Family Support Scale
   Dr. Carl Dunst
   Family, Infant, and Preschool Program
   Western Carolina Center
   Morganton, NC 28655
	Family Resource Scale—thirty items used to assess if family has adequate time, money, and energy resources to meet individual family member's needs and family as a whole. Especially good for low income families.

Parenting Stress Index
   Pediatric Psychology Press
   Idlewood Drive
   Charlottesville, VA 22901
	Parenting Stress Index—one-hundred one items used to assess 2,915 parents' perceptions of parent role and capacity to cope with demands of child care and influence of child care on marital relationship. (Approximately 25 minutes to complete.)

Impact on Family
   Ruth E.K. Stein, M.D.
   Professor of Pediatrics
   Bronx Municipal Hospital Center
   Jacobs Hospital
   Pelham Parkway & Eastecher Road
   Bronx, NY 10461
	Impact on Family—thirty-three items that cover child care; finances; time management; and social, professional, and family relationships. English and Spanish versions. Parent's responses show experience and reactions to living with a handicapped child. (Approximately 15 minutes to complete.)

given a number (e.g., 4 = always, 3 = usually, 2 = sometimes, 1 = never). The interview could then be scored on a numerical scale which could determine the family's perception of effectiveness.

Community Measures

Criteria for measuring the effectiveness of the early intervention programs in the communities include not only the effect the program has on children and their families, but also the effect it has on the community itself. In addition to measuring the program's effectiveness with the children and their families, other members of the community who may be employed to implement the early intervention will be of concern to the community leaders who are doing the evaluation. There will also be concern about the building in which the services are rendered, potential zoning, and traffic concerns. There will undoubtedly be state daycare regulations to be met that include health standards. Some of these issues and concerns are highlighted in Table 6.3.

Although most evaluation of the early intervention program by the community will be the informal opinions of those who live close to the center or those who may hear a talk at a civic club, persons who visit and come away with good or bad things to say about what they saw at the program will also offer opinions. There are official evaluations made by building inspectors, health inspectors, state licensure agencies, and fire marshals. For the most part, these type of evaluations will not be concerned about the quality of the specific intervention techniques or the results of those procedures; however, they will be concerned about health and safety regulations.

For an organization that provides a public service, it is necessary to have public acceptance and the backing of a few community leaders. Advisory boards and public awareness campaigns can help provide structure and support to a community evaluation. The most critical evaluation of the program's effectiveness, however, will be made by the advisory board members.

Advisory Board Evaluation Some early intervention programs currently in existence have advisory boards that consist of active members in the community. Many of these volunteer boards (see Chapter 3) meet infrequently and exert little influence upon day-to-day program activities; however, they usually do examine the budget carefully and are aware of space, equipment, and personnel problems that arise in the program. Since board members do have considerable influence in their individual professions and in their community, favorable and unfavorable observations are highly regarded. By carefully

Table 6.3. Community evaluation issues and concerns

Issue	Concerns
Personnel	Training requirements (i.e., enough to do the job well, but not so much as to exclude potential staff); adequate salary and staff benefits; satisfactory working conditions; staff offer adequate reports about the program's quality; staff are upstanding citizens who fit into the community; no abuse or reports of abuse in the program; volunteers are accepted, trained, and supervised
Physical site	Building meets fire and safety codes; area zoned for buildings for public use; adequate parking is available; place for parents to stop, drop off, and pick up children; property and yard are well maintained
State regulations	Building and staff structure meet day care provider standards
Service provided	Sufficient service for all families, parents satisfied with services

selecting board members, it is possible to have friendly expertise for the program in a variety of pertinent fields including, not only those listed in Table 16.1, but also business and financial leaders in the community. Although few early intervention programs could afford to hire a pediatrician on staff, it is possible to have this input by having an interested pediatrician on the board. Of course, with having such experienced professionals on the board it is important to implement their suggestions. The professional opinions of the advisory board are, perhaps, the most significant community evaluation. A board of advisors that are well-informed and given current information concerning problems as well as successes in the program can make a more accurate professional opinion of the program's effectiveness. It is likely that they will have many official and unofficial opportunities to state their opinions.

Public Awareness   Other community evaluations may be made by persons who have less direct information concerning the project, but who may come to the center as repair or maintenance personnel. Some evaluation of the program will be made by people who may never come to the center, but hear it discussed in a service club presentation by a parent whose child attends, by the bus driver, or by a neighbor. Others may read about the project in a newspaper feature article.

Regardless of how these people have contact with the program, they will be forming opinions concerning the needs of the children and the quality of the services that have been organized to attempt to meet those needs. It is helpful to provide information about the program to the public. Therefore, public awareness planning involves fostering a positive image of the program to community members. Organizing an open house, inviting the public to performances by the children, and other suggestions offer in Chapter 3 to entice volunteers, are also helpful in providing information to the public about the program. If the program is more visible, it has a greater opportunity of creating a positive community image. Programs with positive local image are most likely to have support when the quality needs to be documented for increased, expanded, or continued funding.

Clinical Evaluation

When evaluating the young child, psychologists and teachers frequently use standardized tests and criterion-referenced scales for guidance as to what behaviors to expect a child to perform. Naive observers are hampered by lack of experience and sometimes place too much confidence in both standardized and criterion assessment. Until one has observed and interacted with a large number of infants and children, it is not possible to make appropriate comparisons, to interpret the critical subtleties of movement or response patterns, or to assess the overall effect of delay or immaturity of responses to people. It is also difficult to see early indications of an emerging skill or to recognize a situation that might become a problem in the attainment of a later skill.

Preservice instruction can explain and illustrate some of the critical observations that need to be made, but it is not possible to develop clinical skill from formal instruction. Proud parents of first-born children frequently recognize smiles, hear words, and imply actions in an infant that more experienced infant caregivers only see as random movement or sound rather than early signs of highly intelligent behavior. Reflex behaviors (explained in Chapter 10) are an excellent example of the need for clinical experience for accurate assessment. Until an evaluator has observed a number of children over time, it is difficult to distinguish between what is and is not a normal reaction. Parents and novice early intervention personnel can easily mistake the extended body position of a child with motor problems who is lying on the stomach as controlled head-lifting behavior when actually it is part of a rigid uncontrolled body position that the child needs assistance to overcome.

Some of the behaviors that young children exhibit when they are ill or tired may be mistaken by an inexperienced observer as severe developmental problems if that person has not had the opportunity to watch the same child for some time, under a variety of circumstances. Some under-stress behaviors are similar to ones exhibited by many children, while others are idiosyncratic to a particular child. Therefore, a clinical assessment cannot be made effectively without asking the regular caregiver about a child's typical behaviors.

Clinical expertise can be gained in a variety of ways. All of them, however, require ample observation and interaction with infants and young children. It is absolutely necessary for anyone wishing to improve his or her clinical skills to first observe infants over time, and to pick them up and handle them. Then the person should share his or her observations with someone else who also has had ample hands-on experience. This kind of collaborative comparison can begin in preservice practica and continue in cooperative exchanges with professionals who have already developed clinical expertise.

Although there are a number of routines that many people use in the process of clinical evaluation, clinicians often develop individual preferences for particular observations that they find to be helpful. For example, a pediatrician can complete a developmental evaluation as he or she undresses an infant. Instead of asking the parent to remove the infant's clothing for examination, the doctor performs the task, feeling the muscle tone and noting how the child reacts during the process. The doctor's sensitive response to the child gains the trust of the mother and, in turn, elicits accurate and complete information from her. The mother, too, is then comfortable with asking pertinent questions. In only a few minutes of interaction, the pediatrician has had the opportunity to handle the child, to begin to assess the child's problems, and to develop a rapport with the mother.

Another professional may have a child play with a toy that can create an interaction fruitful to observe (Newson & Newson, 1979). A speech/language therapist, for instance, can use a small wind-up toy to elicit receptive and expressive communication. This can provide the basis for comparison of many children's responses. An experienced psychologist learns more about a child's development by observing his or her behavior during a test than from the test score. It was through decades of this type of observation that Jean Piaget (Flavell, 1963) was able to describe the stages of child development.

One of the problems for skilled professionals in implementing clinical evaluation is finding the time to personally observe each child and, for best results, actually interact with the child. It is also difficult to compare a child's responses today to the responses the child has made in the past. The Early Intervention Research Institute at Utah State University, Logan, Utah, has developed a number of protocols to help overcome these difficulties by capturing a child's behavior on videotape for evaluation. The videotape can be used by someone who does not see the child routinely or for comparison of future skills to current skills. Figure 6.2 is an example of a protocol for videotape assessment of parent-child interaction. There are a variety of methods for summarizing and counting such interactions. Among the most popular are those developed by Jay and Farran (1981); Kogan (1980); Mahoney, Finger, and Powell (1985); and Marfo (1984). Although each of these methods emphasize different behaviors and have different criteria, they all count the number of responses that the child and the adult make, as well as how closely they follow one another.

Clinical expertise cannot be endowed, inherited, or willed in a short amount of time. It must be earned through days and days of careful observation and remembering other observations. Perhaps the most effective strategy for a young professional wishing to develop such skill is to work with someone who has developed clinical expertise and is willing to share their professional life. Sometimes this "sharing" can be part of paid employment. Other times, it must be volunteer work or part of continuing training. If the professional wishing to acquire the knowledge is personally confident and secure enough to keep asking to be told and shown, it is possible to learn more quickly. Good clinical skills come from being a lifelong "student" of human behavior.

Parents can also acquire clinical skills. Sensitive parents who have been around children or have raised other children have daily opportunities for ongoing evaluation. They can clearly see how one child's reactions may differ from the reactions of others. Although most parents have not had the opportunity to observe hundreds of children, they have had the opportunity to intensely observe a few children. Wise professionals will listen to the explanations of parents, particularly to the concerns expressed by parents who have had considerable experience with infants and children.

SETTING

The setting and the individual doing the videotaping should be equally unfamiliar to all caregivers/children, and it should be at a center-based location as opposed to in the home. Set up the videotape equipment in a *small carpeted room* (approximately 12' by 12'). The caregiver may choose to interact with the child on the floor or sitting in a chair. A comfortable adult-sized chair (or sofa) and an end table should be arranged in a corner area.

The camera should be positioned on a tripod approximately 8'–10' from the subjects, should be at the eye level of the caregiver, and should *not* be directed toward a window. Videotape the caregiver and the child so that the frame includes both participants' faces and hands.

MATERIALS

Toys (items from Battelle Kit)
1. Dolls
2. Ball
3. Cloth
4. Fuzzy green bear
5. Play telephone
6. Rattle

Recording equipment
1. Video camera
2. Tripod
3. Cordless microphone
4. Stop watch

INSTRUCTIONS TO PARENTS

"We're interested in observing (*name of child*) in a play session. You will be asked to do several activities during the (16-minute) videotaping sequence.

First, I would like you to simply *relax* and play together (for 10 minutes) as you would at home. You may use the toys in the basket if you want to, or you may spend some time playing your favorite games without using the toys. Save the books for the later reading activity.

After (10 minutes), encourage your child to put away the toys—you may help, if necessary. Do this as you normally would at home.

Next, you'll read a book to your child. There are two books. You may choose either one, or read both. (2 minutes)

Finally, say to (*name of child*), "I will be right back." Leave the room for 45 seconds, closing the door behind you. However, if you hear that your child is in distress, you may return immediately. I'll hand you a stop watch so that you know when the 45 seconds are up.

The videotaping will continue for 2 minutes after you re-enter the room. You may do whatever you like when you return. The toys can be used again if you wish.

I'll let you know when to move on to the next activity, so don't feel that you have to remember all the steps. After videotaping has begun, please try to ignore me and interact only with (*name of child*). Do you have any questions?"

Figure 6.2. An example of a protocol for videotape assessment of parent-child interaction. (From Early Intervention Research Institute. [1987]. *Videotape assessment of parent-child interaction.* Logan: Utah State University.)

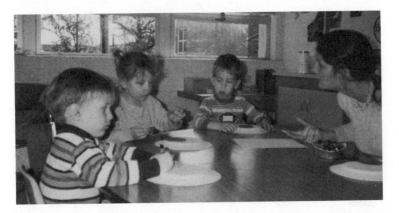

UNINTENDED IMPACT OF EVALUATION ON PARTICIPANTS

No matter how well-intentioned or carefully planned and conducted, even the mere mention of evaluation can cause anxiety for the participant (Glenwick et al., 1985). This anxiety is frequently not abstract worry but directly related to vested interests, such as potential reduction of salary or staff or an emphasis in the evaluation on the more visible parts of a program because they are easier to report on than the less quantifiable (but more substantive) components. For example, the effect of such less visible components of the program, including social work consultation, the information hot line, and support activities for siblings and grandparents, are often extremely difficult to measure. However, these components may have a more positive effect on the families than the easily quantifiable components such as the number of hours of direct service to the child.

If the number of hours served has been identified as a criteria of the evaluation, it is also possible that the number of clients or some other quantifiable aspect of the project may become the focus of the evaluation process, rather than a study of the appropriateness of services for the children and their families (Applegate & Hamm, 1985). To assess individual appropriateness of services, a professional evaluation is required for each child and family (Glenwick et al., 1985). Not only is the process almost always a trying time for those being evaluated, but it is also difficult for the evaluators, especially if they anticipate careful scrutiny by others of the criteria, plans, and data they have collected. It is pertinent also, of course, to review the effectiveness and usefulness of the evaluation process itself. Sometimes this is done by the same evaluation team, while other times an outside party or committee is called in.

Although the response of the evaluators themselves to this review process must be considered in the planning of the evaluation, priority need not be given to the personal reactions of the evaluators. The impact for them can be regarded as part of the stress associated with the job role. Of importance, however, to programs undertaking evaluation are the potential, unintended side effects for the program. These may have an impact on: 1) the program itself, and/or 2) the families who are being served by the program.

Impact on Programs

When time, energy, and other resources are used to evaluate a program, regular program services may be delayed or curtailed. Gathering data by assessing children and families and examining records may consume large quantities of staff time (Hupp & Kaiser, 1986). Additional time is needed to process information into report format. Even the most minimal evaluation requires that meetings be held to discuss procedures and to make staff assignments. Most data collected for the review process must be made available by the staff responsible for maintenance of those records, even if the data are to be summarized by others.

The time it takes to plan and implement evaluation, even if the actual evaluation personnel are supplied through additional resources, must be taken from other program activities. It is thus unavoidable that the evaluation procedure will be disruptive in some measure the agency's routine activities. Consequently, questions concerning how much of a program's resources should be devoted to evaluation need to be asked continually (Marston & Magnusson, 1985).

An evaluation may also create renewed disagreement over philosophical issues or rekindle old arguments about how responsibilities are distributed (Glenwick et al., 1985). Such disagreements can adversely affect the quality and/or level of services being provided to the clients until a resolution is reached. Unfortunately, the handicapped children and their families are the ones who are most jeopardized in these situations.

Unintentional Impact on Families

Most discussions of family needs concentrate on the extra services needed for the child with a handicap and seldom address the additional emotional concerns of the family. Although one unintended effect of an evaluation on a family might be temporary lessening of services during the evaluation procedure, the psychological impact of program evaluation may be more dramatic. Families learn to deal with the emotional stress of having a handicapped member in a variety of ways. Although it is seldom reported in the literature, the coping patterns and mechanisms that parents develop for themselves and their normal children are more related to how parents have learned to deal with altered expectations and increased life stress then they are to loss of self-esteem, and they have little to do with the type or severity of the child's disability (McCubbin, Cauble, & Patterson, 1982).

One of the ways that well-adapted people deal with an overwhelming, life-encompassing problem is to meet the situation "one day at a time" and minimize "worrying" about how things will be in the future (Hall, 1983). For parents of a handicapped child, one significant way to do this is to focus on the skills that the child has learned and to take pleasure in the progress that the child *has* made. Comparison to the progress of other children is avoided. Using this healthy mechanism, it is possible for parents to find additional courage, stamina, and strength to face the day-to-day difficulties caused by handicapping conditions (Tingey, 1987).

Evaluation time, however, brings an abrupt halt to this adaptive procedure. Parents are expected, and sometimes required, to cooperate fully with a procedure that brings them face-to-face with information about their child's progress. The procedure compares other children the same age to their child, giving the parents information they may have already known and tried to "forget." This can be a most stressful situation for the parents and can renew disappointments and concerns about the child's ultimate capabilities.

Evaluation of a program designed to help their child may bring stress to parents in other ways as well. The very process of program evaluation implies that the program might be less than perfect (which, of course, anyone working in the agency already knows). For parents who are generally very concerned about the progress of their child, the implication that the program might have weaknesses may tend to shatter their unconditional faith in the program. For some parents, the program may have been regarded as the means to "saving" their child from a lifetime of difficulty. This questioning of program efficacy may jeopardize the stability of the coping mechanisms they have built around the importance of the program.

Of course, seasoned professionals know that this unconditional faith in the treatment is not well founded. Most children who are enrolled in early intervention programs need continued specialized services well beyond the early intervention years. Indeed, *all* children continue to need at least regular education and child care in order to develop into competent adults. For most handicapped children, it is unrealistic to think that a program, no matter how sophisticated, could save a child from all of the potential effects of a developmental disability.

EVALUATION AS A ROUTINE

If evaluation of program effectiveness is seen not as a one-time procedure but as an ongoing determination of the most adequate use of resources, it can become a more efficient tool for creating continued improvement. In order to use evaluation to improve the program, evaluators should repeatedly address the following questions:

1. Why is the evaluation needed?
2. What questions can reasonably be addressed?
3. What kind of information can be gathered?

4. What will be the responsibilities of planners and staff?
5. What standard of success will be applied to the data? (Glenwick, Stephens, & Maher, 1985)

Answers from these questions guide the ongoing evaluation.

Since early intervention services must meet the needs of a variety of families who are raising young handicapped children services must be tailored to their needs and the community's needs. It is not possible to design a model early intervention program that will be appropriate for all children and all communities. Programs must be modified to meet individual family needs and to respond to changing community needs, as well as responding to evaluation data.

In addition to acknowledging the differences of communities, evaluation processes must also recognize change across time. Although the biological needs of young children are similar across generations and among different cultures, the methods and expectations of meeting those needs change, as does the structure of the family. Many early intervention programs began as in-home training for mothers who then were able to use the procedures with their children. As social and economic changes alter the makeup of the workforce and fewer mothers remain home, this model, no matter how effective in times past, may not meet today's needs. Again, ongoing evaluation is needed.

SUMMARY

As Public Law 99-457 influences early services to handicapped children, the evaluation of the effectiveness of those services will become more important than ever. With ongoing evaluation even today's most successful procedures may be improved. It is critical that the evaluation of program effectiveness be regarded not as an add-on feature, imposed from the outside, but as an integral part of the early intervention program. Instead of addressing the issues raised earlier in this chapter (Who Is Interested and Why?) only when an outside agency poses them, wise program planners will build these questions into their program. Without a questioning attitude, any program can become stale, stagnant, and ineffective.

STUDY QUESTIONS

1. Interview staff members concerning the successful and difficult experiences that they have had in the classroom.

2. Go to a public hearing concerning early intervention in your state/community and write a summary of the discussion.

3. Volunteer to serve as a member of an evaluation team for a local or state program.

4. Observe an early intervention program and write a critique of the activities for children and adults who participate in the program.

REFERENCES

Aman, M. G., Singh, N. N., Stewart, A. W., & Field, C. J. (1985). The Aberrant behavior checklist: A behavior rating scale for the assessment of treatment effects. *American Journal of Mental Deficiency, 89*(5), 485–491.

Anderson, D. R., Hodson, G. D., & Jones, W. G. (1975). *Instructional programming for the handicapped student.* Springfield, IL: Charles C Thomas.

Applegate, R. L., & Hamm, S. J. (1985). Accelerated learning in the resource room. *Accelerated Learning, 21*(1), 71–73.

Bickman, L., & Weatherford, D. L. (1986). *Evaluating early intervention programs for severely handicapped children and their families.* Austin, TX: PRO-ED.

Early Intervention Research Institute. (1987). *Videotape assessment of parent-child interaction.* Logan: Utah State University.

Fewell, R. R. (1986). The management of family functioning. In L. Bickman & D. L. Weatherford (Eds.), *Evaluating early intervention programs for severely handicapped children and their families* (pp. 263–307). Austin, TX: PRO-ED.

Flavell, J. (1963). *The developmental psychology of Jean Piaget.* New York: Van-Nostrand Reinhold.

Fuchs, D., Fuchs, L., Benowitz, S., & Barringer, K. (1987). Norm-referenced tests: Are they valid for use with handicapped students? *Exceptional Children, 54*(3), 263–271.

Glenwick, D. S., Stephens, M. A. P., & Maher, C. A. (1985). On considering the unintended impact of evaluation: Reactive distortions in program goals and activities. *Evaluation and Program Planning, 7,* 321–327.

Goodlad, J. (1984). *A place called school: Prospects for the future.* New York: McGraw-Hill.

Hall, E. (1983). *Psychology today* (Fifth Ed.). New York: Random House.

Hoko, J. A. (1986). Evaluating instructional effectiveness: Norm-referenced and criterion-referenced tests. *Educational Technology, 26,* 44–47.

Hupp, S. C., & Kaiser, A. P. (1986). Evaluating educational programs for severely handicapped preschoolers. In L. Bickman & D. L. Weatherford (Eds.), *Evaluating early intervention programs for severely handicapped children and their families* (pp. 233–261). Austin, TX: PRO-ED.

Jay, S., & Farran, D. C. (1981). The relative efficacy of predicting IQ from mother-child interactions using ratings versus behavioral count measures. *Journal of Applied Developmental Psychology, 2,* 165–177.

Kogan, K. L. (1980). Interaction systems between preschool handicapped or developmentally delayed children and their parents. In T. M. Field (Ed.), *High risk infants and children* (pp. 227–247). New York: Academic Press.

Lamping, D. L. (1985). Assessment in health psychology. *Canadian Psychology, 26*(2), 121–139.

Mahoney, G., Finger, I., & Powell, A. (1985). Relationship of maternal behavioral style to the development of organically impaired mentally retarded infants. *American Journal of Mental Deficiency, 90*(3), 296–302.

Marfo, K. (1984). Interactions between mothers and their mentally retarded children: Integration of research findings. *Journal of Applied Developmental Psychology, 5,* 45–69.

Marrs, L. W. (1984). Should a special educator entertain volunteers?: Interdependence in rural America. *Exceptional Children, 50,* 361–366.

Marston, D., & Magnusson, D. (1985). Implementing curriculum-based measurement in special and regular education settings. *Exceptional Children, 52*(3), 266–276.

McCubbin, H. I., Cauble, A. E., & Patterson, J. M. (1982). *Family stress, coping, and social support.* Springfield, IL: Charles C Thomas.

Newborg, J., Stock, J. R., Wnek, L., Guidubaldi, J., & Svinicki, J. (1984). *Battle Developmental Inventory.* Allen, TX: DLM Teaching Resources.

Newson, J., & Newson E. (1979). *Toys and play things.* New York: Pantheon Books.

Rosenberg, S. A., Robinson, C. C., Finkler, D., & Rose, J. S. (1987). An empirical comparison of formulas evaluating early intervention program impact on development. *Exceptional Children, 54*(3), 213–219.

Shadish, W. R. (1986). Sources of evaluation practice: Needs, purposes, questions, and technology. In L. Bickman & D. L. Weatherford (Eds.), *Evaluating early intervention programs for severely handicapped children and their families* (pp. 149–183). Austin, TX: PRO-ED.

Smith, N. L. (1986). Evaluation alternatives for early intervention programs. In L. Bickman & D. L. Weatherford (Eds.), *Evaluating early intervention programs for severely handicapped children and their families* (pp. 185–207). Austin, TX: PRO-ED.

Swift, C. F., Fine, M. A., & Beck, S. (1985). Early intervention services for young children: National implications from a key informal look at Ohio. *Mental Retardation, 23*(6), 308–311.

Tardy, C. H. (1985). Social support measurement. *American Journal of Community Psychology, 13*(2), 187–202.

Tingey, C. (1987). Cutting the umbilical cord: Parental perspectives. In S. Pueschel (Ed.), *The young person with Down syndrome: Transition from adolescence to adulthood* (pp. 5–22). Baltimore, MD: Paul H. Brookes Publishing Co.

Tingey-Michaelis, C. (1986). Early intervention helps parents too. *The Exceptional Parent, 16*(2), 51–52.

Valus, A. (1986). Achievement-potential discrepancy status of students in LD programs. *Learning Disabilities Quarterly, 9,* 200–205.

Van Hof-Van Duin, J., Mohn, G., & Batenburg, A. M. (1982). Simple tests of visual function of multiply handicapped children. *International Journal of Rehabilitation Research, 5*(2), 239–240.

Weatherford, D. L. (1986). The challenge of evaluating early intervention programs for severely handicapped children and their families. In L. Bickman & D. L. Weatherford (Eds.), *Evaluating early intervention programs for severely handicapped children and their families* (pp. 1–18). Austin, TX: PRO-ED.

Wykes, T., Sturt, E., & Creer, C. (1985). The assessment of patients' needs for community care. *Social Psychiatry, 20,* 76–85.

Chapter 7

Mainstreaming Preschools

A Review of Suggested Procedures

Mary Ann Hanson, Glendon Casto,
Carol Tingey, and Richard A. van den Pol

———————— • ————————

In his opening remarks to the Second Annual Conference of the Division of Early Childhood, Fredericks (1986) provided a 20-year retrospective list of *best practices* in early childhood special education. As one of the top three practices, Fredericks included meaningful integration of handicapped and non-handicapped preschoolers. Other parents agree (Bennett, 1978; Michaelis, 1981; Vyas, 1979). He noted that while his own handicapped son had not received this service, subsequent experiences as a parent and a researcher were sufficiently convincing to cause Fredericks to recommend that integration be included in Oregon state law. Other sources of encouragement for preschool mainstreaming are readily found in *least restrictive* provisions of Public Law 94-142, as well as in literature describing research and demonstration projects implemented during the last two decades.

The legislative mandates of Public Law 94-142 require that school-age handicapped children be guaranteed a free appropriate education in a *least restrictive setting* (McLean & Odom, 1988). A least restrictive setting is generally considered one that is not isolated from nonhandicapped peers (Bellamy, 1987). This requirement has generated a number of questions to be answered,

Work reported in this chapter was carried out in part with funds from the U.S. Department of Education (Contract #s 300-82-0367 and 300-85-0173) to the Early Intervention Research Institute at Utah State University and Grant #G008730535 to the CO-TEACH Preschool Program at the University of Montana.

issues to be resolved, and problems to be solved for educators, administrators, and parents (Irwin & Wilcox, 1987). States have adopted mandates providing for the education of the handicapped preschool population, beginning at either birth or age 3. In most cases, this age group has received services through state education, health, or social services agencies, or under the auspices of a private agency. Historically, specialized services have been provided in settings that include few or no nonhandicapped peers, as most states do not provide preschool educational services for nonhandicapped children. However, as early intervention programs have evolved, there has been more and more concern about social isolation of handicapped children.

Individuals desiring to mainstream children into regular educational or child care settings must deal with such issues as the clarification of responsibilities, how placement decisions are made, and concerns of parents. Parents of nonhandicapped children have voiced concerns about the effects of the handicapped child's presence. In particular, they fear that the quality of education for nonhandicapped children might suffer if staff are busy attending to the special needs of the handicapped child. Parents of handicapped children have been concerned about whether their child's special needs can be met if the child is served in a regular class or day care setting. Professionals have been concerned about development and implementation of curriculum approaches that provide optimal educational opportunities for both populations of children. Moreover, professionals have been challenged with the identification and arrangement of conditions that promote meaningful interactions between handicapped and non-handicapped students in integrated classrooms.

A common theme in reports of research findings and recommendations of service delivery professionals is that meaningful outcomes are likely only when specific mainstreaming goals are targeted, and programs are implemented to address those goals (Faught, Balleweg, Crow, & van den Pol, 1983; Peterson & Haralick, 1977; Striefel, Killoran, & Quintero, 1986; van den Pol, Crow, Rider, & Offner, 1985). Mainstreaming goals might include: 1) integrated social interaction, 2) skill acquisition via integrated educational opportunities, and 3) attitudinal changes on the part of nonhandicapped peers.

Mainstreaming may involve integrating a handicapped child in a *regular* setting, as in Striefel et al., (1986) *Functional Mainstreaming for Success* model. An alternative is *reverse mainstreaming*, where nonhandicapped peers are enrolled in special preschools, as in the Montana Big Sky model (van den Pol et al., 1985). This chapter reviews the outcomes of some of the research studies and model programs, presents the reader with a summary of established *best practices* as well as promising innovative ones, offers guidelines for implementation, and provides suggestions for evaluating the worth of such programs. The authors hope to more fully address the implementation of an "enlightened application of the mainstreaming principle" (Guralnick, 1978).

CRITICAL CONCEPTS FOR MAINSTREAMING

A review of research studies and model programs identified several major areas of critical importance to mainstreaming success: 1) systematic decisionmaking processes to determine each child's program, 2) well-defined management procedures, 3) curriculum approaches, 4) follow-up services to children, and 5) evaluation of the success of the program.

Systematic Decisionmaking

It is agreed by those who have conducted or are conducting research and implementing model programs that a major key to success in mainstreaming efforts is a firm commitment by all involved (Gil & Wend, 1985; Striefel et al., 1986; Taylor, 1982). This commitment must be accompanied by a systematic decisionmaking process by an interdisciplinary team comprised of those individuals concerned with the mainstreaming process in general, and especially with the child being mainstreamed (Allen, 1980; Gil & Wend, 1985; Miesels, 1977; Striefel et al., 1986). Kaufman, Gottlieb, Azard, and Kukic (1975) additionally suggest the need for a "clarification of responsibility among regular and special education administration, instructional and supportive personnel" (p. 4), that is, among the team members.

The Functional Mainstreaming for Success (FMS) Project (Striefel et al., 1986) at the Developmental Center for Handicapped Persons at Utah State University conducted a review of the mainstreaming literature, and found that it was not possible to clearly define or locate research concerning the many variables necessary in successful mainstreaming. The developers of the FMS project isolated the following variables as being of primary importance in the decisionmaking process: selecting appropriate teachers for mainstreamed placements, preparing teachers for mainstream assignments, and preparing normal and handicapped students and their parents for mainstreaming (Striefel et al., 1986, p. 7).

Miesels (1977) provided a series of questions to ask, and listed steps that child care programs should consider when deciding whether to incorporate mainstreaming into their setting. He stressed a sequence of useful steps in exploring the mainstreaming concept, and presented guidelines to consider when the child is in the program. Included in the steps are information gathering, planning, teacher preparation, parent preparation, classroom arrangement, and ongoing in-service training. A similar process is recommended by Gil and Wend (1985), the developers of the Handicapped Children's Early Education Program (HCEEP) model at the Northwest Center for Child Development in Seattle, Washington. These include planning, defining roles, establishing goals and timelines, using a formal intervention model and philosophy, conducting evaluation, ensuring family involvement, and providing ongoing staff training.

Classroom Management Procedures

The concept of mainstreaming has been interpreted, unfortunately, and perhaps too often, as the mere placement of a handicapped child in close proximity with his or her nonhandicapped peers, in the hopes that fortuitous social interactions would occur (see Chapter 12), and that the handicapped child would imitate, learn from, generalize, and make developmental gains as a result of this proximity. It has also been assumed that through the simple proximity of these two groups of children, more positive attitudes on the part of nonhandicapped children and their parents would occur spontaneously. As a result of these assumptions, there has tended to be an emphasis on social interaction alone, with the exclusion of educational integration, resulting in the use of recess or freeplay activities, lunch programs, music, and art in integrated settings as mainstreaming opportunities. There also has been a tendency to fit the child to the program or curriculum approach, rather than making adaptations within settings that accommodate the educational needs of both groups. These mainstreamed activities have resulted largely because there has been a paucity of information available to educators and caregivers on procedures that would promote interaction, or curriculum models that would facilitate educational integration. Some authors are emphasizing the necessity for, and are in the process of, designing program models and curriculum approaches that will assist educators in their facilitation of a "learning and growing environment in which handicapped children interact with nonhandicapped children in a variety of activities . . . related to all areas of development" (Allen, 1980, p.44), and in which handicapped children "participate with their nonhandicapped peers in all aspects of instruction" (Fink & Sandall, 1979, p. 3).

Social Interaction and Peer Imitation   The outcomes of recent studies on social interaction and peer imitation were foreshadowed by Guralnick (1978), who stated that ". . . existing research with preschool children has documented that, especially for widely heterogenous groups of children, spontaneous interactions are not likely to occur . . . " and that "the arrangement of events and other specialized procedures to encourage and support integration may need to take place, especially if peer interactions are intended to serve as an educational and therapeutic resource" (pp. 121–122).

Social Interactions   The following are important considerations for promoting social interactions:

1. Social interactions occur more spontaneously between handicapped children and their nonhandicapped peers when the handicap is mild in nature (Apolloni & Cooke, 1978).
2. Social interactions occur more frequently when the setting is structured to promote interaction (Apolloni & Cooke, 1978; Guralnick, 1978; Ispa & Matz, 1978; Striefel et al., 1986).

3. Structuring the setting to promote interaction leads to more sophisticated and organized play on the part of handicapped children, and an increase in fantasy play (Guralnick, 1978).
4. Teacher praise is an effective tool for increasing social interactions between the two groups, but it must be delivered unobtrusively and without interrupting the flow of play (Apolloni & Cooke, 1978; van den Pol et al., 1985).
5. Dramatic play and role-playing activities are more conducive to promoting social interaction than is continued adult involvement (Shores, Hester, & Strain, 1976).

Peer Imitation   The following are important considerations for promoting peer imitation:

1. Peer imitation studies support the concept of training delayed children to imitate the behavior of nondelayed peers; imitative behaviors were found to generalize, as did increased social interactions (Apolloni & Cooke, 1978).
2. The degree and nature of imitation varies according to age and sex: younger children imitate older; imitation occurs more readily with a child of the same sex.
3. A peer tutoring system and a buddy system can be viable intervention strategies to support interaction (Striefel et al., 1986), and to facilitate positive attitudes of nonhandicapped children toward their handicapped peers.

Curriculum Approaches

Some curriculum approaches may be more appropriate for mainstreaming than others. Anastasiow (1978) reviewed and described four preschool curriculum models that exist as approaches to preschool education: 1) behavioral, 2) normal development, 3) cognitive development, and 4) cognitive learning. He concluded that the behavioral model (alone) is best utilized for treating children with severe behavioral problems, but may not be as appropriate for nonhandicapped children. The normal developmental model places emphasis on specific skill development, readiness, social control (e.g., taking turns, sitting quietly, listening to instructions, and controlling impulses); employs the teaching strategies of group instruction, comparison of the individual child to the group or the norm, or "mean level of achievement in all areas of skill development" (p. 102); and stresses "conformity to the standards of the school" (p. 102). However, it may not be appropriate for the impaired child. Anastasiow concluded, "In my opinion, there are no actual normal developmental models for impaired children, and the model is inappropriate for them" (p. 102). Unfortunately, this model is the standard for the majority of the classrooms in the public school setting, and in many regular preschool and day care settings as well, since many of these programs gear their curriculum approaches to prepare the child for entrance into kindergarten.

Another model, the cognitive developmental, is based on the theories of Jean Piaget, who postulated that the child is an active participant in the learning process (see Chapters 2 and 11 for a discussion concerning Piaget). A curriculum approach and a set of teaching strategies for the education of handicapped children has been developed and implemented by the High/Scope Research Foundation in Ypsilanti, Michigan (Ispa & Matz, 1978). The daily routine, classroom arrangement, teaching strategies, and materials and equipment are coordinated to maximize the child's opportunities to be an active participant in his or her learning process while, at the same time, providing a program that is individualized to meet each child's educational goals. The designers of this model have found that appreciable levels of spontaneous interactions between mildly handicapped and nonhandicapped students did occur in the classrooms. They report that the organization of the classroom, the equal attention paid to both groups by the teachers, and the nondiscriminatory attitude of children at the preschool level are contributing factors to the observed interactions.

Another model that Anastasiow described as the cognitive learning model has been explicated by Bricker and Bricker (1976). The developers of this model combined principles from "operant procedures for lesson strategies and remediation while drawing upon cognitive, psycholinguistic, and perceptual theories to diagnose the child's level of development and to plan intervention programs" (p. 105). Bricker and Bricker also perceived the child as an active explorer of the environment. However, they observed that it may be necessary to teach the impaired child to initiate exploration or play when he or she does not do so spontaneously.

Anastasiow concluded his review by taking the position that the cognitive developmental and cognitive learning models have much to offer. The former, however, would not be appropriate for the severely impaired child, whereas the latter "would be suitable for [the impaired and] the normal preschool child as well" (p. 108). Unfortunately, little research evidence exists to support this assertion (Casto & Mastropieri, 1986). In an integrative review of some 2,000 articles summarizing the effectiveness of early intervention, Tingey-Michaelis (1986) concluded that a high degree of structure, including specific predetermined goals, accompanied progress for handicapped children, but not for nonhandicapped children.

Since all children do not flourish equally well in the same curriculum model, it is highly important that the placement be determined by their needs, as well as the interests of the staff. Since there will likely be a limited number of potential sites at any one location, finding a program with an appropriate curriculum approach for each child will be challenging.

Allen (1980) derived a list of critical components for assisting a child's successful transition from the preschool setting to the kindergarten classroom, based on a review of federally sponsored model programs. She advocated a team approach, emphasizing the following as necessary components: a transition coordinator, visits to public schools, observations in kindergarten classrooms, preschool staff meetings, parent meetings, placement staffings, transition to public school, and support services. She further outlined a sequence of steps and described important activities to be implemented in carrying out the transition process.

Continuing Evaluation

The function of continuing evaluation of mainstreaming activities is at least two-fold: to assess the degree to which specific goals and subordinate objectives have been met, and to guide adjustments in sending and/or receiving environments to allow intended outcomes to be achieved more effectively or efficiently. Because mainstreaming activities are typically contained within IEPs, it is logical that effectiveness should be continually monitored.

Few specific examples are available in the literature on how continuing evaluation procedures can guide adjustments in the preparation of students for transition, or the accommodation of students in integrated settings. Allen (1980) emphasized the need for continuous evaluation and support strategies for teachers in receiving programs. Miesels (1977) and Gil and Wend (1985) included ongoing evaluations as integral aspects of the mainstreaming process, but provided few details as to how this should be accomplished. Ongoing evaluation should be a major feature of model programs to determine the efficacy of the strategies employed and to make revisions based on the outcome of the evaluation (Striefel et al., 1986). Therefore, evaluation strategies are suggested in the final section of this chapter dealing with guidelines for mainstreaming.

Program Models

A variety of curriculum approaches or program models have been developed specifically to facilitate mainstreaming. Several existing models are briefly outlined below as examples.

Guralnick (1978) described the development of a demonstration program for the integration of handicapped and nonhandicapped children at the Experimental Preschool of the National Children's Center in Cincinnati, Ohio, in which children of varying developmental levels were enrolled. He and his colleagues found two approaches to be useful in maximizing interactions. Guralnick suggested that a program pay attention to: 1) the selection of play activities, games, and materials; 2) the flexibility in the design, content, and organization of the curriculum; 3) matching children's interests; 4) classroom arrangements; and 5) the systematic use of prompting activities by the teachers (p. 121). The second approach he suggested is the utilization of specific "reinforcement principles and techniques" to "build the observational, imitative, group involvement, and social interaction skills of the less advanced children" (p. 122).

Allen (1980) presented examples of several curriculum approaches that have been developed over the past several years through funding from the HCEEP model. She reported that "one strong similarity, however, that runs through many integrated preschool curricula is the developmental approach," and concluded that "all handicapped and nonhandicapped children are more alike than they are different, and that the developmental approach is the one with which most preschool teachers feel comfortable" (p. 121). The developmental model utilizes data from normal developmental sequences as a basis for designing tasks that are presented in a hierarchial order of difficulty. Content of the curriculum in this model is based on broad areas of development classified into social, motor, emotional, cognitive, and language domains (Allen, 1980, p. 114). Other evidence for Allen's position can be found in the emphasis on the developmental approach, which is common to most early childhood teacher training programs. Summative research has yet to establish, definitively, which approach or combination yields greatest child progress.

The FMS Project (Striefel et al., 1986) has as a major priority describing models that allow preschool handicapped and nonhandicapped children to be served together, at least on a part-time basis. Aspects of the FMS model that address this issue include: mainstreaming in age-appropriate classrooms; assessing a *best match* between teacher and child, when possible, based on teacher expectations and child skill levels; determining the degree of integration appropriate for each child; and the exploration and utilization of four techniques to foster social interaction. These techniques include a peer tutoring system; a joint teaching activity system; a buddy activity system; and a system in which handicapped and nonhandicapped children are carefully assigned to small groups, and normally occurring teaching opportunities throughout the day in all curriculum areas are used to maximize interaction.

SUMMARY OF CONCEPTS AND MODELS

A number of factors have been found to be critical for educators to consider when deciding on whether and how to place a handicapped child in a mainstream setting. The research cited offers important information on social interaction and peer imitation, emphasizing that for both to occur successfully and to be useful as intervention tools, they require the careful use of certain intervention strategies. Such strategies include attention to what teachers do or do not do, grouping of children, use of materials, and classroom arrangement. Developers of model programs emphasize the importance of commitment by all involved; thoughtful planning; systematic decisionmaking; careful prepara-

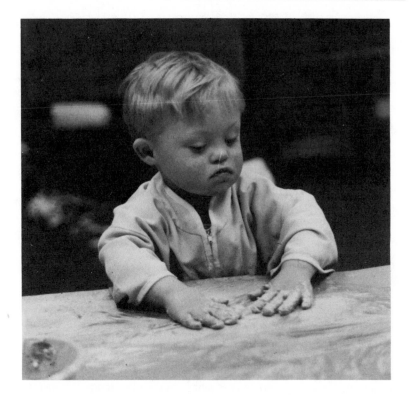

tion for parents, teachers, and administrators; carefully thought-out implementation strategies; and follow-up and evaluation procedures.

The final section of this chapter offers those professionals involved in mainstreaming a set of guidelines based on the literature reviewed. The guidelines are offered in a sequence of three steps, all of which may be considered important aspects of a successful mainstreaming process: 1) planning and preparation, 2) implementation, and 3) follow-up and evaluation. Circumstances within each community will suggest specific strategies, but a basic shared philosophy and a systematic, sequential process must be agreed upon to ensure a successful mainstreaming effort.

GUIDELINES FOR MAINSTREAMING

Planning

Guidelines for mainstreaming apply both when the integration of a handicapped child occurs within a nonhandicapped setting or when it occurs within the handicapped setting (i.e., if *reverse mainstreaming* is being considered).

The first step in planning is to discuss the mainstreaming options with staff members. Helpful questions to ask include:

1. Will the child benefit from mainstreaming?
2. If so, what are the options available? Should existing preschool or day care programs within the community be utilized, or should nonhandicapped children be integrated into a special education setting? Would both options be possible, depending on children's needs?
3. What preschool or day care programs are available? How close or dissimilar are they in their curriculum approach, daily schedule, and so on? What changes would the parents and children have to make if the child were mainstreamed into one of these settings?
4. What are the specific mainstreaming goals and what are the timelines for achieving these goals?
5. What will the staff roles be in the process? Who will be the mainstreaming coordinator?
6. Will supplemental funding be necessary, and if so, how may it be secured?

It is also helpful to have staff members develop a list of questions to discuss. The list of questions could be divided into those that need further exploration, or those that can be translated into assignments. A coordinator can be chosen at this time, and specific responsibilities assigned for staff members to complete.

If programs decide to explore the option to integrate a child or children from an existing setting into one for nonhandicapped children, the next step is to observe those programs that are being considered. Allen (1980) has prepared an observation checklist to be used when observing potential mainstreaming classrooms. This checklist represents an organized means for the observer to look at relevant areas such as teaching staff, classroom arrangement, daily schedule, behavior, self-help, skills, and curriculum approach. However, prior to observation, a meeting with the administrator of the program should be scheduled to discuss ideas and possibilities, and to receive permission to observe. The administrator may want to discuss mainstreaming approaches with the teachers prior to observation. It is important, no matter how the sequence is arranged, to make it clear that the observation is part of a decisionmaking process, that the observer is not an evaluator, and that both teacher's and administrator's ideas and suggestions are an important part of this decisionmaking process.

Other questions that are relevant regarding program options, and which need to be discussed in-depth with program staff and potential sites, include:

1. Which programs observed offer the greatest flexibility in curriculum approach, considering the adaptations that will be necessary to accommodate handicapped children?

2. How readily are the teachers able to individualize programs? What time and skills do they have available? How much training would be needed to help them develop these skills?
3. How receptive are the teachers and administrators to the concept of mainstreaming in their programs? Are they willing to make a commitment to try it?
4. How much in-service training will be necessary? Will it be done by existing staff, or will trainers from other programs, agencies, or a university setting be required?

Following discussion with the program staff, mainstreaming options can be explored, and ideas and options discussed with potential sites.

Next in the planning phase would be a meeting with parents of children in the program to discuss general ideas, and to respond to their questions and concerns. They should be invited to share their ideas and to participate in the exploration and planning process. The emphasis here should be on personal, one-to-one contact designed to increase the probability that they will accept the mainstreaming concept.

When this step of the planning phase has been completed, a meeting with project staff is held to discuss results of observations, parent meetings, and so on. They can then decide whether enough information exists to proceed, or whether further exploration is necessary. If the project is ready to proceed at this time, the nature and scope of the mainstreaming process should be outlined, goals and timelines set, and staff roles and responsibilities discussed and clearly defined. A suggested sequence would be to: 1) return to the mainstreaming site with the plan of action to elicit feedback and approval; 2) meet with the administrator(s) of the receiving program(s) to discuss goals and timelines; and 3) begin the process of the preparation of teachers, parents, and children.

Preparation

Teacher Preparation An initial step in teacher preparation is to meet to discuss the general concept of mainstreaming, as well as specifics such as goals and timelines. A brief overview of handicapping conditions, both written and oral, should be presented, and questions and concerns addressed. Mainstreaming series manuals may be useful. The U.S. Department of Health, Education, and Welfare has produced these manuals, which are available from the Superintendent of Documents, U.S. Printing Office, Washington, DC 20402. More specific information related to the IEP of the child being mainstreamed should be discussed just prior to the child's placement.

Ongoing teacher preparation in the form of in-service training and on-site consultation from sending teachers is helpful. The content of the mainstreaming in-service training can be generated from a survey of teacher concerns and a skills assessment. It can be conducted by staff from the program for handicapped children, using materials from one or more of the model programs listed in this chapter's reference list. On-site consultation would provide necessary support for the teachers, and provide information necessary to help the teachers make program decisions and necessary adaptations.

It is helpful, also, for the receiving teacher to spend some time observing the child in his or her current setting, especially prior to placement. The child will have an opportunity to meet the new teacher in comfortable, more secure surroundings, and the teacher will have the opportunity to observe the child's performance under optimal circumstances.

Parent Preparation   Parents should be active participants in the mainstreaming process. Parents' meetings to discuss the broader issues of mainstreaming give them an opportunity to be introduced to the concept, to share their concerns and ideas with other parents and with staff, and to gain more specific information about the programs into which their child may be mainstreamed. They may want to visit the program being considered, accompanied by the child's teacher. This would be a less intimidating, and likely more comfortable, arrangement for the parents and teachers being visited.

Preparation for parents of nonhandicapped children should include a meeting similar to the one previously mentioned; that is, a combination of providing information and discussing questions, concerns, and ideas. It might be coordinated with a parent potluck dinner at which parents of both groups of children could interact on an informal basis.

Parents of both handicapped and nonhandicapped children like to receive written information. Striefel et al. (1986) have prepared a brochure that addresses the concerns typically voiced by parents and includes questions by both groups of parents about the quality of services each child will receive.

Parents of nonhandicapped children, in both mainstreaming and reverse mainstreaming programs, may want to observe the program. An invitation could be extended, or an open house scheduled, that would include a brief tour and explanation of the program. This would be especially helpful for parents who are considering enrolling their nonhandicapped child in a reverse mainstreaming program.

Specific technical assistance provided by a handicapped child's parents may prove to be a promising support system for teachers. The CO-TEACH Preschool Program at the University of Montana (van den Pol et al., 1985) trains parents to teach preschool staff how to perform certain therapeutic interventions with their child. Future research is necessary to determine the ways whereby parents can effectively assist receiving teachers to work with their child in a mainstreamed setting.

Child Preparation   Information gathered from the observation gives the sending teacher an idea of the similarities and differences in the sending and receiving environments. This information is useful in deciding which is the best placement option (e.g., which is the best match between teacher expectation and child skill level [Striefel et al., 1986], which is the best curriculum approach that best meets the child's needs, or which classroom arrangement is most well suited to the child's needs). Realistically, not all of the *best* is available within one setting. Consequently, some child preparation strategies are likely to be needed to help the child develop readiness skills to enter the new program.

Introductory visits, during which the child is accompanied by his or her teacher, are important in easing the child's transition into a new setting. The visit from the receiving teacher is another way of making it easier for the child to make the change.

Preparation of the nonhandicapped children is also necessary. The FMS project has developed a modification of the *Kids on the Block* puppet show concept, and have found it to be a successful general introduction to handicapping conditions. Discussions with the children, dealing with the specific handicapping condition of the child being mainstreamed, can be helpful for children at the 4–5-year level. This is particularly useful when accompanied with suggestions on how they can help make the child welcome when he or she begins coming to their school.

Implementation

Decisions regarding the nature and scope of the mainstreaming of specific children need to be made next. The child's IEP team should be expanded to include those persons from the receiving program who are involved in the process. A specific plan should be developed that addresses the questions below:

1. Who will be responsible for coordinating the child's program?
2. What are the goals or anticipated outcomes for the child? What specific activities in the new setting will be necessary to meet these goals?
3. When will the mainstreaming program begin?
4. At what times will the child be mainstreamed? Will it be all day, a half-day, or only during certain activities?
5. Who will transport the child? Will it be necessary for a teacher from the existing program to stay with the child during the initial transition stage?
6. Who will evaluate the extent to which the goals are being met (i.e., is the program being effective in meeting the child's needs)?

The plan, when put into operation, includes specific child, teacher, and parent preparation activities as part of the implementation process.

Other important activities during the implementation phase are the setting of goals and timelines, and the defining of roles. These activities must be realistic for the child and family, as well as for special program and regular program personnel. Ongoing observations and support visits from the coordinator or sending teacher are especially important during the intial stages of the implementation. However, the frequency of these visits may be reduced as everyone becomes more comfortable with their roles.

Evaluation

Evaluation of mainstreaming programs is an ongoing process. Several questions must be asked about the general program and about the progress of each child. Specifically, teachers and parents will want to find answers to the questions below:

1. How is the child doing? Is learning occurring? Is the child meeting IEP objectives?
2. Is social integration occurring?
3. Are educational gains resulting from the presence of nonhandicapped peer models?
4. Is the handicapped child's presence interfering in any way with the education of the nonhandicapped students?
5. Is positive attitude change occurring among nonhandicapped children and their families?
6. Is the placement conducive to meeting the IEP goals that were set?
7. What program changes are needed, if any?
8. If changes are needed, what activities are necessary, and who will be responsible for their implementation?
9. Should preparation activities be modified for children prior to mainstreaming?
10. Are *booster sessions* needed to help the mainstreamed child participate?
11. Are parents and mainstream classroom teachers meeting to discuss the child's needs and progress?

It is important to recognize that this ongoing type of evaluation must occur throughout the mainstreaming process. Evaluation is not an activity to be reserved for the child's end-of-the-year IEP meeting because it will be too late to make program adaptations to meet the child's educational needs. It is important to discuss and work out problems that arise with all persons involved both on an informal basis and formally during regularly scheduled meetings.

It is also important to look at the impact of the mainstreaming program on the staff of the sending program, the parents, and the staff of the receiving program. Information on the impact can be gathered through informal visits with administrators, evaluation checklists completed by parents and teachers, and feedback and data gathered from the minutes of the meetings that were held during the mainstreaming process. The information will serve as a guide during the final evaluation procedure, which should take the form, again, of a systematic decisionmaking process that will help answer the questions of whether the program should be continued. The planning, implementation, and evaluation process should then be repeated if the decision is made to continue the program.

SUMMARY

This chapter has attempted, through a review of the literature and an overview of some model programs, to present the reader with what are considered *best practices* to utilize when engaged in the process of mainstreaming a child with handicaps into a setting with nonhandicapped peers. The importance of employing a systematic process of planning, implementation, and evaluation is clearly supported by both research and model programs as the most critical element in the mainstreaming process. Curriculum models, classroom arrangement, grouping of children, and materials and activities are seen as important variables to be considered when choosing a classroom setting. With these variables, the best possible match between teacher expectations and child skill levels is established. To achieve success, a whole-hearted commitment on the part of all persons involved is necessary. All persons should be active participants during the entire process. Teachers and parents should receive careful preparation and be included in the ongoing and final evaluation. The preparation of the children, their educational attainments, and their emotional well-being are of great importance throughout the entire process. Success in mainstreaming is ultimately measured in terms of the growth children make educationally, their ease of adaptation into a new setting, and their general state of well-being. In all stages of the planning and implementation, it is necessary to continually keep in mind that the goal and purpose of mainstreaming is to afford handicapped children the opportunity to learn and practice social skills with other children (see Chapter 12).

STUDY QUESTIONS

1. What experiences with nonhandicapped children do the infants and children have in early intervention programs in your state/community?

2. Interview parents of nonhandicapped preschoolers to discover their attitudes about having their child attend the same day care program as children who are handicapped.

3. Interview a day care provider in a regular nursery setting to discover issues concerning providing programming for a handicapped child in that setting.

4. Interview a neighbor of a handicapped child concerning the interaction of that child with other children in the neighborhood.

REFERENCES

Allen, K. E. (1980). *Mainstreaming in early childhood education.* Albany, NY: Delmar Publishers.

Anastasiow, N. J. (1978). Strategies and models for early childhood intervention programs in integrated settings. In M. J. Guralnick (Ed.), *Early intervention and the integration of handicapped and nonhandicapped children* (pp. 22–41). Baltimore: University Park Press.

Apolloni, T., & Cooke, P. (1978). Integrated programming at the infant, toddler, and preschool levels. In M. J. Guralnick (Ed.), *Early intervention and the integration of handicapped and nonhandicapped children* (pp. 147–165). Baltimore: University Park Press.

Bellamy, G. T. (1987). The OSEP plan for LRE: Schools are for everybody! In M. Irwin & B. Wilcox (Eds.), *Proceedings of the National Leadership Conference, Least Restrictive Environment: Commitment to implementation* (pp. 1–10). Bloomington: Indiana University, Institute for the Study of Developmental Disabilities.

Bennett, J. (1978). Company halt! In A. P. Turnbull & H. R. Turnbull (Eds.), *Parents speak out: Views from the other side of the two-way mirror* (pp. 150–166). Columbus, OH: Charles E. Merrill.

Bricker, W. A., & Bricker, D. D. (1976). The infant, toddler, and preschool research and intervention project. In T. Tjossem (Ed.), *Intervention strategies for high risk infants and young children* (pp. 545–572). Balimore: University Park Press.

Casto, G., & Mastropieri, M. A. (1986). The efficacy of early intervention programs for handicapped children: A meta-analysis. *Exceptional Children, 52,* 417–424.

Faught, K. K., Balleweg, B. J., Crow, R. E., & van den Pol, R. A. (1983). An analysis of social behaviors among handicapped and nonhandicapped preschool children. *Education and Training of the Mentally Retarded, 18,* 210–214.

Fink, W. T., & Sandall, S. B. (1979, February). *Integrated kindergartens: Rationale, curriculum, methodology and data.* Paper presented at the Oregon Conference, Center on Human Development, Preschool for Multihandicapped Children, University of Oregon, Eugene.

Fredericks, H. D. B. (1986, November). *Early intervention.* Plenary address at the annual Division of Early Childhood Conference, Council for Exceptional Children, Knoxville, KY.

Gil, L., & Wend, K. (1985). *Guidelines for development of an integrated program.* Seattle, WA: Northwest Center Child Development Program.

Guralnick, M. J. (1978). Integrated preschools as educational and therapeutic environments: Concepts, design, and analysis. In M. J. Guralnick (Ed.), *Early intervention and the integration of handicapped and nonhandicapped children* (pp. 1–20). Baltimore: University Park Press.

Irwin, M., & Wilcox, B. (1987). *Proceedings of the National Leadership Conference, Least Restrictive Environment: Commitment to implementation.* Bloomington: Indiana University, Institute for the Study of Developmental Disabilities.

Ispa, J., & Matz, R. (1978). Integrating handicapped preschool children within a cognitively oriented program. In M. J. Guralnick (Ed.), *Early intervention and the integration of handicapped and nonhandicapped children* (pp. 169–190). Baltimore: University Park Press.

Kaufman, M., Gottlieb, J., Azard, J. A., & Kukic, M. B. (1975). Mainstreaming: Toward an explication of the construct. In E. L. Meyer, G. A. Vergason, & R. J. Whelon (Eds.), *Alternatives for teaching exceptional children* (pp. 1–12). Denver: Love Publishing.

McLean, M., & Odom, S. (1988). *Least restrictive environment and social integration.* Reston, VA: Council for Exceptional Children.

Michaelis, C. T. (1981). Mainstreaming: A mother's perspective. *Topics in Early Childhood Education, 1*(1), 11–16.

Miesels, S. J. (1977). First steps in mainstreaming: Some questions and answers. *Young Children, 33*(1), 4–13.

Peterson, N. L., & Haralick, J. G. (1977). Integration of handicapped and nonhandicapped preschoolers: An analysis of play behavior and social interaction. *Education and Training of the Mentally Retarded, 12,* 235–245.

Shores, R. E., Hester, P., & Strain, P. S. (1976). The effects of amount and type of teacher-child interaction on child-child interaction during free-play. *Psychology in the Schools, 13,* 171–175.

Striefel, S., Killoran, J., & Quintero, M. (1986). *Functional mainstreaming for success* (A Handicapped Children's Early Education Project). Logan: Developmental Center for Handicapped Persons, Utah State University.

Taylor, S. J. (1982). From segregation to integration: Strategies for integrating severely handicapped students in normal school and community settings. *Journal of The Association of the Severely Handicapped Journal, 8,* 42–49.

Tingey-Michaelis, C. (1986). The importance of structure in early education programs for disadvantaged and handicapped children. *Early Child Development and Care, 23,* 283–297.

U.S. Department of Health, Education, and Welfare. (1982). *Project Head Start Mainstreaming Series.* Washington, DC: U.S. Government Printing Office.

van den Pol, R. A., Crow, R. E., Rider, D. P., & Offner, R. B. (1985). Social interaction research in an integrated preschool. *Topics in Early Childhood Special Education, 4,* 59–76.

Vyas, P. (1979). Just another little kid. In T. Dougan, L. Isbell, & P. Vyas (Eds.), *We have been there* (pp. 53–56). Salt Lake City, UT: Dougan, Isbell, and Vyas Associates.

IMPLEMENTING SPECIFIC INTERVENTIONS

———————————————— • ————————————————

The ultimate effect that a child's intervention has upon his or her future is determined by his or her subsequent quality of interaction. In order to determine this, individual goals must be established and activities for the developmental enhancement must be identified. This requires a sophisticated look at the child's skills and an understanding of how they are developed in children who are not having difficulty. Skills that are developed in the early years are: language, posture and movement, cognitive, social, and self-care. As parents and professionals identify specific problems, individual plans can be made to create appropriate learning environments for each child.

Chapter 8

Individual Goals for Children and Their Families

Carol Tingey, Wendy B. Doret, and
Roberta Rosenblum

•

In 1977, a new educational policy was implemented based on requirements of Public Law 94-142, which states that all handicapped children are entitled to free appropriate public education. This educational policy, which was radically new at that time, requires that school systems alter their educational scope and sequence to include whatever the individual child needs, rather than expecting the child to benefit from the preplanned grade level curriculum for all children. This dramatically democratic concept is a central requirement of Public Law 99-457, and now handicapped or at-risk children, birth through age 5, are entitled to individualized training. In addition, the new law adds another qualitative dimension by recognizing that programs for such children must be formulated in such a way that the services that are provided enhance the daily life functioning of the child. Since an infant or a young child is totally dependent upon the family, it is necessary to recognize that the child is only one element of the family system and that whatever effects him or her effects the entire system (Barber, Turnbull, Behr, & Kerns, 1988). The law, provided for infants and children, encompasses services for the entire family that are coordinated and "managed" in much the same way that a social worker manages a case (Garland, Woodruff, & Buck, 1988) The law does not specify who should be this manager. Some families have the emotional and intellectual resources to manage their own "case," while others may need assistance. Although some families may be in need of a variety of services and may be receiving public assistance for medical, food, and other basic necessities, these services are not seen as early intervention services due to the child's handicap; however, these services are needed due to the fragile condition of the family structure. Individual Family Service Plans (IFSPs) for early intervention must be based upon the identified needs of the child. Services given to strengthen the family system are offered to the family in an effort to enhance the development of the young child. Families whose children are not at developmental risk may need similar assistance, but those families must be served through other structures.

INDIVIDUALIZING FOR INFANTS AND YOUNG CHILDREN

Although implementation of these mandates is a challenge for agencies in even the most progressive states, parents and human services professionals already individualize for infants and preschooler.

Parents of nonhandicapped children can individualize by choosing a nursery school, day care, or care by friends or relatives for their children. The parents are offered a variety of settings, schedules, curriculums, and expectations for their child's care. By establishing their own eating, sleeping, playtime, and nap time habits and routines, infants and young children have unknowingly helped to design their own activities and schedules. Mothers and other careproviders have long had to adjust their daily schedules to meet the active and quiet times of each of the children under their care (Brazelton, 1969, 1974; Sutherland, 1974). However, coordinating the child's schedule with some form of individualized educational program that can be written and followed is a rather new challenge to both serviceproviders and parents (D'Zamko & Raiser, 1986; Mulligan & Guess, 1984). An additional challenge is that this plan must consider the needs of both the child and the entire family. This creates almost limitless possibilities. Programs might need to include training or counseling for siblings, assistance with home feeding equipment, or alternate communication devices. These programs might even provide evening instruction to meet the family's needs. Since plans to provide services to the family system will be more complicated, the challenge of providing service to a number of families simultaneously increases.

Zigler, in his thesis on the importance of individual attention child care for nonhandicapped children, suggests that no adult should be responsible for the care of more than three nonhandicapped infants (Trotter, 1987). Even more adult attention is necessary to establish appropriate individualized care and training for handicapped infants and young children. With careful use of economic resources (see Chapter 3) and supervised volunteers (see Chapter 4), it may be possible to provide ample direct care staff for center-based programming and home treatment of the handicapped child, as volunteers could be trained to assist with the child's treatment plan in the home as well (see Chapter 4).

Two general tasks need to be accomplished when providing an individualized program for an infant or young child. These tasks include: 1) creating the most appropriate individualized plan; and 2) organizing resources to provide consistent supervision, training, and related services as planned for each child throughout the 24-hour day. In order to show how these tasks are an interrelated, ongoing process of the individualized programming, schedules, forms, and implementation routines developed by the Association for Children with Down Syndrome (ACDS—A center-based early intervention project in Long Island, New York, serving children from birth to 5 years of age) provided in the chapter, used as examples.

CREATING AN INDIVIDUALIZED EDUCATION PROGRAM

Assessment of the infant or young child both provides an initial diagnosis and guidelines for goals that might assist the child to develop to his or her full potential. Clinical and psychological assessments (discussed in Chapter 2) yield information about the comparison of the handicapped child with other children, and identify emerging skills that the child may need to develop. The parents' input should also be included in the information gathered about the child's needs. Figure 8.1 is an example of a simple form used by the parents to record their observations.

The parents complete the form, expressing their concerns about their child. This input is then examined by a team of professionals from a variety of disciplines to determine the steps that need to be taken to address these concerns. If the parents ask for assistance with a skill that the child is not ready to perform, it becomes the responsibility of the appropriate professional to explain the developmental prerequisites of that skill (e.g., standing balance before walking). Table 8.1 presents the responsibilities of various professionals involved in the actual writing of the IEP. These responsibilities are also specified in each professional's job description.

In addition to the formalized assessment, each of the professionals is asked to fill out a checklist of skills that might be taught to the child to facilitate a larger goal (see criterion-referenced assessment in Chapter 6). The forms used by ACDS have been developed by the staff and include goals for which daily activities can be created. Figure 8.2 is an example of one such checklist for the child that deals with social skills awareness. Other checklists include function in language, motor, and self-help skills. Although recording the child's daily progress on these skills seems to be tedious, the fine increments of this list make it possible to easily pinpoint the activities that the child has mastered and those still needed so that less paperwork is necessary in the long run. A record-keeping format that provides less detail would require more of the staff's time to complete.

Child's name _____
Date _____
Dear Parents:
    The following information will assist your child's teachers and therapists in planning his or her IEP for this term. Please fill this sheet out and send it back within 1 week. Thank you.
1. What things do you see as priorities or goals for your child during this term?
    a. Gross motor (e.g., large body movement) _____
    _____
    b. Fine motor (e.g., finger or hand movement) _____
    _____
    c. Self-help (e.g., feeding, dressing, toileting, washing) _____
    _____
    d. Social development (e.g., sharing, playing) _____
    _____
    e. Language (e.g., sounds, words, sentences) _____
    _____
    f. Cognition (e.g., thinking, problem-solving) _____
    _____
2. Additional comments or concerns _____
    _____
    _____
    _____

Parent's signature _____

Figure 8.1. Sample parent's input form for an IEP.

Models for Staff Interaction

Adults must work together to create and implement a successful early intervention plan for a child and his or her family. There are a variety of models that have been used in the past that require a different amount of interaction among the professionals planning to serve the child and the family (Garland, Woodruff, & Buck, 1988). The most common models are: consultant, interdisciplinary, and transdisciplinary.

Consultant Model   In the consultant model, professionals evaluate the child and provide a written report prior to the meeting concerning the child's program. Sometimes, due to budget constraints or lack of availability, one or more of the consultants are not regular staff members but hired after the initial meeting due to the needs of this particular child. Most often, records from medical services such as a physical and neurological examination, vision and hearing checkup, nutritional evaluation, and dental screening are only provided in written format, without the professional who examined the child in attendance during the development of the IEP. In some programs speech, physical and occupational, and psychological therapy information is also provided by consultants. Decisions concerning child goals in the consultant model are usually made by the regular program staff sometimes consisting only of educational personnel.

Table 8.1. Specific IEP responsibilities of staff

Staff	IEP responsibility
Teachers	Assessment and establishment of goals: Cognitive Perceptual-motor Perceptual-visual Socialization Self-help
Psychologist	Behavioral observation Behavioral intervention Assessment of goal attainment
Speech/language therapist	Assessment and establishment of goals: Prespeech Feeding Speech and language
Physical therapist	Assessment and establishment of gross motor skills
Occupational therapist	Assessment and establishment of goals: Sensory integration Perceptual fine motor
Social worker	Family needs and concerns Social service needs

Interdisciplinary Model In the interdisciplinary model, professionals assess the child individually, establishing their own hypothesis concerning the child's needs. These professionals then attend a meeting in which they each present their findings and together decide how to use the information in the most effective way. Parents may meet with each of these professionals about their individual recommendation, but programming decisions are made in a team meeting. The teacher is usually the professional who pulls the pertinent information together from each of the professionals' recommendations and includes them in the staffing report.

Transdisciplinary Model As in the interdisciplinary model, each of the professionals in the transdisciplinary model examines the child and attends a staff meeting in which the child's skills and needs are discussed. However, in the transdisciplinary model, the professionals have all been trained to understand and implement the specialized techniques of the various disciplines of other team members. During the course of this assessment, the child is sometimes examined by several professionals simultaneously. Although individual evaluations may be written, the plan for the child is decided together as opposed to each professional submitting an individual report, as in the interdisciplinary model. A single report is written to summarize the child's needs after a consensus concerning these issues is reached during a staff meeting of the participating professionals. One professional is chosen as the team leader for each child. In an educational setting, the team leader is frequently a special educator

Name: _____

**SOCIALIZATION CHECKLIST
OF SELF-AWARENESS**

Date achieved		Comments
	1. Child will demonstrate self-awareness and attempt to make his or her needs known by:	
	a. Quieting when approached by a face or a voice	
	b. Quieting when picked up	
	c. Differentiating between being held and not being held)	
	d. Crying when uncomfortable	
	e. Reacting to hand or washcloth on face	
	f. Looking at own hand	
	g. Bringing feet to mouth when lying on back	
	h. Demanding attention	
	2. Child will demonstrate an awareness of others by:	
	a. Attending to an adult visually (e.g., facial features) for 3–5 seconds during feeding or playtime	
	b. Feeling adult's hand, body, or face with own hand	
	c. Fixating on unfamiliar feature of person (e.g., necklace, hat)	
	d. Attempting to localize the sound of an adult's voice	
	e. Reaching for familiar persons (e.g., visually recognizing caregiver)	
	f. Discriminating between strangers and known adults by clinging to the known adult or stiffening when held by a stranger	
	g. Exhibiting displeasure when caregiver leaves	

Figure 8.2. Socialization checklist of skills and self-awareness.

who is seen as the coordinator of the program intervention. In a hospital setting, the choice of team leader is determined by the participating professionals and the pragmatic needs of the child.

Fulfilling the Program's Needs

There are a number of projects designed to train professionals to work together. The Bridge Project, funded through the Office of Special Education and Rehabilitation Services (OSERS), is perhaps the most comprehensive project. It requires that all of the professionals meet together for a day and a half of training. Other training projects are funded by the Office of Special Education Programs (see Chapter 1, Table 1.1). Although it may be helpful for professionals to work together according to a specific model, it is also possible for the group members themselves to design a combination of cooperative activities found in the various models.

The ACDS program uses an ongoing staffing arrangement in which the speech/language, physical, and occupational therapists; psychologist; and social worker assigned to a particular teacher, meet as a group, weekly, to discuss the changing needs of the children assigned to that teacher. Although needs of each child are not discussed in-depth each week, it is possible to continually update the IEP and discuss details of the implementation. A rather simple listing of topics discussed and decisions made during the meeting provides an ample record of the meeting and can be used as a guide to update child goals (see Figure 8.3). Parents of children in the center-based project come in monthly to observe the child during programming and to talk with those people who work with the child. A summary sheet is completed on the Parent Conference Form. These summary sheets of what was discussed can be used to record follow-up decisions and provide a method to include current parent input and implement the IEP as a working document (see Figure 8.4).

Although complete and detailed IEP records should be kept on file, it may be helpful to have a summary of the plan available for quick reference. This is especially true for complicated therapeutic programs for more involved children. The ACDS program has an Individual Program Plan Summary (see Figure 8.5) that is a shorthand version of the IEP's priority goals and objectives. It can easily be used by all staff.

IMPLEMENTING
INDIVIDUALIZATION IN GROUP SETTINGS

A common concern that exists in both home and center-based programs is "how to deliver services to the child in the most appropriate, individual way and still provide for the needs of other persons." The problem is similar whether the other persons are other children in the program or other people in the child's household. It is rarely possible (and perhaps not even beneficial) for a child to receive the undivided attention of an adult all of the time. Learning appropriate language, social, and cognitive skills requires interacting, sharing, and generally being around other people with varying ideas and actions. Learning self-care skills (e.g., eating, washing, and toileting with as little help as possible) is facilitated by having others around who also need attention to serve as models for achieving independence.

In center-based early intervention programs, children are grouped in such

		STAFFING SUMMARY		

Child's Name: _____ Teacher: _____

Date	Presenting problem	Intervention	Follow-up

Psychologist: _____

Figure 8.3. Sample staffing summary sheet used during weekly meetings.

a way as to maximize the learning potential. At-home children are in the company of family members and others in the neighborhood. In either setting, it is not necessary that the same grouping be used for all activities. Center-based programs may have flexible groupings. Children grouped may be categorized by: chronological age; developmental function; or interest of the children, parents, or families depending on the activity. Families may choose to arrange and modify groupings and responsibilities for various activities in the community. In either setting, however, there is the constant challenge of making sure that all of those who are interacting with the child are aware of his or her program and the particular strategies that need to be used to reach each of the child's goals must be specified.

Communicating Goals to the Staff

A program in which university students are trained, displays each child's goals by writing them in very large letters on posters hung out of the children's reach

Parent Conference Form

Teacher: _____   Date: _____

Child's name: _____

Parent's signature: _____

Professional	Services provided	Suggestions made
Physical therapist		
Occupational therapist		
Speech/language therapist		
Psychologist		
Nurse		
Other contacts		

Follow-up necessary: _____

_____

_____

_____

_____

Figure 8.4. Sample parent conference summary sheet.

around the room. University students are then able to easily see that, for example: "Johnnie is to crawl, alternate legs"; "Jannie is to keep lips closed while eating"; and "Bobbie is to learn to share toys."

This procedure could also be used at home to help parents, older siblings, grandparents, and baby sitters to remember the child's goals. Although large IEP charts may not be an appealing wall decoration, most families of young children decorate the home with crayon drawings and the words from the preprimer. Programs might provide parents with continually updated IEP charts. If they were made to fit the back of a door, they could be kept in sight without offending even the most fussy landlord.

INDIVIDUAL PROGRAM SUMMARY				
Child's name: _____			Date started: _____	
Implementor: _____			Class: _____	
Date	Goals	Methods/materials	Criteria for evaluation	Date evaluated

Figure 8.5. Sample Individual Program Plan summary sheet.

Teachers in the ACDS program communicate the needs of the children to assistants and volunteers by use of a task box. This box contains a task sheet to record the number of times that the child has been "taught" to do the particular skill listed on his or her IEP. Also contained in the box is the toy or other equipment necessary for the adult to implement the task with the child. The task sheet is a backup for the numerous checklists for each child that are kept in a file in the classroom. The task sheet is continually updated by appropriate professionals as the child develops the skill. Volunteers, practicum students, teachers, and teacher assistants can assist the child with the skills that are listed on the sheet and record the responses. During a specific in-service training, staff and volunteers are shown what different types of responses they should be looking for (see Figures 8.6 and 8.7).

A brief description of each task is written on Figure 8.7 in the larger blank spaces on the left and data is entered. As various staff members assist the child with the task, they write their initials in the appropriate block along with the

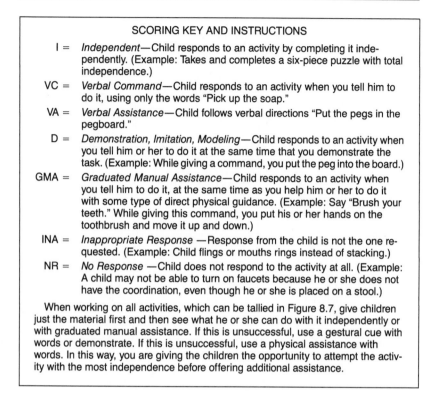

SCORING KEY AND INSTRUCTIONS

I =   *Independent*—Child responds to an activity by completing it independently. (Example: Takes and completes a six-piece puzzle with total
independence.)

VC =   *Verbal Command*—Child responds to an activity when you tell him to
do it, using only the words "Pick up the soap."

VA =   *Verbal Assistance*—Child follows verbal directions "Put the pegs in the
pegboard."

D =   *Demonstration, Imitation, Modeling*—Child responds to an activity when
you tell him or her to do it at the same time that you demonstrate the
task. (Example: While giving a command, you put the peg into the board.)

GMA =   *Graduated Manual Assistance*—Child responds to an activity when
you tell him to do it, at the same time as you help him or her to do it
with some type of direct physical guidance. (Example: Say "Brush your
teeth." While giving this command, you put his or her hands on the
toothbrush and move it up and down.)

INA =   *Inappropriate Response* —Response from the child is not the one re-
quested. (Example: Child flings or mouths rings instead of stacking.)

NR =   *No Response* —Child does not respond to the activity at all. (Example:
A child may not be able to turn on faucets because he or she does not
have the coordination, even though he or she is placed on a stool.)

When working on all activities, which can be tallied in Figure 8.7, give children
just the material first and then see what he or she can do with it independently or
with graduated manual assistance. If this is unsuccessful, use a gestural cue with
words or demonstrate. If this is unsuccessful, use a physical assistance with
words. In this way, you are giving the children the opportunity to attempt the activity with the most independence before offering additional assistance.

Figure 8.6.   Sample scoring key for task sheet.

specific scoring key and instruction that was used (see Figure 8.6 for a description). This procedure was developed so that teachers could train others to implement the specific goals of the children without using teacher time during
programming. By continuing this method of teaching in a home-based program, older siblings, parents, and grandparents could help the child reach his or
her goals.

When selecting the task box items, transdisciplinary team members brain-
storm about various activities that can be used to achieve each objective. This
results in a variety of activities that may be interesting to the child. For example, if the child needs to learn to hold objects in one hand, blocks, rattles, small
stuffed toys, and other objects can be used to create a variety of "put-this-here"
and "pick-up-that" games. Along the same lines, if the child needs to learn to
put things in the mouth, he or she can be asked to use a spoon to pick up cereal
or to hold a cracker and chew it. This teaches children to generalize their newly
acquired skills to different settings with various people.

Some skills, such as toileting, must be functional and do not lend themselves to *task box* teaching. For these skills, the Association for Children with

TASK SHEET

Name of child: _____

Tasks		Criteria and successive trials						Comments
1.	D A T E							
	Initial							
	1.							
	2.							
	3.							
	4.							
2.	D A T E							
	Initial							
	1.							
	2.							
	3.							
	4.							
3.	D A T E							
	Initial							
	1.							
	2.							
	3.							
	4.							
4.	D A T E							
	Initial							
	1.							
	2.							
	3.							
	4.							

Figure 8.7. Sample task sheet. (I = independent; VC = verbal command; VA = verbal assistance; D = demonstration; GMA = graduated manual assistance; INA = inappropriate response; NR = no response.)

Down Syndrome (ACDS) program has developed charts to keep track of the teaching that is being implemented. Figure 8.8 is a chart for an individual child's toileting skills.

This chart could be kept on the wall close to the toilet. The teacher, teacher assistant, volunteer, or parent writes the date on the blanks on the left. The time of day is written across the top and dry, D; dry, urinated, DU; wet, W; and wet, urinated, WU are written to indicate the circumstances in each trial. General comments can be written on the right side of the chart. Toileting skill charts for both home and school would not only help adults remember to keep up the training but could show child progress more efficiently. Of course, for children who are physically handicapped or severely delayed, more specific information concerning toileting skills could be incorporated into the charts. Also, for each child, it is necessary to know exactly how much independence in undressing, dressing, and handwashing to expect. Charts could also be designed to show more specific details.

For a program just beginning service delivery, it may be helpful to secure copies of the forms used by other programs. However, an even more effective procedure would be for program staff to design a system that fits the level of detail needed for the children in that particular program. It is important to remember that information on the forms should be as complete as possible, and that forms should be organized to require as little writing as possible; thus, making it possible for staff or parents to keep everything updated by making only a few marks.

Grouping and Regrouping Schedules

Once it has been determined which skills and tasks need to be accomplished by each child to enhance his or her present development, small and large group activities can be planned and a regular routine established. For a center-based program, this routine can resemble preschool activities designed for handicapped children. A possible schedule could be as follows:

9:00 A.M.—greeting and singing time
9:15 A.M.—story time
9:30 A.M.—large motor activity
10:00 A.M.—snack time

Children are then programmed in the classroom group activities. Children are pulled out of the classroom group when a therapist needs to work with one child or several children in a smaller group activity designed to increase specific social communication, or other skills that can most readily be developed in cooperation with others or for other training specified in the child's individual program.

Preschool-like activities such as playing house, molding with clay, or building with blocks can also be implemented as an activity base over which

Toileting Chart

Name _____

Toileting Task _____

Time Interval _____

Reinforcement Used _____

Date	Time													Comments

Figure 8.8. Sample toileting chart for an individual child. (D = dry; DU = dry, urinated; W = wet; WU = wet, urinated.)

specific training can be superimposed of the child's goals (see Chapter 15 for description of incidental teaching). This procedure can also be used at home, where the routines are more functional and include the whole family, during eating, grooming, housekeeping, and other household routines (Tingey, 1987). For the most part, young children, and even the adults who supervise them, function best when the general configuration of each day is the same (Tingey-Michaelis, 1983).

EVALUATING THE IEP

Although it is important that the child perform the skill at the time it is being trained, it is more important that he or she spontaneously perform the skill when it is appropriate to do so. In order to know if this is happening, the child must be observed continually. This continual observation is the basis for updating the IEP. Due to legal requirements, the IEP is annually updated at formal meetings, usually held in the spring. The child's goals are reviewed at this time and updated if needed.

It has been found, however, that waiting an entire year to evaluate the appropriateness and progress of the young child's designated goals is simply too long. Since there are a number of different skills that young children learn in only a few months, the goals can change almost daily. If careful observation of the child's continued development is not regularly made, it is possible to lose valuable learning time by not selecting new, more appropriate goals for the child. The appropriate degree of difficulty, the amount of training, and the practice needed for any one child to accomplish the task is based solely on that individual child's progress. Therefore, it is not possible to suggest a learning time and sequence for any handicapped child by using the progress made by other children as a guide (Johnson & Mandell, 1987).

Continuing Review with Appropriate Forms

The Association for Children with Down Syndrome (ACDS) program finds that rather than having only one formal annual meeting to update the IEP, it is more appropriate to have a formal mid-year IEP review as well as one later in the year. In order to be sure that information is continually gathered for the IEP, a regular testing/observation/visiting schedule is kept each year. Two home visits made by the teacher during the year to determine the child's functional progress at home, and to receive input from the parents on their child's skill development. Figure 8.9 presents a school-year calendar for continuing assessment and updating IEPs. Staff and parents are aware of conferences and home visits in ample time for scheduling. Giving tests to a number of children is a time consuming task and staff members need to be able to plan ahead in order to have all protocols finished on schedule.

IEP PROCESS SCHEDULE

September
— Update all checklists and assessments for IEP
— Pretest, criterion-referenced assessment begun by last week in this month

October
— Pretest, criterion-referenced assessment finished by second week in this month
— IEPs due early in the month
— Parent-teacher conferences
— First home visit

January
— Update all checklists and assessments for IEPs
— Mid-year evaluations due

February
— Updated IEPs due mid-February

March
— Parent-teacher conferences

May
— Second home visit
— Year-end developmental testing due end of month
— Posttest, criterion-referenced assessment begun by last week in this month

June
— Posttest, criterion-referenced assessment finished by second week in this month

---

Figure 8.9. Sample yearly calendar of continuing assessment and IEP updating.

In preparation for the IEP, each professional completes a therapy goal sheet for his or her discipline that includes specific goals and physical settings appropriate for that goal (see Figure 8.10). The form has space allotted for the specific goal as well as the description of the most appropriate place for training to occur. For example, a child cannot learn to climb stairs using alternate feet unless the training and practice occurs on a stairway. A rough draft of the IEP is reviewed by the educational director before the final form is written. The ACDS form used for the completed IEP is shown in Figure 8.11. It provides space for short-term goals, for materials to be used, and for methods for evaluating success. This form also has space for information regarding the data achieved. This is necessary when the IEP is to be updated.

Even though goals may be suggested for a variety of development areas, specific goals should be selected based on the child's particular needs. If the child develops maladaptive behavior such as temper tantrums that might interfere with acquisition of other skills, it may be wise to forego training of developmental skills until the behavior is under control. By doing this, the personnel in the early intervention program and the family can then concentrate on teaching an adaptive behavior to replace the behavior that is inhibiting development. Since it is not possible to emphasize training on all possible skills at the same time, it is important that the decision concerning the child's ongoing developmental needs be evaluated and re-evaluated continuously (Tjossem, 1976). Task sheets for each of the children are updated daily by the teacher, and

THERAPY GOALS FORM					
Date	Name of child	Teacher	Goal of therapy service	Physical setting	Time

Discipline: _____   Signature: _____

Figure 8.10. Sample therapy goal form.

	IEP		For year ☐
			Update ☐

Name of student: _____ Date of birth: _____

Implementation date: _____ Evaluation date: _____

Class placement: _____ Concentration: _____

IEP prepared by: _____ Discipline: _____

Parent/guardian signature: _____

Present level of educational performance

Goal	Short-term objective	Method and materials	Method of evaluation	Date achieved

Figure 8.11. Sample ACDS form used for completed IEPs.

frequent observation is made by the psychology staff to quantify the child's progress. With updated task sheets, current information concerning the child's functioning at school is available.

Information about the child's activities at home may not be easily obtained if staff visits do not occur frequently enough to gather accurate observational data concerning behaviors that occur at home. To correct this situation, however, the ACDS employs a frequently used method to communicate daily with the parents. A tote bag is sent back and forth to school each day with the child. In the bag is a notebook in which correspondence between the staff and parent are kept. Figure 8.12 is an example of a form developed for children who may

Daily Activities for_____**(Name)**_____**(Date)**

Morning	Afternoon	Activity	Evening	Nite	Morning
		Meals			
		Sleep			
		Snack			
		Liquid			
		Bowel Movement			
		Bath			
		Seizure			
		Medication Given			
		Teeth Brushed			
		Unusually Happy			
		Unusually Fussy			

Special Notice: (Change in Medication, Diarrhea, Special Activity, Amount Eaten, Unusual Amount of Sleep - etc.)

Figure 8.12. Sample form developed for home/school communication. (Adapted from Michaelis [1980].)

be experiencing medical problems that possibly interfere with their daily functioning. This information, concerning medical needs, may be vital for caregiving as well as understanding the functioning of the child at that time.

In order to keep the records of the child's functioning current, input from home- and center-based programs is necessary. For home-based programs, the information is even more vital. If home visits are more than a week apart, the information could be relayed over the telephone. For evaluations of children with working parents, it may be helpful to talk to the daily careprovider as well as the parent. Of course, it will be necessary to have the parent's permission before such a contact is made.

Communicating Child Needs to Staff

In a center-based program, both the summary IEP form and accessible information should be readily available and perhaps even displayed on the wall close to the teacher's desk. Each child's folder should be current, with a summary sheet located in the front. Since the child's learning process must be reinforced continuously, it is important that all care-providing professionals be aware of the specific skills that need to be developed and the procedures that are to be employed in teaching.

It may be helpful to share portions of the child's IEP goals with nonteaching staff, especially bus drivers, to ensure consistency. It might also increase staff morale if nonteaching staff understood the need for individual goals. (See Chapter 5 concerning staff morale for suggestions about in-service training.)

BASIC GOALS FOR CONTINUAL INSTRUCTION

Early intervention goals for infants and young children are basic, personal, and central to the child's life. The goals include such things as independence in feeding and toileting skills as well as the ability to maintain eye contact and to ask for assistance. Instruction must be ongoing and should be incorporated in all the child's activities. The instruction should occur naturally in the environment, and the goals should be clear, understandable, and incorporated into all care providing activities.

The early intervention goals should be geared toward what is frequently described as the "career of life" (Kokoska, 1985; Kokoska & Brolin, 1985). This concept is usually considered to be related to the provision of vocational goals for normal and handicapped teenagers. In actuality, it is concerned with making sure that the skills taught to a child are functionally important to that person. For example, Latin has been taught in some schools not because there was expectation that the children would be able to use the langauge, but because the drill would help them "learn how to think." Sometimes early intervention personnel choose to teach "Standing on one foot" or making the "b" sound, not because these skills are functionally useful, but because they appear as items on a developmental assessment instrument.

A handicapped child cannot waste valuable learning time on tasks that are unrelated to daily life and must "learn to think" about the day-to-day skills that he or she faces. These skills must be applicable to the daily routines of eating, sleeping, taking care of the body, playing appropriately, interacting with others, and adapting to all social and educational environments. A poorly structured drill that is not functional in the classroom or at home is of no use to children who are experiencing difficulties in learning.

Sometimes, early intervention programs primarily provide instruction in general skills that may be listed only on standardized tests or in criterion-referenced assessments (e.g., turns to sound of noise, stands on one foot for 3 seconds, attends for 3 seconds). These skills do not relate to the basic needs of the child. However, being able to turn to your name, to balance on one foot while participating in children's games, and to attend to instruction are functional skills and are geared specifically to the needs and activities in the child's typical day-to-day activities (Chapter 15 discusses naturalistic teaching).

It is only possible to use naturalistic teaching to teach specific skills that are natural or common occurrences for the child. Many of the goals in assessment materials are generalized skills that are more useful for making statements concerning comparative functioning than for identifying the most specific training needs. In order to be useful to the child, the skills taught must be those required in his or her own home and community. For example, children who are growing up in the country may need to relate to farm animals and children growing up in the city may need to learn to cross the street when the light is green.

It is important for all children to learn to relate to others socially, and to adapt to a variety of environments. For instance, sharing a room with another child for the first time could be a social learning experience for the child who has always had his or her own room. Also, it may be helpful for all children to learn to climb stairs with alternate feet even if their environment does not call for such skills.

Ideally, of course, it would be nice if children were able to learn all possible skills; however, this is functionally impossible for even nonhandicapped children and adults. The "basic" skills are usually taught; however, the definition of basic is not always clear. Even general educational personnel do not agree on which skills are basic, other than reading, writing, and arithmetic. It is clear that for the handicapped child, some skills may be even more basic than the "three R's" and must be learned first.

Prewritten Goals

Since the implementation of Public Law 94-142, numerous lists of goals for children have been created (Gardner & Breuer, 1985; IEPs Unlimited, Inc.,

1988). Although such lists might be used as a reference, each child should be considered a unique individual who has his or her own set of individualized needs, depending on the specific handicapping conditions and the constellation of family strengths and needs (Deno & Minkin,1977). Although the various needs and skills of young children are basically similar, difficulties in the development process make it necessary to recreate a list of potential goals for each child by implementing a problem identification and problem-solving process for each child. This process should be independent of the one used for another child, even though he or she may be the same age and have a similar label for the handicapping condition.

The guiding philosophy used by many human service professionals when selecting goals for the young child who is either handicapped or at risk for handicaps is "no two children are alike." This philosophy should be coupled with the knowledge that families vary even more than children. Contributing factors to the differences in families include: size of family, religion, and health concerns. All of these factors have an effect on the family's day to day activities and on the belief systems and values that guide the lives of family members, both at home and in the community.

Accomplishing the Selected Goals

Although it is important for any teacher to plan stimulating activities, the early intervention teacher enters the center- or home-based program with some very specific constraints. The daily activities of the child must be geared toward his or her special needs as identified by the goal selection. In the process of monitoring the implementation of Public Law 94-142, evaluation teams have sometimes found that the goals selected for the child are appropriate and written after considerable assessment and discussion of prioritizing those goals. However, the day-to-day teaching activities actually implemented have little relationship to the goals. If the child's individual goals are not the primary focus of the daily intervention activities, the efforts of the goal selection process are wasted. The activities become an academic exercise that is often frustrating for both staff and parents and provides no real advantage for the child.

After the individual goals for each child are identified, intervention is planned. The teacher can only begin to devise preliminary plans for the child after goals have been identified. The preliminary plans consist of actual intervention activities for the child (Sugai, 1985). These activities can be either informally or formally structured according to the proposed activity. Some activities are very similar to informal preschool activities, while other activities must be formally structured, in which the teacher's behavior is almost scripted. Of course, it is important that children receive service during the process of goal selection, but this early service should be considered part of the assessment. During the assessment process, the child's strengths and weaknesses should be carefully observed (see Chapter 2).

In addition to establishing planned activities after goal selection, the teacher has the added challenge of providing an opportunity for one child to share, another to go to the restroom alone, and another to simultaneously develop fine motor coordination. Teachers must provide continuous, appropriate activities for each child. Once again it is important to remember that "no two children are alike." Although the general description of children may be the same, individual strengths and weaknesses may require a variety of different activities. For example, the profiles of four handicapped children from the ACDS program show varying scores on the Uniform Performance Assessment Profile (see Figures 8.13). Although each of these children is showing progress, it is in different areas of development and at varying rates. The general progress of these children is similar, but the individual strengths and weaknesses differ even though they all have the same handicap. Obviously, each of these children has different individual goals, resulting in a different emphasis even when participating in the same activity. This tends to create difficulties when planning routine activities for a group of children. (See Chapter 15 for a discussion of structured teaching during regular activities.) Home intervention implementation has the same difficulty, since the parent must be able to provide appropriate activities for all family members, not just the child who is experiencing problems.

Early Intervention Activities at Home

The Early Intervention Research Institute has developed several methods of documenting for research the amount of time that parents spend in early intervention activities at home with their children. These include weekly telephone calls to parents to ask about the amount of at-home training time spent with the child, calenders in which the amount of time is recorded and sent to school with the child, and post cards addressed to the center on which the amount of time could be marked. All methods have thus far been less than successful because it is very difficult to teach parents how to separate regular caregiving time from time spent implementing goals. This is particularly difficult for the parents when the goals relate to toileting, feeding, or other activities outside of the early intervention program with which the child may need assistance. It is also difficult for the parents to determine how to classify activities such as reading stories to a child when one of his or her goals is to increase interest in communication. In this case, the story is used as a basis for an interaction episode.

It is also possible that the time spent may not accurately measure effectiveness. Mastering a specific skill makes it possible for the skill to be performed in less time. With the support of an early intervention program, parents could possibly provide more appropriate care to the child in less time.

Most early intervention programs do not need to document parent time spent training the child at home; rather, they need to organize goals that parents want to implement at home. When goals are selected, the time and interest of

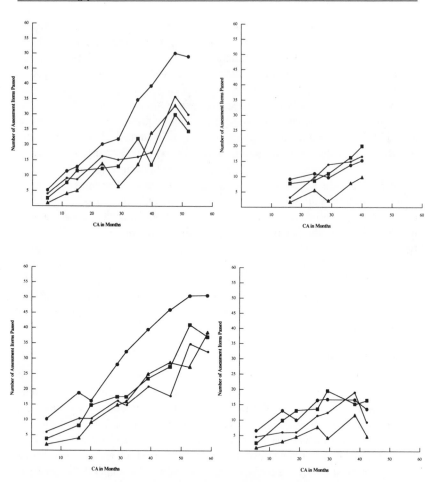

Figure 8.13. Uniform Performance Assessment Profiles for four children with the same handicap. (CA, chronological age; PREACA [●——●], preacademic skills; COMM [■——■], communication skills; SOC/SH [▲——▲], social/self-help skills; G. MOTOR [●——●], gross motor skills.)

the parent(s) must be a prime factor. For example, the book by Azrin and Foxx (1974) addresses the issue of toilet training, and describes when both the parents and the child are ready for this step. An inopportune time to address the task of toilet training would be when the family has a new infant or is in the process of moving. Selection of the child's goals and the procedures for implementation must be something that parents see as vital for the child. Parents must have the time and equipment necessary for home implementation. For example, unless the family has a wedge for use in providing posture support or a communication board for use in practicing language, they cannot assist with their child's training with these devices. When parents are aware of their child's day-to-day activities they can more easily pinpoint the goals their children need to accomplish. For instance, a father, who did not have input into his son's early intervention goals, was pleased that the program helped the boy stack blocks but the father wanted help with what the boy really needed, to be able to feed himself.

Since more and more parents are both working, having children's training continued in the daily care setting becomes more complicated. This can be an additional challenge to the early intervention staff. Although day care providers are not required by law to be involved in the selection of IEP goals, it is not an unreasonable suggestion. Parents of young handicapped children frequently have difficulty finding appropriate day care, let alone someone who will be willing to implement special training goals.

Factors that Complicate the Goal Selection Process

On the surface, it appears quite simple to select goals for young handicapped children or children at risk for handicapping conditions; however, this is not true. There are several sets of assessment materials that list skills in sequence and according to what most children learn during the early years (see Chapters 2 and 6 for lists of specific tests containing skill development lists). Even without seeing the child, it is common knowledge that a 1-year-old child is usually learning to walk, and a 2-year-old is usually being toilet trained.

The difficulty with selecting IEP goals for infants and young children who are handicapped is in determining the most appropriate activity for a particular child to learn at a specific time. The nuances of the effects of the disability and all the needs and concerns of the parents and other children in the family should be considered by the professional when planning the IEP. This requires enough experience on the professional's part, with children of similar disabilities, to know how children develop as they grow older and how disabilities affect such things as later reproductive capacity and ability to perform abstract reasoning skills. The list of general skills pertains to children who grow and develop in a normal sequence and time line. These lists show that children learn to move about before they talk and to undress themselves before they ask to go to the toilet. For children with physical impairments, this order of learning may be reversed. When a developmental disability alters this pattern, it becomes less probable that a normal developmental progression for this child will occur (Warren, Alpert, & Kaiser, 1986). Too often, early intervention programs use preplanned curriculum models and choose goals for the children that seem appropriate according to the published curriculum without ample observation of the behaviors and skills that the child spontaneously displays and without consideration of the effect of the child's disability.

The planning of a young child's IEP is divided into two parts. The first part is to listen carefully to the parent's concerns. The second part is to repeatedly observe the child in natural settings to identify his or her learning style and needs. Although early intervention model programs have existed for many years, the profession itself is only in its infancy in regard to knowing how to train staff to observe children. Such observation can identify clearly what each child needs to learn at any given time.

SUMMARY

Identifying problem areas, designing goals, and implementing treatment for handicapped infants and preschoolers requires formal and informal observation by a number of individuals that represent a variety of disciplines. Input from the child's parents is also vital. Documentation of the process, assessment results, and goals created during staff meetings is essential to successful planning. The process and timelines used to provide for smooth communication of information among professionals are also necessary. However, the careful planning is of no value unless each child's goal is translated into day-to-day interaction with the child that is guided by the specific techniques identified for him or her and that continued progress is monitored. Programs are challenged to provide all of these individual services, concurrently, to a large number of families and to individualize the activities for each child continuously.

STUDY QUESTIONS

1. Make arrangements, obtain parental permission, and observe the assessment of a child.

2. Obtain permission from the parents to study the development of a child's IFSP.

3. Observe in an early intervention program as the teacher/therapist works with a child on a specified goal.

4. Observe how several different children are expected to use the same or similar objects.

REFERENCES

Azrin, N. H., & Foxx, R. M. (1974). *Toilet training in less than a day.* New York: Simon & Schuster.

Barber, P. A., Turnbull, A. P., Behr, S. K., & Kerns, G. M. (1988). A family systems perspective on early childhood special education. In S. L. Odom & M. B. Karnes (Eds.), *Early intervention for infants & young children with handicaps* (pp. 179–198). Baltimore: Paul H. Brookes Publishing Co.

Brazelton, T. B. (1969). *Infants and mothers.* New York: Dill Publishing.

Brazelton, T. B. (1974). *Toddlers and parents: A declaration of independence.* New York: Dill Publishing.

Deno, S. L., & Minkin, P. K. (1977). *Data based program modification: A manual.* Minneapolis, MN: Minneapolis Leadership Training Institute, Special Education Department.

Dunkin, M. J., & Biddle, B. J. (1974). *The study of teaching.* New York: Holt, Rinehart, & Winston.

D'Zamko, M. E., & Raiser, L. (1986). A strategy for individualizing directed group instruction. *Teaching Exceptional Children, 18,* 190–195.

Gardner, J. M., & Breuer, A. (1985). Reliability and validity of a microcomputer assessment system for developmentally disabled persons. *Education & Training of the Mentally Retarded, 20*(3), 209–213.

Garland, C., Woodruff, G., & Buck, D. M. (1988). *Case Management.* Reston, VA: Council for Exceptional Children.

IEP's Unlimited, Inc. (1988). *Teaching Exceptional Children, 20*(3), 84.

Johnson, R., & Mandell, C. (1987). A social observation checklist for preschoolers. *Teaching Exceptional Children, 20*(2), 18–21.

Kokoska, C. (1985). Position statement on career development. *Career Development for Exceptional Learners, 2,* 125–129.

Kokoska, C. J., & Brolin, D. E. (1985). *Career education for exceptional learners* (2nd ed.). Columbus, OH: Charles E. Merrill.

McGonigel, M. J., & Garland, C. W. (1988). The individualized family service plan and the early intervention team: Team and family issues and recommended practices. *Infants and Young Children, 1,*(1), 10–21.

Michaelis, C. (1980). *Home and school partnerships in exceptional education.* Rockville, MD: Aspen Systems.

Mulligan, M., & Guess, D. (1984). Using an individualized curriculum sequencing model. In L. McCormick & R. L. Schiefelbusch (Eds.), *Early language intervention* (pp. 128–142). Columbus, OH: Charles E. Merrill.

Sugai, G. (1985). Case study: Designing instruction from IEPs. *Education & Training of the Mentally Retarded, 20*(3), 232–239.

Sutherland, J. (1974). *Child care.* Van Nuys, CA: Sutherland Learning Association.

Tingey, C. (1987). *Helping parents meet the practical demands of daily life.* Paper submitted for publication, Early Intervention Research Institute, Utah State University, Logan.

Tingey-Michaelis, C. (1983). Repetition, relaxation, and routine. *The Exceptional Parent, 13*(3), 52–54.

Tjossem, T. D. (1976). *Intervention strategies for high risk infants and young children.* Baltimore: University Park Press.

Trotter, R. J. (1987). Project day care. *Psychology Today, 21*(12), 32–38.

Warren, S., Alpert, C. L., & Kaiser, A. P. (1986). An optimal learning environment for infants and toddlers with severe handicaps. *Focus on Exceptional Children, 18*(8), 1–11.

Chapter 9

Atmosphere
for Language Learning

DeAnna Horstmeier and Carol Tingey

●

A visitor to a preschool for children with developmental delays might see children playing in a rich environment of toys and equipment, and teachers facilitating the children's learning in a positive, caring way, but notice something different about this school as compared to other preschools. The early intervention classroom might seem almost too quiet. Although there are activity sounds in the room, the conversations, the short quarrels about "my toy," the commands by the "bossy" child, the quick yell from one area to another, and the joyful, spontaneous noises from the children are missing.

IMPORTANCE OF LANGUAGE

The absence from the early intervention classroom of joyful noises is the result of the prelanguage and language deficits frequently present in children with delays. Communication is an integral part of a normal child's life at home, at school, and in the community. Each person needs to be able to communicate basic wants, needs, and ideas. When a child is unable to communicate effectively, the quality of life for that child is restricted. The child's inability to communicate can become a continual source of frustration not only for the child but for family and concerned others as well. A child who cannot communicate lacks an important tool for social interaction. Without language, the child will be unable to make specific requests or respond clearly to others. Difficulty in learning from the environment may follow (Bates, 1976; Bruner, 1975). Growth in such areas as cognition can also be affected by lack of an ability to communicate (Clark & Clark, 1977).

Helping children to develop the ability to communicate is difficult when left to speech/language therapists who only operate in short, individual sessions a few times a week. Family, teachers, and other concerned professionals need to understand and use effective ways of facilitating communication development so that the child's learning experience may be continuous (Cherry, 1979; Horstmeier & MacDonald, 1978; Raver, 1987).

NORMAL LANGUAGE DEVELOPMENT

Knowledge of normal language development provides the framework for planning early language/communication intervention. Language development is more than acquiring a variety of words; it involves the acquisition by the child of a *system* for:

Comprehension—understanding others' language
Production—producing symbolic labels
Content—relating ideas
Structure—creating meaningful word phrases
Social use—using language appropriately

Language also includes any nonverbal communication that has a system of rules underlying its use.

Although there are some variations in speed of acquisition by various children, the complicated subskills of language are learned by normal children in a remarkably similar sequence. The process begins with the cry of the newborn and continues to build into one word, then two words, and on to more complicated communication. Table 9.1 provides a summary of normal language development.

Several authorities have produced charts of phonological (sound) development in young children (Olmsted, 1971; Poole, 1934; Prather, Hedrick, & Kern, 1975; Sanders, 1972; Templin, 1953). The ages and order of acquisition do not agree, mainly because the standards for acquisition and the methods of eliciting the sound are different. Although most parents and teachers can recognize the levels of language skills of a child, articulation assessment usually must be made by a speech/language therapist who has experience and training in developmental articulation and phonology, and who can bring clinical experience to the task. The approximate order of acquisition of sounds in children is given in Table 9.2.

ADULT ROLE IN LANGUAGE ACQUISITION

Since the 1970s, research focused on the communicative environment provided by parents and others to young children who are still learning language. Studies have shown that adults adjust their language when interacting with children.

Table 9.1. Sequence of language skills

Level	Average age acquired	Behaviors	Description
Preverbal	Newborn	One type of cry	Cry of desperation, strong intensity.
	1–5 months	Differentiated cry	Cries of hunger, pain, discomfort, and need for attention can be distinguished by familiar adults.
		Comfort sounds	Sounds made with an open mouth, often vowels, may be practiced (not for communication purposes).
	5–8 months	Babbling	Plays with different combinations of consonants and vowels, often repeated (e.g., "ba," "da," and "baba").
		Gestural communication	Uses facial expressions and sounds for communication and play with others.
	8–12 months	Beginning jargon	Mimics adult varieties in pitch in longer phrases; often sounds like an unknown foreign language.
		Imitation	Imitates new sounds and gestures (e.g., "bye, bye" word and gesture).
		Understands commands	Can use some gestures, words, and situations to understand directives (e.g., "Open your mouth," "Come here").
Beginning word	12–18 months	First words	Labels important items or activities in own world meaningfully and consistently.
		Additional words	Words are added relatively slowly (from approx. 10 to 50 words).
	18–24 months	Increased understanding	Rapid increase in comprehension.
		Word strings	May put words together without a relationship between them (e.g., "Daddy, Mommy, Kevin, Lynelle").
Two word	24–26 months	Two-word combinations	Uses two-word combinations that relate to each other (e.g., "More juice").

(continued)

Table 9.1. *(continued)*

Level	Average age acquired	Behaviors	Description
		Increased vocabulary	Rapid increase from approx. 200 to 1,000 words.
		Improved intelligibility	Only 25% of speech unintelligible to those unfamiliar with child.
		Word endings	Uses ending of "s" for plurals, "ing" for present progressive.
Conversation	36–48 months	More complex sentence construction	Formulates rules of words and sentence construction (e.g., "ed" for past tense, "'s" for possession, "n't" for negation, use of *to be* verbs, simple "wh" questions, and simple clauses).
		Uses speech for range of functions	Beginning to explain and verbally describe in addition to asserting, requesting, replying, and so on.
		Good intelligibility	Still may have problems with *l, r, s, z, sh, ch, j, th*.

Adapted from Cherry (1979), Clark and Clark (1977), Leitch (1977), and McCormick and Schiefelbusch (1984).

Adult conversation with children is simpler, has shorter phrases, and is more concrete and immediate. It has a greater variation of pitch and emphasis than conversation with adults (Broen, 1972; Cross, 1977; Garnica, 1975; Nelson, 1975; Phillips, 1973). Researchers are now trying to relate various features of mother's speech to the acquisition of child language (Chapman, 1981; Jones, 1977; Moerk, 1980).

Table 9.2. Simplified order of consonant sound acquisition

Age	Sounds	How made
Before 3 years	*p, b, m, w*	Front of mouth, lips together
	h	Lips open, airway open
	k, g, d, t	Air stopped suddenly
	n, ng	Nasal sounds
Before 4 years	*f, s, z, v, j*	Hissing sound
Before 5 years	*sh, ch, th*	More difficult hissing sounds
	r, l	Tongue slides to another position (may not be acquired until age 6)
After 5 years	*st, str, bl, fl, br,* and other combinations	Blend, especially those of sound combining r and l with other sounds

Adult conversation with language learning ("normal") children has been compared to adult conversation with children with developmental delay. At first, the researchers compared the normal and delayed children on the basis of chronological age. Mothers of children with delays were then shown to be providing a deficient language environment (Buim, Rynders, & Turnure, 1974). However, when the children were matched for the expressive language measure of *mean length utterance* (MLU) or amount of speech produced, the language environment provided by both groups of mothers was strikingly similar (Horstmeier, 1985; Lombardino & MacDonald, 1978; Rondal, 1977). It seems that most adults are providing a language environment for children with developmental delay at least as facilitating as is provided normal children at the same language learning level.

Children also play an important role in their own language learning by cuing parents and others to supply the appropriate language experience necessary for growth. However, regardless of similar input from adults, delayed children are not learning language as quickly and completely as normal children. Further intervention is needed to facilitate better communication skills.

LANGUAGE INTERVENTION

The strategies and activities that are discussed below can be used by all adults who interact with children, whether they are professionals in early intervention or parents. Some activities are more suitable for a classroom than a home setting. Parents usually maintain different levels of involvement with their child's formal learning experiences depending on the situations and their attitudes toward parenting. Most parents, however, can weave these language facilitating strategies into their daily routines.

INFORMAL AND FORMAL INTERVENTION STRATEGIES

Formal intervention is that instruction that is specifically preplanned to teach certain language skills. Informal intervention facilitates language growth by interweaving learning opportunities into other routine activities (see Chapter 15).

Informal language intervention has several advantages. One of the major benefits of informal language intervention is that skills learned by the child in an open, common setting are frequently used by the child in his or her natural daily interactions. Language skills taught informally, as part of naturally occurring events, have a greater chance of being used regularly by the child. Skills learned as part of a regularly occurring dialogue between child and adult, or as part of a routine task, do not require extra time after the adult has learned the strategy and objective.

Most of a person's life is spent in informal social interactions with others, not in formal classroom settings, therefore, it would seem important to learn communication skills in a social setting. In addition, learning language from the environment, even when adults *beef up* the approach, is more like the natural way that normal children learn language. However, informal language learning does have problems. As the child progresses, it becomes increasingly more difficult to weave the learning into routine activities because there are increasingly more complicated things for the adult to remember. Teachers and parents of several children are also challenged to remember each child's individual learning level and to provide various simultaneous incidental teaching activities (see Chapter 15).

In the milieu of the ongoing activity, it may also be difficult to both interact with the children and keep data for accountability of child growth. If the teacher or parent has a person available to do observations, it is possible to have data taken on several children at one time. However, if personnel for observation are not available, it is usually easier for a teacher or parent to take data to measure child growth in a formal teaching situation.

It may also be difficult for the child to know what aspect of the informal situation is being emphasized. The child may be confused and wonder, "Does the adult want me to talk about what is happening in this pumpkin carving experience or to talk in longer sentences?" An alert adult may be able to recognize the child's dilemma and create a brief formal session in a natural setting. Consider, for example, Scott's learning of the plural:

> Scott was talking in 4–5 word sentences but had not learned the early concept of plurals formed with an "s" ending. When a plural was modeled for him in a conversational setting, he would imitate the word, carefully reproducing the adult's emphasis of the "s" ending, but continued to omit the ending in his spontaneous speech. From the child's other activities, the adult was aware that Scott understood the concept of more than one. The adult then planned a specific formal teaching session. Using a variety of objects familiar to Scott, she was able to teach the concept in one session. Especially effective was the demonstration of one cookie, two cookies. After this session, Scott was much more accurate with plurals in regular conversation. When he did omit the plural, a questioning look from the adult was all that was required for him to correct himself.

Articulation training may also need specific planned intervention. The teaching of signing and other forms of alternative or augmentative communication can also be facilitated by initial formal training. Formal situations should be planned as closely as possible to the natural setting. Real objects should be used when possible. Pictures should be used only when the teacher knows that the child understands pictorial representation of an object or an action. Formal teaching should be followed up with training in natural life situations.

LANGUAGE CONCEPTS TO CONSIDER

Comprehension and Production Skills

Language is not a one-sided activity but a highly sophisticated method for sending and receiving messages. Therefore, children's language learning needs must be addressed in both the areas of comprehension and production. For children experiencing developmental difficulties, it appears that although both areas need facilitation, production skills are typically more difficult than comprehension skills (Miller, 1987), and the child comprehends more than he or she is able to produce.

Even though the difference for normal children is not as great, in general, all young children understand more than they are able to say. Parents and teachers of preverbal children often lament, "He understands everything that I say. Why doesn't he talk?" However, the children may not understand all the *words* that are said. Young children are very adept at getting cues from the situation to help them understand. For example, when an adult says "Put the box on the table," the child sees the adult point to the table, giving him or her the box, so he or she puts the box on the table. The adult's gesture and the presence of the box and the table have helped the child understand the command. Adults should introduce ideas and objects by naming them and explaining their use and characteristics. An example of this would be when an adult says "Feel this basket. Here, carry the basket on your arm. This basket can carry your toys. I have baskets for the wash."

A useful technique that can help show what a child understands is that of asking the child to touch the item you have named without giving cues by gesture. One such example of this would be when an adult says "Sean, please touch the pillow."

Most parents and teachers give the names of objects quite naturally, but action words are frequently not taught. Actions may be more difficult to learn because the child has to decide what is being labeled. While the adult is saying, "run," the child may be thinking, "Is *run* the name of the man? Is it the man's legs and feet? Is *run* where the man is going? Or is *run* the action?" Action words should be taught using the actual actions. Simple location action words such as "up" and "down," and adjectives and adverbs such as "big" and "fast," are appropriate to teach.

Some of the same singing games described later in the chapter for imitation can be used for comprehension training. The adult must *not* do the action, but clearly call out the action word. Puppets can help a physically immobile child make the movement, or he or she can be physically assisted to demonstrate the action, if necessary.

IMITATION AS A LANGUAGE SKILL

Physical Actions

Imitation is also an important skill for language learning and has long been valued in the development of intelligence. Most of the words that we speak were originally learned by imitating someone's sounds. Later, we learned to combine those words in our own unique way. Imitating gestures may also be a necessary preliminary skill for a child who uses signs to communicate. Some children who have difficulty learning to imitate sounds may need to learn physical imitation to get the concept of "do-as-I-do." It is also possible to physically assist a child in making motor movements, something that cannot be done with sounds.

Teaching motor imitation to toddlers and preschoolers can be a pleasant activity using songs, finger plays, and stories with motor actions. Many nursery rhymes can be adapted to allow gestures to accompany the words. One caution, however: if children hear a song or finger play over and over, they may learn the action and repeat it from memory. In this case, they are no longer imitating when they make the motions.

Children who have difficulty learning physical imitation can be helped to make actions by using toys that have an obvious expected action (e.g., put hat on doll, knock blocks over, or push toy off table). The adult can do the action, wait for the child's response, then physically assist, if necessary. It is important that children who may need to sign have frequent pleasant experiences imitating actions.

Sounds and Words

If a child easily imitates sounds, it is not necessary to teach motor imitation for the sake of language. If physical imitation has been established and the child does not yet imitate sounds, it may help to teach actions that include closely linked sounds such as: 1) toy falls—"oh, oh"; 2) rub stomach—"Mmmmm"; 3) arms up—"so big"; and 4) hand on mouth—make Indian war whoop.

At certain stages in a child's development, when the mother frequently imitates the child's sounds, he or she will often repeat that sound (Folger & Chapman, 1978). This feedback technique can be used for establishing new sounds. The adult imitates the child's own sounds and the child often repeats the sound, setting up a turn-taking chain. Sometimes the adult can change the sounds slightly so the child is imitating the adult's sounds. An example of this is when the child says "Pah" and the adult answers "Pah." The child then again says "Pah" but this time the adult answers "Pah, dah." The child will then repeat the newly created word.

Some children go through a babbling stage where they stop if an adult answers. They seem to practice by themselves and stop to listen if the adults speak. In this situation, it is not helpful to imitate the child's babbling as it makes the child stop babbling. Usually, practice babbling becomes babbling-for-dialogue in a short time. It is not necessary for a child to imitate or produce an extensive vocabulary of isolated sounds before those sounds can be paired with objects to begin saying words. Adults can help by repeating words for familiar objects with the same simple sound patterns.

EXPERIENCE AND EXPLORATION FOR LANGUAGE

Before children communicate with words or signs, they need to explore and experience the world around them. Activities done for fun or in a home or pre-school environment provide children with the raw material that they need to develop language (Piaget, 1963). For example, a trip to the supermarket with a baby can help provide meaning for the concepts of riding, lights, and colors. An older child would learn concepts about types of food, money, following directions, and, perhaps, sitting still. Experiences planned for cognitive growth often have great potential for language development as well. A trip with a young girl's class to the baby animal farm, for example, produces the experiences that she needs to understand the language concepts behind the words *lamb, wet, suck,* and *hold on.* The young girl also has an opportunity to answer a request from an unfamiliar adult in a strange setting.

DIFFERENT STRATEGIES FOR VARIOUS LANGUAGE LEVELS

Preverbal Language Level

A parent took her child to a speech/language therapist because he was 3 years old and did not speak. The therapist tried some assessments and then said, "I don't know what to do with him. Bring him back when he talks."

What do you do when a child isn't speaking? How does a child develop language before he speaks? Meaningful experiences, imitation, social dialogues, and comprehension occur even before speech and are all vital to speech and language development.

Social Dialogue

A child begins to communicate long before any words are expressed. A cry of hunger or for attention serves to alert the caregiver that something is needed. Children participate actively in their own language learning. Children and the adults who respond to them form a language learning team.

Adults treat babies who make comfort or practice sounds as if they are trying to communicate. Examples of such instances could be when a child says, "Kaaa" and the adult answers, "Oh, you like that, do you?", then, the child blows a "raspberry" and the adult answers "Well, the same to you!", *or* when the child blows a "raspberry" and the adult tickles the child, then the child begins to giggle and the adult answers "I saw that. You did like it." The adult is helping the child set up a back-and-forth sequence (turn-taking). Many of the play activities that adults share with babies have language teaching value, or they *can* have teaching value if adults are aware of their possibilities. "Patty Cake," "So-o-o Big," "Peek-a-boo," and "This Little Piggy" can be valuable in teaching back-and-forth dialogue (turn-taking) and the concept of "do-as-I-do" (imitation). Both of these skills are essential to social conversation. Certainly, the fun in the activity and the caring bond between the adult and child make the prelanguage learning rewarding (MacDonald & Gillette, 1982).

Children with developmental delays may not have acquired these prelanguage skills when they were infants. Therefore, adults may need to assist them with added emphasis in these areas.

Strategies for Adults when Talking to Preverbal Children

The following are some strategies that adults may find helpful when working with preverbal children:

1. Get the child's attention.
2. Talk about things important to the child.
3. Use simple, short, clear sentences.
4. Treat the child's sounds as if they were communications.
5. *Wait* for the child to respond. Don't be afraid of a little silence.
6. Label actions as well as objects and people.
7. Make the learning as much fun as possible.
8. Pause between sentences or phrases.

(Adapted from Horstmeier & MacDonald, 1978)

Beginning Word Level

When a child begins imitating consonant-vowel combinations consistently, it is possible to pair the sounds with objects or people to teach the concept that sounds can have meanings. For example, when a child says "Pah" the adult can ask, showing the child the can of pop, "You want pop? Pop?" If the child says "Pah" again, the adult hands the child a small cup of pop saying, "Yes, you did want pop." The adult models the correct form of the words while accepting the child's sounds. The adult can also begin the dialogue by asking the child to imitate the word "pop." Many words are learned by direct imitation; however, it is important that the child learn to label the can of pop with the word "pop" *without* the adult model.

A word is not learned until a child can use it appropriately without imitating. Once a child has clearly learned a word, she or he should be required to use it in routine situations. It may help to use new words in play and game situations first.

When children have a beginning vocabulary of words, it may be helpful to arrange some of their routine experiences so they are likely to initiate language. A favorite or new toy may be placed out of reach, but visible, so the child needs to ask for it. At snack time, a child must verbally make a choice of which treat to receive from the many offered. An adult should not be too quick to assist, unless safety is an issue, so that the child is given a chance to use his or her new words. If the child is puzzled about what is required, the adult can cue him or her to ask with words. A good example of this could be when a child pulls on an adult's hand and sticks out his or her untied shoe. The adult then asks "What?", waits 10 seconds or so, then asks "Tell me what you want. Use your words." The child is then forced to use his words to communicate and blurts out "Sooo" which results in an "Oh, your shoe!" reply from the adult. It is important that a child's first words are about things that are vitally interesting to him or her. All children's first words are not the same words (Nelson, 1973), but they are always words about the child's immediate world and things that interest him or her.

> A child being taught sign language (total communication) was making very little progress. The therapist asked the parents what foods the child liked. The parent replied, "He really doesn't like any food, but he does put ketchup on everything." The therapist quickly learned to make the sign, found a ketchup bottle, and the delighted boy learned a symbol for his favorite *food* which he used appropriately and very frequently. Once the idea of a sign standing for an object was understood, the child learned quickly.

Parents and teachers can use family photos, favorite toys, and situations to elicit beginning language, spoken or aided (see later section in this chapter on aided communication). As with understanding of language, words taught should serve a variety of functions. Besides just naming objects, Horstmeier and MacDonald (1978) found that children also use words to:

1. Express actions and existence (e.g., *run, is*).
2. Show locations (e.g., *up, here*).
3. Get attention and be social (e.g., *hi, thanks*).
4. Describe things (e.g., *more, wet*).
5. Express negatives (e.g., *no, all gone*).

Two-Word Phrase Level

When children have mastered a variety of meaningful words, their next step is to combine them into two-word phrases. The two words must have a relationship to each other, like *kick ball* (Bloom, 1970; Brown, 1973; MacDonald, Blott, Gordon, Spiegel & Hartmann, 1974). Both normal children and children with developmental delay put two words together as if they are operating under a set of rules. Professionals often have a difficult time assisting children with developmental delay in progressing from the one- to the two-word semantic level. MacDonald (1978) stresses using meaningful experiences, having a basic vocabulary of words that serve different functions, and having parents who can do the training or help with the follow-through. Children may need a carrier word such as "want" that can be used with many nouns until they are secure and ready to move on to a variety of two-word phrases.

Children who are secure with two-word phrases in therapy should be required to use them, especially in requesting situations. Adults should encourage children to use longer phrases by asking questions that take longer replies, such as "Tell us about that monkey," rather than questions that can have one-word answers, such as "Do you like the monkey?"

Conversation Level

Children who use phrases of three or more words have often developed to the point where others respond to them and continue building their conversations. The following is an example of how Bobby was able to create a better language environment for himself:

> Bobby was getting intensive language therapy in preschool. The school had not been able to get the family involved because they seemed very sure that Bobby wouldn't really talk. The preschool intervention had just established some two-word combinations when Bobby became ill and missed almost a month of school. To the school's surprise, Bobby returned speaking in three- to four-word sentences. The professionals were puzzled and wondered whether maturity had produced the change. Then his parents gave them the clue. His father said that when he heard him talking "little sentences," they decided he might talk after all, and they all "talked up a storm with him." Bobby had reached the point where his environment took over the teaching role.

Routine activities at home and in the preschool create a wealth of opportunities for developing and encouraging language. Raver (1987) discusses three strategies for encouraging language in children at the conversational level that can be easily woven into regular activities. These strategies include: changing routine events, withholding objects or turns, and violation of object functions.

Changing Routine Events　A child can be stimulated to initiate language by protesting a change in an expected routine. A change in schedule, such as changing outdoor playtime, could elicit some surprise or protest that would be encouraged and expanded by the instructor. Calling a student by the wrong name, wearing a blouse backwards, changing a bulletin board, moving furniture, hiding chairs, building a pile of the trash cans, and hanging streamers around the room are suggestions that might elicit language from the child.

Withholding Objects or Turns　Withholding objects until the child asks for them can be an effective language stimulant as early as the age when a child begins imitating. If the child is capable of naming what he or she wants, he or she should be required to do so. Teachers and parents who wait a short period of time before giving help encourage a child to verbalize. Of course, safety, frustration, or cleanliness may preclude use of the time-delay strategy in some situations. For example, if a child is spilling chocolate milk on the other children in the room, the adult may have to assist before the child asks for help; however, waiting when a child is trying to open a package may encourage a verbal request for help.

Violation of Object Functions The violation of object functions strategy can both elicit spontaneous language and teach object and action use. This strategy can also be an enjoyable one for adults and children. The adult may put a mitten on a child's foot, comb a book, wear a spoon in his or her hair, put a clock in the oven, and similar actions to stimulate conversation and highlight appropriate functions.

Strategies for Adults Interacting with Children at Various Levels

The following are a few useful strategies for adults who interact with children at the beginning word, two-word, and conversational levels. The strategies include:

1. Use repetition to teach new words. Use a new word in several meaningful sentences.
2. Use more descriptive words than at the preverbal level.
3. If the child doesn't pronounce the words correctly, *expand* his or her sentence into a more complete one, pronouncing the child's words correctly. For example, if the child says "Man fall," the adult should say "Oh, your man falls down?".
4. If the child is understandable, comment on the content of his or her sentence. For example, if the child says "Man fall," the adult could repeat by saying, "You pushed him off the table. Where is he?" (Horstmeier & MacDonald, 1978).
5. Have the child watch your face as you teach new words (for better articulation).
6. If the child cannot be understood at all, repeat his or her exact sounds with a questioning voice. For example, if the child says "Baa am ee," the adult should repeat what the child said. The child may then make a modification in the sound of his or her words and give additional information, "Barkee dog."
7. Use an incomplete sentence and pause so the child can finish it (Moerk, 1974).

STRUCTURE AND INTELLIGIBILITY CONCERNS

Children with developmental delay who speak in short phrases may have difficulty with word order and sentence construction (Weigel-Crum, 1981). Even if children know how to make sentences with clauses, they may use simpler forms. Rather than saying, "After dinner, I'll watch Star Trek," they are more likely to say, "I eat dinner. I watch Star Trek." Intervention at the preschool level should only be to possibly model the more advanced sentence construction after the child's comment.

When children have established language, it is time to start paying attention to intelligibility. Intelligibility problems can arise because the children have not learned the consonant sounds, or because of difficulties that arise when the sounds are combined. Sounds are produced and combined according to phonological rules that are modified as children get closer and closer to adult speech. Children with developmental delay often use immature phonological patterns much longer than normal children. Final consonant deletion (leaving off the last consonant of each word in a phrase) is quite common in children with delay (Ingram, 1978). An example of this is: "Ge my boo" instead of "Get my book."

The child may be able to produce individual sounds when tested, but may have difficulty forming them in connected speech. Speech language therapists can effectively work on an entire phonological process such as deletion of final consonants instead of teaching individual sounds.

It is important that a child's hearing be tested regularly. Children with Down syndrome often have unsuspected hearing losses. Balkany, Downs, Jafek, and Krajicek (1979) found that 64% of individuals with Down syndrome had significant (more than 15 dB) losses in both ears. Children with cerebral palsy and other handicapping conditions frequently have hearing problems as well. Language learning is a difficult enough process for children with developmental delay without a compounding hearing loss.

AUGMENTATIVE AND ALTERNATIVE COMMUNICATION

In the 1980s, professionals have increasingly looked at alternatives to speech for children at risk for speech development. As some children learn to speak, signs and communication devices are used to aid communication (augmentation). For other children, the alternative form is taught because the likelihood of understandable speech is low. No one would deny a system of communication to someone who had no other way to make needs and desires known. However, it is often difficult to determine whether a young child will develop speech. Silverman (1980) details 40 studies showing that teaching nonspeech communication does not appear to reduce the person's chances for improving actual speech. Almost 40% of the studies reported an increase in verbal output. It seems to prove that an alternate form of communication used with speech does not seem to hurt and may even enhance eventual speech development. In addition, the child has been saved the frustration of being unable to have his or her wants and needs known during the crucial preschool years.

Alternative forms of communication are often divided into two forms: unaided (using hands and body in signing) or aided (using communication boards and devices, including computers). Several factors must be considered. The following are considerations for total communication, whether it be signing or speaking:

1. Can the child make the necessary hand and finger movements?
2. Are the family and the staff willing to at least learn to read the child's signs?
3. Can the child imitate movement patterns? (Children with autism may develop imitation while learning to sign.)
4. Does the child communicate now with facial gestures? (Not a prerequisite, but a good sign.)

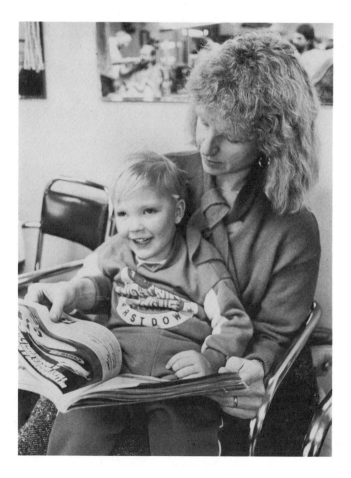

COMMUNICATION DEVICES FOR AIDED COMMUNICATION

Children who have not developed verbal language because of physical or perceptual reasons, often surprise concerned others with their display of understanding. The touch-on-command skill is very important for children who need communication boards or other communication aids. These aids can be anything from a few pictures for functional needs (e.g., a glass for drinking), to elaborate electronic dictionaries. The following is an example of the touch-on-command skill:

> A physical therapist in a rural area was working with a 4-year-old girl with cerebral palsy. On a whim, she got out some picture cards and positioned the girl so she could touch them. "Touch the house," she said. The girl did this correctly and continued on, identifying picture after picture. The girl's mother, who was observing, got tears in her eyes. "I always believed she was learning things in that head of hers. Now I know."

A teacher or speech/language therapist observing the above incident would quickly see the need for a well designed communication board or device so that the girl would be able to communicate. The example also illustrates that adults frequently do not use the touching response to indicate comprehension of language in an informal situation. Once alerted to the possibility, adults could have the child touch the named item in a variety of situations. When reading to a child, a parent can ask the child to touch a named picture before a page is turned.

DETERMINING THE NEED FOR AIDED COMMUNICATION

There are many ways of determining whether or not aided communication is needed. The following questions will help determine the need:

1. Has a method been found for the child to respond, such as pointing or head movement?
2. Is the device portable?
3. Does the child need pictures, or can symbols or written words represent ideas?
4. Is the device expensive? What resources for payment are available? (Adapted from McCormick & Shane, 1984)

There are many communication devices, including computers, with a variety of features that cannot be mentioned here (Silverman, 1980). A brief comparison of aided and unaided systems is presented in Table 9.3.

Alternate ways of communicating can be taught in much the same way that preverbal and verbal language is taught. If signs are going to be taught to one or two children, that entire preschool class should be able to understand and

Table 9.3. Comparison of aided and unaided systems

Total communication (Signing plus speech)	Communication devices
Advantages	
No cost	No special learning to communicate
Needs no equipment	Can be used for person with severe
Quite fast	physical disabilities
Disadvantages	
Others need to know signs to communicate	Need to carry equipment
Needs fairly good hand and finger	Can be expensive
movement	Usually slow

make, if possible, the signs being taught. Children need to communicate with each other as well as with adults. Teachers need to be at least a few signs ahead of the children and be handy with a dictionary of signs. All the children should understand how a child's communication device works. They should also be urged to wait while the other child responds, since operating a communication device may be a slow process.

USING COMPUTERS TO FACILITATE LANGUAGE

The availability of computers has revolutionized record keeping and analysis of data. It is no wonder that the excitement of the use of these devices has overflowed into other forms of information storage. Computers are seen by professionals and the public as an exciting new way to facilitate language development. This excitement has generated research projects and computer programs for use with young handicapped children (Meyers, in press). Although computers can be effective devices to facilitate speech and language, it is important to remember that for any young child, language is always based upon the concepts learned through personal interaction with people, and through objects that can be touched, carried, and explored. Speech sounds, in their basic form, are modeled after the sounds of others language (Michaelis, 1978). Therefore, even though computers may be used, there is no substitute for personal interactions with people who are speaking and with objects that the child can handle and move.

PLANNING FOR INDIVIDUALIZATION

Even though children are at different language levels, they can receive language training in both small and large groups. Teachers need to select language goals and make sure all the staff know and promote them. Sample teaching goals for five children might include:

Nathan: Request demonstration of comprehension of simple words.
Sean: Require one-word and encourage two-word combinations.
Cheryl: Encourage initiations.
Justin: Encourage short, complete sentences.
Kevin: Encourage production of sounds that are close to word sounds.

Then, when general activities are planned, language goals can be integrated into the activity. One example of such an activity follows:

> The teacher had read the story "The Three Bears." He starts it for the second time, telling the children they must be storytellers this time.
> Teacher: "And Momma Bear said . . . " (looking at Cheryl)
> Cheryl: "Too hot!" (initiating)
> Teacher: "Nathan, will you put your finger on Baby Bear's bed?"
> Nathan: Touches the picture of the bed (shows understanding)
> Teacher: (Holds up picture of bears walking) "What do you see here?"
> Sean: "Bear"
> Teacher: "Right, bears walk."
> Sean: "Bears walk" (two-word phrases)
> Teacher: "Kevin, who found Goldilocks?" (Holding up picture of Baby Bear)

Some questions that teachers and parents of several children must continually be asking are: Do all of the adults in the classroom speak to the children? Do all of the adults wait at least 1 second for the child to respond? Are some adults frequently talking to each other in rapid, sophisticated speech and not giving the children the attention and modified speech models that they require (Michaelis, 1978)? Are there ample opportunities for the children to talk to each other?

SUMMARY

In conclusion, the following points are important to remember:

1. Adults enhance the language learning of children with developmental delay by modifying how they talk to them.
2. Many language-learning activities can be woven into routine activities. Other activities may be specifically tailored for a child and chosen when needed.
3. Augmentative or alternative means of communication should be available to a child who shows delay in speaking, even though he or she may eventually speak.

STUDY QUESTIONS

1. Obtain permission from a child's parents to observe as a therapist explains to the parents how to facilitate language for their child.

2. Observe an interaction between the teacher and a child and how the teacher uses objects to help the child communicate.

3. Examine a language assessment instrument for young children.

4. Observe a child using an alternate communication technique or device and describe the technique or device and the interaction created.

REFERENCES

Balkany, T., Downs, M. P. , Jafek, B. W., & Krajicek, M. J. (1979). Hearing loss in Down's syndrome. *Clinical Pediatrics, 18*(2), 116–118.

Bates, E. (1976). *Language and context: The acquisition of pragmatics.* New York: Academic Press.

Bloom, L. (1970). *Language development: Form and function of emerging grammars.* Cambridge: MIT Press.

Broen, P. (1972, December). The verbal environment of the language-learning child. *American Speech and Hearing Association Monographs, 17.*

Brown, R. (1973). *A first language: The early stages.* Cambridge: Harvard University Press.

Bruner, J. (1975). The ontogenesis of speech acts. *Journal of Child Language, 2,* 1–19.

Buim, N., Rynders, J., & Turnure, J. (1974). Early maternal linguistic environment of normal and Down syndrome language-learning children. *American Journal of Mental Deficiency, 79,* 52–53.

Chapman, R. S. (1981). Mother-child interaction in the second year of life. In R. L. Schiefelbusch & D. Bricker (Eds.), *Early language: Acquisition and intervention* (pp. 203–249). Baltimore: University Park Press.

Cherry, L. (1979, September). *Theoretical bases of language and communication development in preschool children.* Paper presented at the Symposium on Developmental Disabilities in the Preschool Child: Early Identification, Assessment, and Intervention Strategies, Chicago.

Clark, H., & Clark, E. (1977). *Psychology and language.* San Diego: Harcourt Brace Jovanovich.

Cross, T. G. (1977). Mother's speech adjustments: The contribution of selected child listener variables. In C. E. Snow & C. A. Ferguson (Eds.), *Talking to children: Language input and acquisition* (pp. 151–183). Cambridge: Cambridge University Press.

Folger, J. P., & Chapman, R. S. (1978). A pragmatic analysis of spontaneous imitations. *Journal of Child Language, 5,* 25–38.

Garnica, O. K. (1975, September). *Nonverbal concomitants of language input to children.* Paper presented at the Third International Child Language Symposium, London.

Horstmeier, D. (1985). *The mother-child communicative interactions of educationally advantaged Down syndrome and normal children matched for auditory comprehension.* Unpublished doctoral dissertation, Ohio State University, Columbus.

Horstmeier, D., & MacDonald, J. D. (1978). *Ready, set, go: Talk to me.* Columbus, OH: Charles E. Merrill.

Ingram, D. (1976). *Phonological disability in children.* New York: Elsevier/North Holland.

Jones, O. H. M. (1977). Mother-child communication with prelinguistic Down syndrome and normal infants. In H. S. Schaffer (Ed.), *Studies in mother-infant interaction* (pp. 379–401). New York: Academic Press.

Leitch, S. M. (1977). *A child learns to speak: A guide for parents and teachers of preschool children.* Springfield, IL: Charles C Thomas.

Lombardino, L., & MacDonald, J. D. (1978). *Mother's speech acts during play interaction with nondelayed and Down syndrome children.* Unpublished doctoral dissertation, Ohio State University, Columbus.

MacDonald, J. D. (1978). *Environmental prelanguage inventory.* Columbus, OH: Charles E. Merrill.

MacDonald, J. D., Blott, J. P., Gordon, K., Spiegel, B., & Hartmann, M. (1974). An experimental parent-assisted treatment program for preschool language-delayed children. *Journal of Speech and Hearing Disorders, 39,* 395–415.

MacDonald, J. D., & Gillette, Y. (1982). *A conversational approach to language delay: Problems and solutions.* Columbus: Ohio State University.

McCormick, L., & Schiefelbusch, R. (1984). *Early language intervention.* Columbus, OH: Charles E. Merrill.

McCormick, L., & Shane, H. (1984). Augmentative communication. In L. McCormick & R. Schiefelbusch (Eds.), *Early language intervention.* Columbus, OH: Charles E. Merrill.

Meyers, L. (in press). *The language machine.* San Diego, CA: College-Hill Press.

Michaelis, C. T. (1978). Communication with the severely and profoundly handicapped: A psycholinguistic approach. *Mental Retardation, 16*(5), 346–349.

Miller, J. (1987). Language and communication characteristics of children with Down syndrome. In S. Pueschel, C. Tingey, J. E. Rynders, A. Crocker, & D. Crutcher (Eds.), *New perspectives on Down syndrome* (pp. 233–262). Baltimore: Paul H. Brookes Publishing Co.

Moerk, E. L. (1974). Changes in verbal mother-child interactions with increasing language skills of the child. *Journal of Psycholinguistic Research, 3,* 101–116.

Moerk, E. L. (1980). Relationships between parental input frequencies and children's language acquisition: A reanalysis of Brown's data. *Journal of Child Language, 7,* 105–118.

Nelson, K. (1973). Structure and strategy in learning to talk. *Monographs of the Society for Research in Child Development, 38*(1–2, Serial No. 149).

Nelson, K. (1975). The nominal shift in semantic-syntactic development. *Cognitive Psychology, 7,* 461–479.

Olmsted, D. (1971). *Out of the mouths of babes.* The Hague: Mouton.

Phillips, J. (1973). Syntax and vocabulary of mother's speech to young children: Age and sex comparisons. *Child Development, 44,* 182–185.

Piaget, J. (1963). *The origins of intelligence in children.* New York: Norton.

Poole, I. (1934). Genetic development of articulation of consonant sounds in speech. *Elementary English Review, 11,* 159–161.

Prather, E., Hedrick, D., & Kern, C. (1975). Articulation development in children aged two to four years. *Journal of Speech and Hearing Disorders, 40,* 179–191.

Raver, S. A. (1987). Practical procedures for increasing spontaneous language in language-delayed preschoolers. *Journal of the Division for Early Childhood, 11*(3), 226–232.

Rondal, J. A. (1977). Maternal speech to normal and Down's syndrome children matched for mean length of utterance. In P. Mittler (Ed.), *Research to practice in mental retardation: Vol. 2: Education and training* (pp. 239–243). Baltimore: University Park Press.

Sanders, E. (1972). When are speech sounds learned? *Journal of Speech and Hearing Disorders, 37,* 62.

Silverman, F. H. (1980). *Communication for the speechless.* Englewood Cliffs, NJ: Prentice Hall.

Templin, M. C. (1953). Norms on a screening test of articulation for ages 3 through 8. *Journal of Speech and Hearing Disorders, 18,* 323–331.

Weigel-Crum, C. A. (1981). The development of grammar in Down syndrome children between the mental ages of 2–0 and 6–11 years. *Education and Training of the Mentally Retarded, 16,* 24–30.

Chapter 10

Posture and Movement

Philippa H. Campbell

●

Normal, full-term infants acquire the essential posture (position or alignment of body parts) and movement skills that are used throughout their lifetimes during their first years. Little is known about the processes that underlie these developments, but a great deal of information is available about the ages at which typical children are able to demonstrate specific posture and movement skills, such as sitting or walking (Gesell & Amatruda, 1941; Illingworth, 1983). A sequence of acquisition of posture and movement skills that appears to be typical across normally developing children is implied in standardized developmental assessment instruments, such as the *Bayley Scales* (1969) (see Chapter 2). A similar sequence also appears in the extensive descriptive studies of infant motor behavior conducted by Gesell and others more than 50 years ago (Halverson, 1931; McGraw, 1935). Recent theorists have concluded that motor development is probably one of the predetermined hereditary characteristics carried in the genes. However, motor development is strongly influenced and modified as an infant begins using motor behavior, such as locomotor and grasping or holding skills, to interact with various objects and people in his or her particular environment (Bower, 1982; Kopp, 1979) (see Chapter 13 for a discussion of development of self-care skills).

THE IMPORTANCE OF POSTURE AND MOVEMENT

The importance of posture and movement skills can be viewed from several different perspectives. Of primary importance is the relationship between posture and movement skills and thinking (or problem solving) abilities (see discussion of sensorimotor learning in Chapter 11). Movement enables infants to explore their physical environments as they choose, and investigate the people and objects that make up that environment. Infants can move themselves to different locations to explore different types of objects and their properties, to interact with people, and to learn about social and physical contingencies (Piaget, 1952). This use of movement as a means for self-directed learning is only possible when movement skills are easy for the child to accomplish and when the child has a reason for doing them. Thus, movement is an important link to learning only when infants are capable of directing their movement for specific purposes.

Few studies have explored the development of postural skills acquired in infancy. Studies that have investigated the importance of movement skills differentiate between abilities that occur before and after the point at which infants are able to use these skills for their own purposes (Bower, 1977, 1982; Wolff, 1982). Infants' initial motor learning is focused on acquiring the skill itself with sufficient coordination and control, these skills can be used for movement for an intended purpose (Bruner, 1973; Kopp, 1979). The initial process of acquiring coordinated and controlled movement skills is not well studied. Initial acquisition can be explained as genetic preadaptation, a theory that is substantiated by the invariance in sequential performance of these skills across normally developing infants of all cultures (Kopp, 1979). It can also be explained as the inability of researchers to significantly alter the sequence of the skills performed (Bower, 1979) (see Chapter 2). The quickly learned sequence of these initial skills, as well as the skills themselves, provide infants with a fundamental repertoire of posture and movement skills for use in interaction with people and objects in the environment.

Competencies in Posture

Postural skills, such as sitting or standing, are the first skills that the infant uses to gain motor control over the physical environment. One primary feature of the posture of newborns is a lack of sufficient control over muscles and parts of the body to move against or withstand the pull of gravity. The young infant's typical postures of stomach (prone) or back (supine) lying are those that do not require holding a position or moving against the pull of gravity (Campbell, 1987b; Scherzer & Tscharnuter, 1982). Antigravity postures at this age are possible only with the support of an adult. Sequentially greater independent control over gravity occurs during the first year of life as the infant acquires at least basic competence over this feature of the physical world.

Infants learn central postural control by developing the ability to maintain a posture against gravitational influences. They do this without adult support or without using their own arms for balance by developing efficient use of the trunk muscles (Campbell, in press-a; Scherzer & Tscharnuter, 1982). In the beginning, infants maintain central postures for very short, often momentary, periods of time, gradually increasing the length of time that central control can be maintained. Central postural control is a dynamic process that results from movement within the trunk and central body axis and allows infants to: 1) adjust the body position for comfort; and 2) control the head, limbs, or total body against the influences of gravity. Increasing competence in central postural control allows maintenance of posture(s) in increasingly more difficult situations.

Head and Extremity Control Initially, control over gravity occurs with one limb or with the head, using a sequence of: 1) *movement against,* 2) *sustained control over,* and 3) *movement with control* as presented in Table 10.1. Head lifting provides an example of this sequence. The infant first lifts the head against the force of gravity but is unable to hold the head up for any length of time. With practice, the infant acquires the necessary muscular control to maintain the head in an upright position for indefinite periods of time. Initially, the head is upright but *locked into* the position, and the infant is unable to turn the head while holding it up. The final step is achieved when the infant is able to lift the head and hold it in position while using head movement, such as rotation, for a functional purpose such as looking around the environment.

Total Body Control A slightly different sequence occurs in learning to control total body postures against gravity (e.g., sitting or standing). Infants are typically positioned and maintained in postures by adults or through the use of pillows and other supports that help the infant to *maintain with external support.* Less external support becomes necessary over time, and the infant is able to use his or her arms to balance and *maintain with extremity support.* As control of the muscles of the trunk is achieved, the infant is able to achieve postures such as sitting and standing and *maintain posture with no supports* for brief periods of time.

The Link between Posture and Movement Central postural control allows the infant to maintain antigravtiy total body, head, and limb postures without supports. The ability to move the head or a limb that is maintained in an antigravity posture is a first link between postural control and movement. Links between total body postures and movement occur through balance. The coordinated movement patterns used to restore or maintain balance against gravity, link postural control and movement to allow an infant to maintain a posture

Table 10.1. Development of postural control

Body part	Sequence
Extremity and head	Movement against (away from) gravity
	Sustained control over gravity
	Movement with control over gravity
Total body	Maintain with external support
	Maintain with extremity support
	Maintain with no supports
	Movement into and out of a posture

indefinitely without use of external supports. A second link occurs when an infant has sufficient postural control and balance to not only hold a position, but to move in and out of that position.

Sitting postures provide an example of the importance of central postural control in linking posture and movement skills. Initially, infants sit for short periods of time, alternating the use of their arms and hands between support of the trunk (or posture) and the manipulation of objects. Increased ability to use the muscles in the trunk shifts control of the posture from the arms to the trunk and allows central maintenance of the posture. The infant is able to sit and use the arms without falling or losing control. Well controlled and practiced movements of the trunk musculature, in combination with head and extremity movements, result in the ability to maintain a posture through balance. The infant is able to sit for long periods of time under all conditions. With this degree of competence *while* sitting, the infant learns ways to move *into and out of* sitting, moving from back or stomach lying to sitting, sitting to lying, sitting to an all-four's position, and so on.

Sensorimotor Aspects of Posture and Movement

All posture and movement occur on the basis of sensory inputs that provide information to the muscles concerning the amount and type of contraction (tension) required.

Sensory Input for Posture   Postural control is the directly observable outcome of sensory input that precedes the production of muscle contractions. The sensory input is provided largely through the tactile (touch), vestibular (balance), proprioceptive (internal), and kinesthetic (movement) senses. These are internal sense organs, for the most part, and, therefore, the input is not directly observable. However, use of these systems is a focus in many types of therapeutic programming for infants with dysfunctional posture and movement skills.

Basic Movement Patterns   The relationship between sensory input and motor output in coordinated movement can be represented by levels, as presented in Figure 10.1. These levels range from simple to complex (Campbell, 1987a; Dunst, 1981; Feurstein, 1980). At the simplest level, motor skills are reflexes (see Chapter 2 for a list of reflexes) and the result of hereditarily determined links between sensory input and motor expression (Bower, 1979; Piaget, 1952). Thus, an infant stimulated with the edge of a nipple or by a finger turns the head to seek the stimulus (i.e., rooting reflex) or begins sucking when something is placed in the mouth (i.e., sucking reflex). These responses occur each time the stimulus is presented and stop when the stimulus is removed. They are the simplest forms of motor expression and are common across all infants except those with the most severe impairments (Kopp, 1979).

Specific Use   Several processes of development enable an infant to expand upon basic patterns of movement and to use these patterns more selec-

Level	Representation	Purpose
Basic patterns	S→R	Survival Protection
Differentiated use	S→(M)→R	Practice Expansion Contingency awareness
Functional use	S→(M)→R→S→R	Problem solving Self-direction Acquisition of new information

Figure 10.1. Relationship of sensory input to motor input.

tively to interact with environmental stimuli (Piaget, 1952). Repetition of the same response across similar stimuli allows practice of basic movements. These responses are practiced across a variety of eliciting situations, allowing for general use. Finally, an infant learns to produce the movement when the object or person associated with the response is present (Dunst, 1981).

Grasping provides an example of how these various processes allow an infant to achieve competence in the use of movement patterns for a specific purpose. Initially, anything placed in an infant's hand results in a grasping response that is reproduced each time a stimulus is provided. This response quickly becomes generalized to a variety of objects and situations such as grasping a rattle, mother's finger, or a shirt. Later, the infant begins grasping after seeing the rattle. The infant is now capable of producing a specific response without a direct touch and is able to produce that response consistently across a variety of objects and people.

This process allows an infant to learn to adapt more selectively and discriminatively to environmental stimuli. Movement performed in relation to different types of stimuli produces different types of responses. The different responses, in turn, if interesting to the infant, result in different rates of response in relation to different stimuli. Thus, an infant learns to suck a bottle more often (and slightly differently) than a pacifier or a finger, or learns to shake a rattle that has interesting consequences more frequently than a nonnoisemaking object. Later responses become directed away from the infant toward objects and people in the environment. The stimulus then becomes intertwined with the movement response. When this happens, the response and its action function as a stimulus for the infant to repeat the movement. These circular situations provide opportunities for an infant to learn how actions and objects are related (Dunst, 1981).

Functional Use of Posture and Movement Skills The combination of several self-directed movement patterns allows the infant to solve environmental problems or to acquire new information. At this point, the cognitive processes learned in infancy become linked to motor system expression, enabling an infant to use specific postures and movements as a means for individual expression of thoughts, ideas, feelings, and intentions. Coordinated movements are a means for obtaining information from interactions as well as for initiating those interactions with the physical and social world. The coordinated movements also allow response to environmental stimuli (Campbell, 1987a, 1987b; Dunst, 1981). These abilities take on greater importance in infancy, before a child is able to use language for initiation, response, and expression. When linked with cognition, posture and movement skills become *intentional* or *functional* because the movement is directed by the infant for a specific purpose. Posture and movement skills are no longer simply an expression of the motor system but involve a synthesis of cognitive direction with motor output for functional purposes (Kopp, 1979) (see Chapter 11 for a discussion of cognitive development).

IMPACT OF DISABILITY ON DEVELOPMENT OF POSTURE AND MOVEMENT

A number of different types of disorders affect posture and movement skills (Campbell, 1984; Hanson & Harris, 1986). Some disorders impair performance, some delay acquisition, and others result in both impairment and delay (Campbell, 1987b). Conditions such as generalized developmental delay or Down syndrome result in a delayed rate of acquisition of posture and movement skills (Cowie, 1970; Hanson & Schwarz, 1978; Harris, 1981; Molnar, 1978), while cerebral palsy and other major neurological conditions impair motor coordination and delay acquisition of posture and movement skills (Bobath & Bobath, 1984). Infants with severe visual impairment acquire postural skills at the same rate as infants without impairment, but show delays in acquisition of movement skills, particularly those requiring movement in space (Fraiberg, 1968).

What is less clearly understood is the impact of impaired and delayed posture and movement skills on other areas of development. A limited number of studies have documented abilities to acquire cognitive concepts in the absence of sensorimotor competence (Fraiberg, 1971; Kopp & Shaperman, 1973), and clinical studies report normal to above average intelligence in children with severe forms of cerebral palsy (Bigge, 1982; Cruikshank, Hallahan, & Bice, 1976). Competence in posture and movement may be less important to self-direction, cognition, and other developmental skills when impairments are present than in the normally developing infant with an intact motor system (Bricker, Macke, Levin, & Campbell, 1981). "Motor behaviors need to be considered as one of many of the child's resources. Motor functions should be examined as a channel to social, cognitive, and emotional growth, not as entities in and of themselves" (Kopp, 1979, p. 30).

Impairments in Posture and Movement

A number of factors contribute to impaired or delayed posture and movement skills. Some disorders result from damage to the neurological system; others are the result of congenital malformations or genetic abnormalities.

Muscle Tone Predominant among these factors are discrepancies in muscle tone that characterize cerebral palsy (Bobath & Bobath, 1976; Campbell, 1987a, 1987b; Scherzer & Tscharnuter, 1982; Wilson, 1984) and result from such etiologies as prematurity (Stanley & Alberman, 1984), intraventricular hemorrhage (Bennett & Chandler, 1980), periventricular leukomalacia (Calvert, Hoskins, Fong, & Forsyth, 1986), porencephalocele, or full-term asphyxia (Susser, Hauser, Kiely, Paneth, & Stein, 1985). Muscle tone is defined as the degree of tension in the muscles of the body. Discrepancies in muscle tone range from mild to severe, increased (hypertonic) to decreased (hypotonic), and may be pathological as in cerebral palsy, or something the child may outgrow, as is the case with many very low birth weight infants. Many infants with significantly low tone at birth may develop increased tone (hypertonus) as they get older. Still others, such as infants with Down syndrome or those diagnosed with overall delays in development, may have low tone (hypotonia) throughout life.

Coordinated Patterns of Movement Contraction of muscle groups provide the basis for both posture and coordinated patterns of movement. While postures such as sitting or standing appear to be relatively static, muscle groups are constantly contracting to keep the body in alignment and to provide adjustments in posture necessary for comfort. Even the most simple movement patterns require coordinated contractions of muscle groups necessary to produce the movement. An infant's use of movement for specific intentions or purposes is a result not only of coordinated muscle actions, but also of cognitive direction of the movement pattern. Initial attempts to use movement for functional purposes may be random and poorly coordinated. Coordination and accuracy improve through repeated use of the pattern (practice) that establishes a motor sequence that can be reproduced automatically (Connolly, 1981). Thus, for example, when an infant first begins to use a spoon, the accuracy and efficiency of the movement pattern are poorly coordinated but improve with practice as the motor sequence for eating with a spoon becomes established. The older child can reproduce the motor acts required in eating automatically, without thinking about how to do it.

Various types of coordinated movement patterns are necessary for competence in posture and movement skills. They include: 1) total body postural control involving the ability to control the head and limbs in various positions, 2) simple motor patterns, and 3) functional movement patterns. Infants with neurological disorders, such as cerebral palsy, are likely to have significant difficulty with each of these aspects of coordinated patterns of movement. However, infants whose acquisition of skills is delayed may have less pronounced problems that are more often associated with coordinated movement rather than with postural control.

Atypical Development of Posture and Movement Skills

Figure 10.2 illustrates a developmental sequence for atypical posture and movement that represents the possible progressive changes in muscle tone that may occur as an infant begins to achieve antigravity posture and patterns of movement (Campbell, 1987b). The figure illustrates the development of secondary handicapping conditions, such as changes in muscle length or orthopedic deformities, that were not present in early infancy but were caused, in part, by the child's inability to move normally. A concept of *primary* (or original) and *secondary* handicaps is critical to understanding impairments in posture and movement abilities that are directly related to significant discrepancies in muscle tone. Many infants who are born only with hypotonia eventually demonstrate hypertonus; permanent changes in the muscles, joints, and soft tissue of the body; and orthopedic deformities. The primary problem of hypotonia is present during early infancy; the secondary problems are acquired as a function of interaction with the environment (Campbell, in press-b).

Infants born with low muscle tone have difficulty achieving the co-contraction of muscle groups necessary to maintain postural alignment against the influences of gravity. The degree of low tone present may not *prevent* an infant from achieving the postures themselves, but may significantly influence the

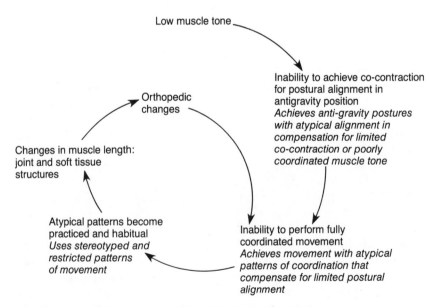

Figure 10.2.   A developmental sequence for atypical posture and movement.

alignment of the spine. Thus, antigravity postures of the head and limbs or total body are frequently achieved with various degrees of malalignment in the spine that are the result of biomechanical adjustments between body parts or increased tone (in response to gravitational stimuli). The distribution of hypertonus is more likely to be distal (arms and legs) than proximal (head and trunk), although tonal changes may occur in proximal areas as well.

This lack of normal alignment, in turn, influences the type of movements that may be possible in specific parts of the body. In essence, the possibility of performing specific coordinated movement patterns may be eliminated by either the tonal changes or the malalignment among body parts. However, because most infants are motivated to move, an atypically coordinated movement pattern that *compensates* for inability to produce a normally coordinated movement pattern may result. Compensatory movement patterns may be problematic in that if these patterns are functionally used and successful in achieving the desired intent of the child, the patterns will be frequently repeated. Thus, the compensatory movements become patterns highly practiced by an infant, and automatically and habitually used. They may not be recognized as potential problems by someone who has been trained to observe motor milestones but has not developed clinical skill in assessment (see Chapters 2 and 6). Highly used patterns that are characterized by high tone result in the development of changes in the muscles, joints, and soft tissue structures that are not only secondary to the original problem of hypotonia but are also disabling. These physical changes, in turn, may directly lead to the development of deformities that are only correctable through orthopedic surgery or other intrusive means. The orthopedic deformities, whether corrected through surgery or not, reinfluence a child's ability to move and result in further restrictions in postural alignment and coordinated movement.

INTERVENTION WITH INFANTS

Many types of delays or disorders in posture and movement skills are diagnosed and classified on the basis of atypical muscle tone, distribution throughout the body, and degree of severity. This system of diagnosis and classification allows physicians to identify an infant with cerebral palsy, as well as to generally describe the extent of the condition (Gorski, 1984). A diagnosis of *severe spastic hemiplegia,* for example, describes an infant who has severe hypertonus on one side of the body, whereas an infant with *moderate congenital hypotonia* is one with moderately low muscle tone throughout the body.

This type of classification system is an effective means for describing muscle tone deviations for the purpose of categorizing groups of children, but is less effective when used as a basis for planning intervention. A classification system for use in planning intervention for infants with atypical muscle tone has been proposed by Campbell and Forsyth (1987). Seven types of infants have been described on the basis of disordered or delayed posture and movement skills. This system, briefly summarized in Table 10.2, provides a general basis for differential treatment procedures that derive from a neurodevelopmental perspective of intervention. It is important to note, however, that although classification may be helpful in the general focus of planning for treatment, each child must be examined individually to determine appropriate treatment.

Principles of Intervention

The most effective treatment interventions for all infants with impaired or delayed performance of posture and movement skills are guided by a set of principles. These principles include specific methods and techniques that facilitate optimal development of these skills (Campbell, 1987c, in press-a; Campbell & Stewart, 1986). These include: an emphasis on family functioning, the use of least to most intrusive intervention approaches, and clear identification of infant goals and objectives.

An Emphasis on Family Functioning   The family is a key variable in the growth and development of their infant. Well designed interventions are those that can be easily implemented within the routines of a family (Turnbull & Turnbull, 1986; Washington & Gallagher, 1986). Enabling families to implement caregiving routines, such as holding, feeding, bathing, and playing, in ways that maximize the capabilities of their infants and prevent the development of secondary disorders (e.g., changes in muscles and joints, orthopedic impairments) is the focus of infant intervention (see Chapter 16 for a discussion of family needs).

Use of Least to Most Intrusive Intervention Approaches   Many infants have only mild problems and family members can be taught skills and competencies necessary to optimize development of posture and movement skills. An infant who receives various individual therapy sessions, that are isolated from the environment of the family, may be receiving intervention that impedes (rather than optimizes) the development of posture and movement abilities. The most beneficial services are well coordinated and provide care within the context of what is appropriate for individual family and infant needs. Physical therapy alone may be the most appropriate service for one infant and family, whereas an integrated therapy approach that includes education and physical, occupational, and speech/language therapy, as well as other disciplines, may be the structure that best addresses the needs of another infant and family. Unique needs can best be met through flexible systems of intervention (see Chapter 8 for a discussion of individual programming).

Clear Identification of Infant Goals and Objectives   The major purposes of intervention with infants who have neurological and other impairments that result in dysfunctional posture and movement skills are different from those with infants with delayed acquisition of these skills (Campbell, in press-a). Goals for infants with dysfunctional posture and movement must be directed toward: 1) altering postural tone, in combination with facilitating de-

Table 10.2. Overview of categorical classifications of infants with posture and movement difficulties

Type	Characteristics	Treatment aims
Severe hypotonia	Very low tone in head, trunk, extremities; limited antigravity posture; small repertoire of antigravity movement; poorly coordinated patterns of movement with low rate.	Develop activation of antigravity muscles; use supports to enable antigravity postures; facilitate coordinated upper extremity movement.
Severe hypertonia	Increased tone in the trunk and extremities; antigravity hypertonus in posture and movement; may adapt to sensory stimuli with increased tone; few movements that are functional.	Decrease increased tone in combination with facilitation of antigravity tone for functional alignment; facilitate coordinated upper extremity movement.
Central hypotonia with distal hypertonia	Increased tone in the extremities; limited antigravity posture; small repertoire of antigravity movements that may be performed with increased tone; increase central tone/decrease extremity tone.	Increase central tone/decrease extremity tone; develop activation of antigravity muscles; facilitate coordinated movement in head, trunk, and limbs.
Hypertonus on one body side	Increased tone on one body side; asymmetrical antigravity postures; coordinated movement on the nonaffected side, paucity of movement on the affected side, difficulty with bilateral movements.	Decrease tone in affected side while increasing symmetrical posture and alignment; develop coordinated bilateral movement patterns.
Slight hypotonia	Low tone throughout the body; poor alignment in antigravity postures; poorly coordinated movements—may be restricted in variety.	Develop alignment in antigravity postures through increasing tone in proximal muscles; develop coordinated and self-directed movement patterns.
Atypical muscle tone in combination with other physical disorders	Severe hypertonus or hypertonus throughout the body; vision and/or hearing impairment; limited antigravity posture; poorly coordinated and directed movement, restricted rate of movement; poor use of movement for directed functions.	Alter muscle tone through aligned posture and specific techniques; identify stimuli that are reinforcing to the child; develop self-directed and functionally coordinated movement.

velopment of posture and movement abilities; 2) preventing the use of hypertonus for functional posture and movement skills by inhibiting high tone and facilitating posture and movement abilities; 3) preventing the development of compensatory postural and movement patterns, while facilitating the development of coordinated patterns of intentional or functional movement; 4) preventing development of secondary physical changes (e.g., changes in muscle length or orthopedic changes); and 5) remediating any delays in performance. Remediating delayed performance is the least important focus when postural tone and posture and movement skills are impaired, but is a more important focus with infants who have only motor delay. Facilitating continual acquisition and use of functional posture and movement skills, while remediating any existing delays, is the focus of intervention with infants with delays in skill performance.

Intervention Methods

Three general methods are most often used to provide direct intervention for infants with delayed or disorders of posture and movement abilities. The first of these methods is the Neurodevelopmental Treatment (NDT), originated by Dr. Karel and Mrs. Berta Bobath and used by physical, occupational, and speech/ language therapists and teachers with infants and children with cerebral palsy (Bobath & Bobath, 1984; Campbell, 1986; Scherzer & Tscharnuter, 1982). A second approach is to provide pediatric physical and/or occupational therapy where therapists, for the most part, use remedial and eclectic approaches to assist in overcoming disabilities and facilitating developmental skills. The third approach is one of directed infant stimulation. The focus of intervention with infant stimulation is to identify the developmental skills that an infant cannot perform, and provide activities designed to stimulate development in these identified skill areas. This approach is the least effective, but one that can be used by any type of professional. Positioning and exercise are incorporated into most methods that are used to influence posture and movement abilities.

Positioning The primary purposes of positioning are to: 1) maintain postural alignment to prevent the development of secondary deformities, and 2) compensate for the infant's inability to control the trunk in order to allow use of the head and arms to interact with objects and people (Campbell, 1987d). Equipment is often used to enable an infant to be upright against gravity. Standard equipment, used with all infants, such as car seats, high chairs, and strollers, just to name a few, is adapted for use with infants with disabilities. More specialized equipment such as wheelchairs is seldom necessary for infants. However, prone boards or supine standers that allow infants to stand are necessary when infants have severe disorders in posture and movement. Proper positioning is an important first step in assisting infants to engage in activities that are not specifically directed to posture and basic coordinated movement abilities. Equipment enables those infants with particularly low tone (hypotonus) in the head and trunk to be less dependent on adults for antigravity postures. In combination with other intervention methods, the equipment can also facilitate independence in essential developmental skills (e.g., self-feeding, mobility, communication).

Exercise Methods that are directed toward altering postural tone and facilitating aligned posture and coordinated movement abilities are fairly specific techniques that can be incorporated into play activities or caregiving routines such as diapering. The primary purposes of these activities are to: 1) increase and/or decrease muscle tone in specific muscle groups, 2) develop muscle strength, 3) change the amount of movement in a joint, and 4) facilitate independent posture and movement skills. Methods and techniques are not isolated exercises but are unique combinations designed to meet the specific characteristics of an infant with impaired posture and movement skills. Not all techniques are necessary for all children. Those that are appropriate for an infant can be taught by physical and occupational therapists to parents and other non-therapists who are involved with the family and infant. For example, consider the techniques selected for use with Laura:

Laura is a 5-month-old infant who was born prematurely and suffered a severe intraventricular hemorrhage. She was enrolled in early intervention on discharge from the neonatal intensive care unit at 2 months of age. Her muscle tone has been hypotonic in the head and trunk since birth. Goals related to posture and movement skills have included: 1) altering postural tone and facilitating aligned antigravity postures; and 2) facilitating use of the arms to interact with objects through use of discriminated movement patterns, performed without hypertonus.

Laura's motor programming has been with NDT techniques. Activities have been designed to improve aligned posture in sitting and to sufficiently stabilize the trunk to allow Laura to use her arms for functional movement. The focus of her intervention is not only to improve motor skills, but also to ensure that growth in cognitive areas is not hindered due to current difficulties with posture and movement.

Laura receives intervention for posture and movement skills on a once-per-week basis. Activities such as lifting the pelvis (to bring her feet toward her trunk) when back lying, supported movement into sitting from both lying on her stomach and her back, and shifting weight from side to side in a supported sitting position, have been used to activate tone in the trunk muscles while establishing a properly aligned sitting position.

Laura's mother incorporates the lifting pelvis activity into diaper changing and clothes changing so that Laura has an opportunity to practice this skill (and therefore activate the correct muscle groups) at least 30–40 times per day. Laura's mother also holds Laura at the rib cage when she is playing with her on her lap in order to ensure alignment of the trunk in a supported sitting position. She has noticed that Laura can hold her head up much better when the trunk is first held in an upright position. In addition, Laura's mother has learned to shift Laura's weight from side to side and front to back when she is holding her in sitting, and although she sometimes just picks Laura up, she is trying to remember to use the sequence of back or stomach lying to sitting in order to give her daughter even more practice in activating the correct muscle groups.

Suggestions were initially made to limit the number of times per day that Laura was placed on her stomach. Laura's mother could see that her baby's trunk "sunk into gravity," and she noticed that Laura stiffened her legs when trying to raise her head while on her stomach. Now she positions Laura in her infant seat with towel rolls to align her trunk, and gives her toys that are easy to grasp.

Key Concepts Underlying Posture and Movement Intervention

Several common concepts are incorporated into positioning and exercise. The following are a few of the concepts.

Process Versus Product   Many approaches that are labeled as developmentally focused (e.g., stimulation, remediation) place emphasis on performance of specific skills (e.g., sitting, walking, manipulation) and ignore posture and movement patterns used to perform the skill. Aligned posture and coordinated movement are the result of interaction between muscle contractions. Infants with atypical muscle tone can achieve postures that are not aligned (but that compensate for hypotonus or hypertonus) and perform discriminated or functional (intentional) movements that are poorly coordinated and compensate for problems with muscle tone and postural malalignment. Proper positioning and active *exercise/activity* programs are designed to place equal emphasis on the underlying components that result in skill performance. This focus is directed toward postural tone, aligned antigravity posture, and coordinated patterns of movement, rather than toward achieving the motor milestones listed on standardized assessment charts (see Chapter 2).

Gravity   Inability to move in ways that counteract gravitational influences is a common problem for both infants with *impaired* and *delayed* acquisition of posture and movement abilities. Those infants with impairments require methods that are specifically directed toward the underlying problems (e.g., tone) in order to develop the competencies necessary to become upright and move against gravity. Infants with delays in these areas can be helped through therapeutic interventions of positioning and *exercise,* but eventually learn these skills even without such specifically focused intervention (Harris, 1981; Molnar, 1978).

Planes of Space   Posture and movement skills are performed within physical space that is divided spatially into several planes, including those in which the body moves forward and backward (e.g., leaning forward from sitting to retrieve an object from the floor), side to side (e.g., reaching sideways), and top to bottom (e.g., how *straight* an individual sits). Postural alignment and coordinated movement result from shifts of body weight within these general places of space. Thus, in order to lift the head when lying on the stomach, for example, body weight has to be shifted from the head and trunk onto the pelvis. Walking results when weight is shifted from one leg to the other, then forward off of the weight-bearing leg, and so forth. Shifting the body weight in the desired planes of space can help an infant to learn how to move with coordinated and aligned patterns. Thus, to teach an infant to lift the head, hands could be placed over the infant's buttocks to shift weight and enable the infant to lift

the head. Toys or interesting objects could be used to motivate the head movement, but, if used without facilitation of the required weight shift, the infant
will have extreme difficulty performing the skill, or will learn to do so using
patterns of movement, such as neck extension, that compensate for lack of
weight shifting. Postural misalignment results when the body is out of alignment within these planes of space. Thus, an infant who is positioned in sitting
on the sacrum (rather than directly over the pelvis and hips) is out of alignment
in the frontwards-backwards plane of space. It is difficult to describe facilitation methods with words. They must be demonstrated in order to ensure understanding of the concept.

Static Versus Dynamic Infants with impaired or delayed acquisition of
posture and movement skills don't need therapy, per se, but require intervention that can teach posture and movement abilities that are as normal as possible. An infant has to be moved (or move independently) in order to learn how to

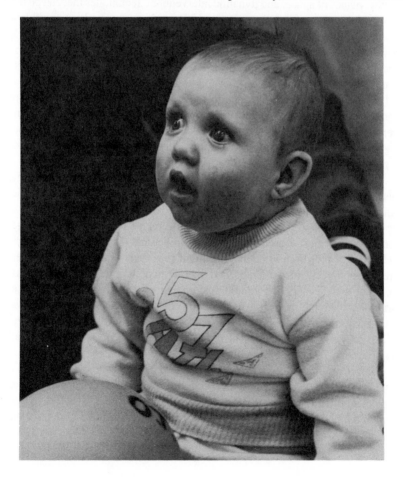

move with better alignment or more coordinated patterns of movement. Positioning is a *static method* that is often required to maintain alignment and prevent deformities. This static method is not an effective method in improving posture and movement abilities. Rather, only *dynamic intervention approaches,* where the infant and adult move together, have effectiveness in influencing posture and movement skills.

Linking Posture, Movement, and Cognition

Positioning and *exercise* approaches, such as those just described, are methods and techniques designed to influence underlying components necessary for an aligned posture and coordinated basic and discriminative movements. Functional movement, or the ability of an infant to use his or her movement abilities for an intended purpose, results only when cognition is linked to concepts of gravity, planes of space, and dynamic intervention. Techniques that can be used to provide *exercise* that influences specific muscle groups make it possible for an infant to generate a specific movement pattern. However, such exercises are ineffective by themselves as a means for enabling an infant to use that pattern in a goal-directed manner (Campbell, 1987b, in press-a). Some infants lack sufficiently sophisticated cognitive concepts to direct movement patterns that are well within their performance repertoire. Others understand the cognitive concepts, but lack sufficient tone and coordinated patterns of posture and movement to direct movements for intended purposes. Still others may lack both cognitive and motoric competence. Approaches for each of these combinations of problems would differ.

The goal of any intervention is to enable infants to use posture and movement skills for intended purposes. Well coordinated posture and movement skills are of little value to an infant or child who does not understand how to use them or is not allowed to use them for a self-directed purpose. Early intervention specialists must work carefully with families and their infants to determine the extent of the disabilities that an infant may have in each of these areas. Creative approaches are often needed in order to determine the extent to which an infant with severely disordered posture and movement is able to solve environmental problems, using means-end, causality, object permanence, and other early cognitive abilities. Too often, a child with severe disabilities is unable to demonstrate understanding of these concepts when tested through traditional means (Bricker et al., 1981; Zelazo, 1982) (see Chapter 11).

Information about posture and movement, as well as knowledge of an infant's abilities or disabilities in basic cognitive skills, is necessary to plan and implement effective programming. In most instances, the most effective intervention methods combine this information in order to ensure that infants learn not just to move better, but to move for their own purposes.

INTEGRATED PROGRAMMING FOR INFANTS

The ways in which infants and children with impaired movement compensate for inabilities to use movement to initiate and respond to the physical and social world are not clearly understood. One mechanism that has been suggested is the development of language skills that can be used to self-direct people in the environment (Kopp, 1979). Others have suggested that children may learn from observation when unable to learn through physical interaction with objects.

Many infants have multiple handicaps that may include disorders in vision, posture, and movement (Campbell, 1987a) or that may combine posture and movement disorders with multisensory impairments. These infants, as well as those with less challenging program demands, as more likely to benefit from intervention approaches that *integrate* the expertise of a variety of professionals in ways that compensate for the degree of disability that may be present in the motor, visual, and auditory systems. An infant with disorders in only one of these areas is at risk for acquiring a number of secondary handicaps such as cognitive, language, or social-emotional disorders. Well integrated team programming is a necessity if secondary problems are to be prevented in infants with combined disorders (see Chapters 5 and 8). Physical or occupational therapy or intervention provided by someone who is NDT trained or who has competence in motor programming using other methods is not enough. The likelihood of making a dramatic difference in the development and future of an infant with posture and movement disorders becomes greater when methods for intervening with postural tone and coordinated patterns are combined with other approaches (Campbell, 1987b).

SUMMARY

The purpose of this chapter is to describe the importance of posture and movement skills in the development of infants and young children and to differentiate between children with *impaired* performance of these skills and those with *delayed* skill acquisition. This essential difference is important when planning appropriate services for families and their young children. A second purpose is to describe the types of intervention that are used with infants and young children when focusing on posture and movement abilities. Infants with impaired performance require programming that prevents secondary handicaps from developing while focusing on optimizing functioning in those areas that enable skill performance. In contrast, infants with delayed abilities can be helped through strategies designed to remediate delays in performing essential gross and fine motor skills. Occupational or physical therapy services that are delivered in isolated environments are less likely to be effective with both groups of infants than therapeutic strategies that are incorporated into functional activities and caregiving routines appropriate for each individual family and infant.

STUDY QUESTIONS

1. Observe nonhandicapped infants who are playing on the floor and describe their movements.

2. Observe infants with posture and movement difficulties who are playing on the floor and describe their movements.

3. Examine and make diagrams with measurements of the supportive equipment used for a child with motor impairment.

4. Obtain parental permission and hold an infant with a severe motor problem.

REFERENCES

Bayley, N. (1969). *Bayley Scales of Infant Development*. New York: Psychological Corporation.

Bennett, F. C., & Chandler, L. S. (1980). Spastic diplegia in premature infants: Current etiological and diagnostic considerations. *Developmental Medicine and Child Neurology, 22*, 124.

Bigge, J. L. (1982). *Teaching individuals with physical and multiple disabilities*. Columbus, OH: Charles E. Merrill.

Bobath, B., & Bobath, K. (1976). *Motor development in the different types of cerebral palsy*. London: Whitefriars Press, Ltd.

Bobath, B., & Bobath, K. (1984). The neurodevelopmental treatment. In D. Strutton (Ed.), *Management of the motor disorders of children with cerebral palsy* (pp. 6–18). Philadelphia: J. B. Lippincott.

Bower, T. G. R. (1977). *A primer of infant development*. San Francisco: W. H. Freeman.

Bower, T. G. R. (1979). *Human development*. San Francisco: W. H. Freeman.

Bower, T. G. R. (1982). *Development in infancy* (2nd ed.). San Francisco: W. H. Freeman.

Bricker, W. A., Macke, P., Levin, J., & Campbell, P. H. (1981). The modifiability of intelligent behavior. *Journal of Special Education, 15*, 145–163.

Bruner, J. (1973). The organization of early skilled action. *Child Development, 4*, 1–11.

Calvert, S. A., Hoskins, E. M., Fong, K. W., & Forsyth, S. C. (1986). Periventricular leukomalacia: Ultrasonic diagnosis and neurological outcome. *Acta Paediatrica Scandinavica, 75*, 489–496.

Campbell, P. H. (1987a). The integrated programming team: An approach for coordinating professionals of various disciplines in programs for students with severe and multiple handicaps. *Journal of The Association for Persons with Severe Handicaps, 12*(2), 107–116.

Campbell, P. H. (1987b). Integrated programming for students with multiple handicaps. In L. Goetz, D. Guess, & K. Stremel-Campbell (Eds.), *Innovative program design for individuals with dual sensory impairments* (pp. 159–188). Baltimore: Paul H. Brookes Publishing Co.

Campbell, P. H. (1987c). Physical management and handling procedures with students with movement dysfunction. In M. Snell (Ed.), *Systematic instruction of persons with severe handicaps* (3rd ed.) (pp. 176–187). Columbus, OH: Charles E. Merrill.

Campbell, P. H. (1987d). Programming for students with dysfunction in posture and movement. In M. Snell (Ed.), *Systematic instruction of persons with severe handicaps* (3rd ed.) (pp. 188–211). Columbus, OH: Charles E. Merrill.

Campbell, P. H. (in press-a). Sensorimotor-based programming. In M. J. Wilcox & P. H. Campbell (Eds.), *Communication programming from birth to three: A handbook for public school professionals*. San Diego: College-Hill Press.

Campbell, P. H. (in press-b). Service delivery approaches. In M. J. Wilcox & P. H. Campbell (Eds.), *Communication programming from birth to three: A handbook for public school professionals*. San Diego: College-Hill Press.

Campbell, P. H., & Forsyth, S. (1987). *A system for linking assessment-intervention for infants with motor disabilities*. Unpublished manuscript.

Campbell, P. H. (1986). *Introduction to neurodevelopmental treatment* (rev. ed.). Akron, OH: Children's Hospital Medical Center of Akron.

Campbell, P. H., & Stewart, B. S. (1986). Measuring changes in movement skills with infants and young children with handicaps. *Journal of The Association for Persons with Severe Handicaps, 11*(3), 153–161.

Campbell, S. (1984). *Pediatric neurologic physical therapy* (Vol. 5). New York: Churchill Livingstone.

Connolly, K. J. (1981). Maturation and the ontogeny of motor skills. In K. J. Connolly & H. F. Prechtl (Eds.), *Maturation and development: Biological and psychological perspectives*. Philadelphia: J. B. Lippincott.

Cowie, V. A. (1970). *A study of the early development of mongols*. Oxford: Pergamon.

Cruikshank, W. M., Hallahan, D. P., & Bice, H. V. (1976). Assessment of intelligence. In W. M. Cruikshank (Ed.), *Cerebral palsy: A developmental disability* (pp.123–174). Syracuse: Syracuse University Press.

Dunst, C. J. (1981). *Infant learning: A cognitive-linguistic intervention strategy*. Hingham, MA: Teaching Resources.

Feurstein, R. (1980). *Instructional enrichment: An intervention program for cognitive modifiability*. Baltimore: University Park Press.

Fraiberg, S. (1968). Parallel and divergent patterns in blind and sighted infants. *Psychoanalytical Study of the Child, 23*, 264–300.

Fraiberg, S. (1971). Intervention in infancy: A program for blind infants. *Journal of American Academy of Child Psychiatry, 10*, 381–405.

Gesell, A., & Amatruda, C. S. (1941). *Developmental diagnosis*. New York: Hoeber.

Gorski, P. A. (1984). Infants at risk. In M. J. Hanson (Ed.), *Atypical infant development* (pp. 57–80). Baltimore: University Park Press.

Halverson, H. M. (1931). An experimental study of prehension in infants by means of systematic cinema records. *Genetics Psychology Monographs, 10*, 107–286.

Hanson, M. J., & Harris, S. (1986). *Teaching your children with motor delays*. Rockville, MD: Aspen Systems.

Hanson, M. J., & Schwarz, R. J. (1978). Results of a longitudinal intervention program for Down's syndrome infants and their families. *Education and Training of the Mentally Retarded, 13*(4), 403–407.

Harris, S. (1981). Effects of neurodevelopmental therapy on improving motor performance in Down syndrome infants. *Developmental Medicine and Child Neurology, 23*, 477–483.

Illingworth, R. S. (1983). *The development of the infant and young child: Normal and abnormal* (8th ed.). Edinburgh: Churchill Livingstone.

Kopp, C. B. (1979). Perspectives on infant motor system development. In M. H. Bornstein & W. Kessen, *Psychological development from infancy: Image to intention.* Hillsdale, NJ: Lawrence Erlbaum Associates.

Kopp, C. B., & Shaperman, J. (1973). Cognitive development in the absence of object manipulation during infancy. *Developmental Psychology, 9,* 430.

McGraw, M. (1935). *Growth: A study of Johnny and Jimmy.* New York: Appleton-Century-Crafts.

Molnar, G. E. (1978). Analysis of motor disorder in retarded infants and young children. *American Journal of Mental Deficiency, 83*(3), 213–222.

Piaget, J. (1952). *The origins of intelligence in children.* New York: International Universities Press.

Scherzer, A., & Tscharnuter, I. (1982). *Early diagnosis and therapy in cerebral palsy.* New York: Marcel Decker.

Stanley, F., & Alberman, E. (1984). Birth weight, gestational age, and the cerebral palsies. In F. Stanley & E. Alberman (Eds.), *The epidemiology of the cerebral palsies.* Philadelphia: J. P. Lippincott.

Susser, M., Hauser, W. A., Kiely, J. L., Paneth, N., & Stein, Z. (1985). Quantitative estimates of prenatal and perinatal risk factors for perinatal mortality, cerebral palsy, mental retardation, and epilepsy. In J. M. Freeman (Ed.), *Prenatal and perinatal factors associated with brain disorders* (pp. 359–440). (NIH Publication No. 85-1149) Washington, DC: U.S. Department of Health and Human Services.

Turnbull, A. P., & Turnbull, H. R. (1986). *Families, professionals, and exceptionality: A special partnership.* Columbus, OH: Charles E. Merrill.

Washington, V., & Gallagher, J. J. (1986). Family roles, preschool handicapped children, and social policy. In J. J. Gallagher & P. M. Vietze (Eds.), *Families of handicapped persons: Research, programs and policy issues* (pp. 261–272). Baltimore: Paul H. Brookes Publishing Co.

Wilson, J. (1984). Cerebral palsy. In S. Campbell (Ed.), *Pediatric neurologic physical therapy.* New York: Churchill Livingstone.

Wolff, P. H. (1982). Theoretical issues in the development of motor skills. In M. Lewis & L. Taft (Eds.), *Developmental disabilities: Theory, assessment, and intervention* (pp. 117–134). New York: Spectrum Publications.

Zelazo, P. R. (1982). An information processing approach to infant cognitive assessment. In M. Lewis & L. T. Taft (Eds.), *Developmental disabilities: Theory, assessment, and intervention.* Jamaica, NY: SP Medical & Scientific Books.

Chapter 11

Cognitive Development

Glendon Casto

•

Jean Piaget has dramatically expanded our knowledge of cognitive development, perhaps more than any other scientist to date. His qualitative studies were begun by observing French children as he assisted with standardization of early intelligence tests (see Chapter 6). Piaget continued his studies at the Institute Roussen in Geneva, Switzerland, and later with his own children as subjects (Flavell, 1963). His lifelong studies, and those of numerous students he supervised in several institutes, provide a rich conceptual framework for looking at the process of cognitive development.

In this chapter, Piaget's basic conceptions of how cognitive skills develop are presented, followed by an examination of current theories of cognitive deficit as seen in mental retardation. The relationship of cognitive development to other areas of development are then explored, followed by a discussion of the course of cognitive development in handicapped children. The chapter concludes with a discussion of systems for stimulating cognitive development to prevent possible mental retardation.

For Piaget, cognitive development occurs in stages. Piaget did not see these stages as directly related to age. Instead, he perceived them as ordinal progressions of difficulty. His theory of cognitive development identifies the period from birth to about 2 years of age as the *sensorimotor stage,* the period of about 2 to about 7 years of age as the *pre-operational stage,* the period from about 7 to 11 years of age as the *concrete operations stage,* and the period from about 11 on as the *formal operation stage* (see charts in Chapter 2).

In the sensorimotor stage, the reflex patterns that are present in the infant

Work reported in this chapter was carried out in part with funds from the U.S. Department of Education (Contract #s 300-82-0367 and 300-85-0173) to the Early Intervention Research Institute at Utah State University.

at birth enable the infant to interact with the environment. These patterns, or *schemas* in Piagetian terms, link with other behavior patterns, and become coordinated and generalized. As infants interact with their environments, they begin to repeat behaviors that produce certain results. Hunger, for example, may produce certain cries and gestures that, in turn, are the means for securing food. Subsequently, most infants discern that certain cause and effect relationships exist, and they develop a complex series of repertoires based on this knowledge. At this time, infants also expand their knowledge base by looking at, grasping for, and mouthing objects. Objects are thus experienced concurrently through a variety of sensory modalities. Watching a baby with a favorite toy provides a good lesson in the many ways in which infants gain experience with objects in their environment. Piaget's prolific writings contain detailed, dated notes of his observations of infants.

Next, the infant acquires the concept of object permanence. "Out of site and gone forever" is replaced by "Where is it?" Infants, for example, displace blankets placed over familiar toys and actively search visually for interesting objects placed out of their reach. When infants develop the concept of object permanence, they are then able to replace problem-solving physical activity with mental operations.

As children enter the pre-operational stage, they become increasingly able to deal with their environment in abstract ways. Children begin to lose interest in trial and error approaches to problem-solving and begin to develop metacognitive approaches. At this time, children also become adept at imitating the actions of others in solving problems. Two characteristics of the pre-operational stage, however, are that children's immediate perceptions dominate the problem-solving efforts, and both speaking and points of view are egocentric, that is, centered about themselves. For example, if two balls of clay of equal size are placed before children in this stage, and then formed in such a way that one appears to be larger or smaller, their immediate perception dominates reality and they insist that one is larger or smaller.

When children enter the concrete operation stage of thinking at about age 7, their cognitive processes become increasingly logical. Now, if presented with two balls of clay of the same size that are then reformed, the child remembers the first exposure and correctly says that they are the same size. Children in this stage also begin to understand number operations and general concepts of sorting and classifying. The child's egocentrism also gives way to consideration of the points of view of others.

The period of formal operations begins in adolescence. In this stage, adolescents acquire the ability to think in abstract terms, including the manipulation of abstract symbols, the formation of testable hypotheses, and deductive reasoning operations.

For years, researchers have tested Piaget's theories with both normal and mentally retarded children. Weisz, Yates, and Zigler (1982), after reviewing studies testing Piagetian stages in retarded persons, concluded that they progressed through Piagetian stages in the same sequence as persons with normal intelligence, but at a much slower rate. In other words, while the order of progression may be fixed, individual differences determine the rate of progression.

For Piaget, cognitive skills develop out of indirect interchanges between the experiences of the individual and maturation caused by these experiences and physical development. Cognition involves the progressively organized adaptation to one's environment with both experience and maturation playing key roles.

COGNITIVE DEVELOPMENT AND MENTAL RETARDATION

Some children appear to have more than the usual difficulties in development of cognitive skills. Depending on the degree of difficulty, these children may

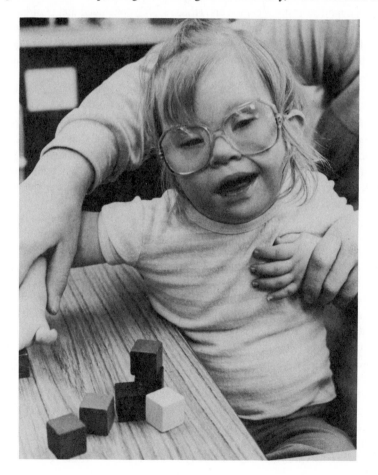

show deficits in cognitive functioning on standardized tests (see Chapter 6) and, therefore, be labeled mentally retarded. A frequently asked question has been, "How do mentally retarded persons differ from others in regard to cognitive skills?" There are currently three concepts concerning cognitive development in retarded persons. Stated simply, there are: 1) the deficit theory, 2) the developmental theory, and 3) the separate but equal theory. These views are discussed briefly in the following paragraphs.

Deficit Theory

The deficit theory to explaining mental retardation is proposed in the work of Ellis (1963). The theory is based on the premise that there are specific deficits in retarded persons' cognitive functioning, and that these deficits can be identified and experimentally isolated. Ellis originally suggested, for example, that short-term memory deficits account for the retarded person's poor performance on certain cognitive tasks. Zeamon and House (1963) concluded that retarded persons fail to attend to relevant stimulus dimensions in discrimination learning.

The deficit theory has also guided recent research attempts to identify and manipulate differences in information processing strategies between retarded and normal subjects (Bray, 1979).

Developmental Theory

The developmental theory (Zigler, 1967) states that individuals who are at the same cognitive levels perform the same on cognitive tasks. Developmental theorists downplay the notion that retarded persons have deficits in cognitive functioning, but suggest that cognitive functioning is the same on both groups. There has been some lively debate in the literature between deficit and development proponents.

Also central to the developmental position is the Piagetian notion that development proceeds in an invariant sequence, with all children proceeding through stages in a similar order, but at a different rate. Developmental theorists frequently site Piagetian lines of research in support of their position.

Baumeister (1984) has asserted that a principle distinction between deficit and developmental theories is the way they view IQ. For the developmentalists, IQ is a measure of the rate of cognitive development, while for the deficit theorists, differences in IQ reflect both rate and process.

Baumeister (1984) has also pointed out that developmental theories have excluded mentally retarded individuals with organic brain damage from their conceptualizations, and he chided them for: 1) believing that two different theories of mental retardation are required (organic versus nonorganic), and 2) implying that organicity is detectable with any degree of accuracy. It could be argued, of course, that for infants born with identified congenital conditions or certain chromosal disorders, or infants who have birth injuries that cause obvious neurological problems, organicity can be detected with accuracy.

Separate but Equal Theory

A third, more recent, conceptualization of mental retardation is *the separate but equal theory* of Detterman (1987). Like Meeker (1969), who detailed the existence of many types of cognitive skills, Detterman claims that retarded individuals possess a normal range of abilities across many cognitive areas, but are deficient in certain critical areas that are highly valued in society. That is, individuals may be considered to be mentally retarded because they are deficient in certain verbal abstract problem-solving skills that are valued in society, when, in fact, they may be well equipped in skills unrelated to what Neisser (1976) calls *academic intelligence*. It is interesting to note that prevalence figures for mental retardation are highly correlated with ages, increasing each year until age 12 or 13, and declining in a marked fashion after age 15. The prevalence figure thus suggests that the 6-hour retarded person (thus described since the child functions adequately except in academically related activities at school) does, in fact, exist. Individuals may lack certain verbal abstract skills that make succeeding in school problematic for them, but a lack of these skills does not prevent them from living fruitful lives when they leave educational settings.

STERNBERG'S TYPES OF INTELLIGENCE

Sternberg (1984) proposed a theoretical foundation for understanding cognitive abilities in all people that shows great promise for explaining observed differences in cognitive skills between retarded and normal individuals. He suggests that several large-scale information processing components make up human intelligence. These include a *general factor* that generally cuts across all cognitive areas, an *academic intelligence* that has been discussed earlier (an area where retarded persons have particular difficulty), and a factor called *practical intelligence* that corresponds to what others have called social intelligence or fluid intelligence. A final factor, *crystallized intelligence,* comprises abstract thinking and reasoning skills. Thus, intelligence is composed of the sum of all experiences that an individual has accumulated that can be used in problem-solving tasks. Sternberg also sees a motivational component in intelligence, an attribute largely ignored by theorists, but certainly an important contributor to performance of cognitive tasks.

The inner relationships among the principle components have been conceptualized by Sternberg (1984) in Figure 11.1.

Sternberg has further added to the understanding of cognition by identifying metacomponents that are used for planning and decisionmaking. He has identified six problem-solving areas that include:

1. Identifying the problem (For the retarded person, knowing the problem to be solved presents difficulties.)

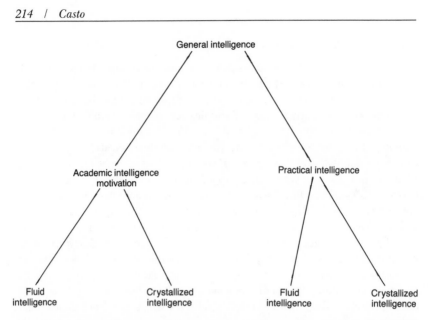

Figure 11.1. Relationships among macrocomponents of intelligence (From Sternberg, R. J. [1984]. Macrocomponents and microcomponents of intelligence: Some proposed loci of mental retardation. In P. H. Brooks, R. Sperber, & C. McCauley [Eds.], *Learning and cognition in the mentally retarded.* Hillsdale, NJ: Lawrence Erlbaum Associates; reprinted by permission.)

2. Selecting lower-order learning strategies
3. Selecting the proper representatives or organizers
4. Selecting a strategy for combining components
5. Making decisions about the amount of time to spend on subtasks
6. Monitoring progress toward problem solution

In addition to the higher order planning and executive components, Sternberg identifies the mental processes that are used in information processing, including: 1) encoding, combining, and comparing of stimulus elements; and 2) selecting and emitting a response. Retarded persons have difficulty with all of these problem-solving tasks.

The final element in Sternberg's view of information processing relates to how individuals acquire (learn in the first place) and retain or remember information, and how information learned by an individual in one setting may be transferred for use in other problem-solving activities.

Brown and Campione (1977) are two of the pioneer investigators in the training of acquisition, retention, and transfer components. Like Sternberg, they also see the necessity of training individuals in basic problem-solving functions, a sort of *learning how to learn approach* (Wight & Casto, 1979).

In summary, Sternberg has made an important contribution to the understanding of cognitive development in retarded persons, and his model suggests questions for future research.

COGNITION RELATED TO GENERAL DEVELOPMENT

The relationship between the development of cognitive skills and the development across other domains has also intrigued researchers. Infant IQ tests, for example, contain items that heavily tap motor, language, self-help, and social/emotional areas as part of assessment of cognitive functioning. Similarly, infant curriculum developers have shown a tendency to blur distinctions between the domains as if they are substantially interrelated. If one examines curriculum objectives across various types of intervention programs, what seems to be a cognitive objective in one program may well be a language objective in another program. It does seem true that progress in each developmental domain is highly influenced by occurrences in other domains. Indeed, especially for infants, it may be difficult to separate skills into the various developmental domains frequently seen in older children. Sroufe and Waters (1977) found that the development of self-esteem and secure attachment (social/emotional domain) are associated with better problem-solving strategies (cognitive domain). This interrelationship suggests that when cognitive development is examined, there must also be concern with other developmental domains. Development proceeds as part of a co-adapted set of reciprocal influences across developmental domains.

COGNITIVE DEVELOPMENT IN HANDICAPPED CHILDREN

The course of cognitive development in handicapped children can be viewed from many different perspectives. In this chapter, the focus is on the perspectives of Jean Piaget and Benjamin Bloom.

As described earlier, Piaget claims that development proceeds through invariant stages, with development in each stage building on the skills acquired in a previous stage. Piaget has described the stages of cognitive development, while Bloom has compiled a taxonomy of educational objectives to guide instruction. Both individuals have had a tremendous effect on the conceptualization of cognitive development.

Uzgirus and Hunt (1975) have developed an ordinal scale for assessing cognitive development that is based on Piaget's theory. Basically, they broke the stages of Piagetian development into steps that could be observed and assessed. This enables the determination of an infant's position on a developmental trajectory and perhaps suggests the type of instructional programming that could be provided.

Bloom, however, identified the cognitive objectives (as well as other objectives), that were written in the form of educational objectives. Bloom, in fact, has heavily influenced the development of curriculum programs designed to accelerate cognitive development. An example of cognitive objectives found in an intervention program derived from principles of Bloom's taxonomy and from the developmental milestone literature (Casto, 1979) are presented in Figure 11.2.

STIMULATING COGNITIVE DEVELOPMENT

To stimulate cognitive development in handicapped infants and young children, a variety of approaches have been used. A few of these approaches are described in the following paragraphs.

Fuerstein (1980) has described *cognitive functioning* as being composed of process variables that are compounds of native ability, attitudes, work habits, learning history, motive, and strategies (Haywood, 1979). Fuerstein has further identified cognitive functions that may be deficient in individuals by virtue of their educational experiences or social class backgrounds. Table 11.1, which is adapted from Arbitman-Smith, Haywood, and Bransford (1984) provides examples.

0 - 6 Months

___ YES	___ NO	1 - THE CHILD ATTENDS TO SOUNDS
___ YES	___ NO	2 - THE CHILD MOVES HIS EYES ACROSS THE MIDLINE
___ YES	___ NO	3 - THE CHILD LOOKS AT HIS HANDS FOR 3 SECONDS
___ YES	___ NO	4 - THE CHILD GRASPS A TOY WHEN TOUCHED ON FINGERS
___ YES	___ NO	5 - THE CHILD BRINGS HIS HANDS TO HIS MOUTH
___ YES	___ NO	6 - THE CHILD SWATS AT A DANGLING OBJECT
___ YES	___ NO	7 - THE CHILD EXPLORES TOYS BY MOUTHING THEM
___ YES	___ NO	8 - THE CHILD REACHES FOR AN OBJECT
___ YES	___ NO	9 - THE CHILD MAKES EYE CONTACT WITH SPEAKER

7 - 12 Months

___ YES	___ NO	10 - THE CHILD TRANSFERS A BLOCK FROM ONE HAND TO THE OTHER
___ YES	___ NO	11 - THE CHILD REMOVES A CLOTH PLACED ON HIS FACE
___ YES	___ NO	12 - THE CHILD LOOKS IN THE DIRECTION OF A DROPPED OBJECT
___ YES	___ NO	13 - THE CHILD IMITATES A SIMPLE MOTOR RESPONSE (PLAYS PEEK-A-BOO)
___ YES	___ NO	14 - THE CHILD MOVES ONE OBJECT TO OBTAIN ANOTHER OBJECT
___ YES	___ NO	15 - THE CHILD IMITATES ACTIONS HE SEES OTHERS DO
___ YES	___ NO	16 - THE CHILD FINDS AN OBJECT WHICH HAS BEEN REMOVED FROM HIS SIGHT
___ YES	___ NO	17 - THE CHILD PUTS A SMALL BLOCK INTO A CUP
___ YES	___ NO	18 - THE CHILD DUMPS A BLOCK FROM A CUP

13 - 18 Months

___ YES	___ NO	19 - THE CHILD REMOVES 3 PEGS FROM A PEGBOARD
___ YES	___ NO	20 - THE CHILD GIVES FAMILIAR OBJECTS TO THE TEACHER
___ YES	___ NO	21 - THE CHILD PLACES 2 PIECES IN A PUZZLE
___ YES	___ NO	22 - THE CHILD POINTS TO FAMILIAR PEOPLE/OBJECTS
___ YES	___ NO	23 - THE CHILD USES ONE OBJECT TO OBTAIN ANOTHER ONE
___ YES	___ NO	24 - THE CHILD BUILDS A TOWER OF 3 BLOCKS
___ YES	___ NO	25 - THE CHILD IMITATES BODY ACTIONS ON A DOLL
___ YES	___ NO	26 - THE CHILD MATCHES LIKE OBJECTS
___ YES	___ NO	27 - THE CHILD POINTS TO FAMILIAR OBJECTS (IN A BOOK/ON CARDS)

19 - 24 Months

___ YES	___ NO	28 - THE CHILD PLACES 5 PEGS IN A PEGBOARD
___ YES	___ NO	29 - THE CHILD IMITATES SIMPLE MOTOR AND LANGUAGE MODELS
___ YES	___ NO	30 - THE CHILD TURNS PAGES IN A BOOK ONE AT A TIME
___ YES	___ NO	31 - THE CHILD STACKS RINGS ON A PEG IN ORDER
___ YES	___ NO	32 - THE CHILD FINDS A HIDDEN OBJECT

(continued)

Figure 11.2. (*continued*)

___ YES ___ NO 33 - THE CHILD USES AN ALTERNATE ROUTE TO REACH AN OBJECT
___ YES ___ NO 34 - THE CHILD TOUCHES SEVERAL ARTICLES OF CLOTHING
___ YES ___ NO 35 - THE CHILD NAMES FAMILIAR PICTURES (IN A BOOK/ON CARDS)
___ YES ___ NO 36 - THE CHILD MATCHES SIMPLE SOUNDS WITH PICTURES

25 - 30 Months

___ YES ___ NO 37 - THE CHILD MATCHES OBJECTS BY COLOR
___ YES ___ NO 38 - THE CHILD PUSHES AND PULLS OBJECTS
___ YES ___ NO 39 - THE CHILD IMITATES ACTIONS FROM MEMORY
___ YES ___ NO 40 - THE CHILD MATCHES OBJECTS BY SHAPE
___ YES ___ NO 41 - THE CHILD FOLDS PAPER IN IMITATION
___ YES ___ NO 42 - THE CHILD OBEYS A TWO-PART COMMAND
___ YES ___ NO 43 - THE CHILD DEMONSTRATES THE CONCEPT OF ONE
___ YES ___ NO 44 - THE CHILD INDICATES HIS AGE BY SHOWING CORRECT NUMBER OF FINGERS
___ YES ___ NO 45 - THE CHILD MATCHES OBJECTS BY SIZE

31 - 36 Months

___ YES ___ NO 46 - THE CHILD POINTS TO ONE OF THREE OBJECTS THAT DOES NOT BELONG
___ YES ___ NO 47 - THE CHILD DEMONSTRATES THE CONCEPT OF "ONE MORE"
___ YES ___ NO 48 - THE CHILD SORTS OBJECTS BY COLOR
___ YES ___ NO 49 - THE CHILD COUNTS TWO OBJECTS AND STATES HOW MANY THERE ARE
___ YES ___ NO 50 - THE CHILD MATCHES AN OBJECT TO A PICTURE OF THAT OBJECT
___ YES ___ NO 51 - THE CHILD SORTS OBJECTS BY SHAPE
___ YES ___ NO 52 - THE CHILD REPEATS 3 SINGLE DIGITS IN THE SEQUENCE PRESENTED
___ YES ___ NO 53 - THE CHILD DISCRIMINATES BETWEEN WET AND DRY
___ YES ___ NO 54 - THE CHILD SORTS OBJECTS BY SIZE

37 - 48 Months

___ YES ___ NO 55 - THE CHILD FORMS CLAY INTO SIMPLE SHAPES
___ YES ___ NO 56 - THE CHILD IDENTIFIES LOUD AND SOFT SOUNDS
___ YES ___ NO 57 - THE CHILD IDENTIFIES 6 BASIC COLORS
___ YES ___ NO 58 - THE CHILD PUTS TOGETHER TWO PARTS TO MAKE A WHOLE
___ YES ___ NO 59 - THE CHILD GIVES HIS AGE
___ YES ___ NO 60 - THE CHILD IDENTIFIES SHAPES
___ YES ___ NO 61 - THE CHILD DISCRIMINATES BETWEEN SHORT AND LONG
___ YES ___ NO 62 - THE CHILD MATCHES A SEQUENCE OF BLOCKS OR BEADS
___ YES ___ NO 63 - THE CHILD SORTS OBJECTS BY SHAPE AND COLOR
___ YES ___ NO 64 - THE CHILD DISCRIMINATES OBJECTS BY TEXTURE
___ YES ___ NO 65 - THE CHILD NAMES 6 COLORS
___ YES ___ NO 66 - THE CHILD SORTS OBJECTS INTO CATEGORIES
___ YES ___ NO 67 - THE CHILD COUNTS 5 OBJECTS
___ YES ___ NO 68 - THE CHILD NAMES HIS FIRST AND LAST NAME
___ YES ___ NO 69 - THE CHILD NAMES 3 SHAPES
___ YES ___ NO 70 - THE CHILD NAMES ONE OBJECT REMOVED FROM A GROUP OF THREE
___ YES ___ NO 71 - THE CHILD DRAWS THE FACE OF A PERSON

49 - 60 Months

___ YES ___ NO 72 - THE CHILD PUTS A 5-PIECE PUZZLE TOGETHER
___ YES ___ NO 73 - THE CHILD IDENTIFIES HIS FIRST NAME IN PRINT
___ YES ___ NO 74 - THE CHILD IDENTIFIES THE MISSING PART OF A PICTURE
___ YES ___ NO 75 - THE CHILD MATCHES OR IDENTIFIES BASIC SYMBOLS
___ YES ___ NO 76 - THE CHILD IDENTIFIES A PICTURED OBJECT WITH ITS USE
___ YES ___ NO 77 - THE CHILD NAMES 4 OBJECTS FROM MEMORY
___ YES ___ NO 78 - THE CHILD PUTS 3 PICTURES IN SEQUENCE TO TELL A STORY
___ YES ___ NO 79 - THE CHILD DISCRIMINATES FIRST, MIDDLE, AND LAST
___ YES ___ NO 80 - THE CHILD DISCRIMINATES BETWEEN "MORE" AND "LESS"
___ YES ___ NO 81 - THE CHILD IDENTIFIES AND TELLS THE USE OF COMMON OBJECTS
___ YES ___ NO 82 - THE CHILD GIVES HIS ADDRESS
___ YES ___ NO 83 - THE CHILD DISCRIMINATES BETWEEN "FARTHER" AND "CLOSER"
___ YES ___ NO 84 - THE CHILD POINTS TO A PENNY, NICKEL, DIME, QUARTER
___ YES ___ NO 85 - THE CHILD GIVES HIS TELEPHONE NUMBER
___ YES ___ NO 86 - THE CHILD DISCRIMINATES BETWEEN FASTER-MOVING AND SLOWER-MOVING
              OBJECTS
___ YES ___ NO 87 - THE CHILD COMPLETES ANALOGIES
___ YES ___ NO 88 - THE CHILD DISCRIMINATES MORNING, AFTERNOON, AND NIGHT ACTIVITIES
___ YES ___ NO 89 - THE CHILD LOCATES RIGHT AND LEFT
___ YES ___ NO 90 - THE CHILD DRAWS A STICK FIGURE OF A PERSON

Figure 11.2. Preacademic objectives.

Table 11.1. Examples of deficient cognitive functions

Input:
— Unplanned, impulsive, and unsystematic exploratory behavior
— Lack of, or impaired, spatial orientation, including the lack of stable systems of reference that impairs the organization of space
— Lack of, or impaired, temporal orientation

Elaboration:
— Inability to select relevant, as opposed to irrelevant, cues in defining a problem
— Lack of orientation toward the need for logical evidence as an interactional modality with one's objectal and social environment
— Lack of, or restricted, inferential-hypothetical thinking
— Lack of, or impaired, planning behavior

Output:
— Trial and error responses
— Lack of, or impaired, verbal tools for communicating adequately elaborated responses
— Lack of, or impaired, need for precision and accuracy in communicating one's responses

Fuerstein has developed a set of instructional procedures designed to modify deficient cognitive functions and to enhance the development of a set of critical cognitive functions. Although these procedures have been utilized more extensively with school-age children, they have important implications for early intervention.

What Fuerstein accomplishes through a set of curriculum guides is to teach a set of problem-solving or cognitive skills. First, individuals are taught problem definition and the use of strategies. Problem definition involves being able to identify relevant cues as opposed to irrelevant ones in defining a problem. Fuerstein asked students to verbally define the task when given a problem, then to justify their definition. By doing this, the students learn to separate essential elements from nonessential ones. Next, they evaluate the strategies that they use, and are instructed in meta-cognitive or executive strategies. They are also asked to identify the executive functions used as an aid to remembering these strategies and keeping them in their repertoire. Then, basic concepts of cognitive problem-solving are introduced as strategies that can generalize to other problem-solving efforts. Finally, some generalization training is provided so that students are able to utilize problem-solving principles in other environments, with other problems. What Fuerstein is actually teaching may be the set of cognitive strategies that Sternberg calls meta-components.

If one were to use the Fuerstein approach to stimulating cognitive development, the first task would be to identify the important learning-how-to-learn strategies that infants would need to master their environment, and then to teach them these strategies. Unfortunately, the identification of these strategies for infants is still a task for the future.

PRESENT TECHNIQUES

The present techniques for stimulating cognitive development in handicapped infants and toddlers are based upon a variety of major premises. Peterson (1987, pp. 4–5) has identified eight major premises to be considered:

1. During the early years, the initial patterns of learning and behavior that set the pace for and influence the nature of all subsequent development are established.
2. Research suggests the presence of certain critical periods, particularly during the early years, when a child is most susceptible and responsive to learning.
3. Intelligence and other human capacities are not fixed at birth, but, rather, are shaped to some extent by environmental influences and through learning.
4. Handicapping conditions and other factors that render a child at-risk for developmental disabilities can interfere with development and learning so that the original disabilities become more severe and secondary handicaps will appear.
5. A child's environment and early experience, particularly the degree to which these are nurturing or depriving, have a major effect upon development and learning; both greatly influence the degree to which a child reaches his or her full potential.
6. Early intervention programs can make a significant difference in the developmental status of young children and can do so more rapidly than later remedial efforts after a child has entered elementary school.
7. Parents need special assistance in establishing constructive patterns of parenting with a young handicapped or at-risk child and in providing adequate care, stimulation, and training for their child during the critical early years when basic developmental skills should be acquired.
8. Early intervention implies some economic-social benefits in that prevention or early treatment of developmental problems in young children may reduce more serious, burdensome problems for society to cope with later, including their accompanying costs.

Each premise, in turn, has spawned different intervention approaches or models. The models used have all included cognitive development as one of their key components. A brief discussion of two well-known preschool models follows.

Preschool Models and Cognitive Development

High/Scope Cognitively Oriented Curriculum The *High/Scope Cognitively Oriented Curriculum Model* is based on certain Piagetian principles. The educational emphasis in the program is to develop children's thinking skills

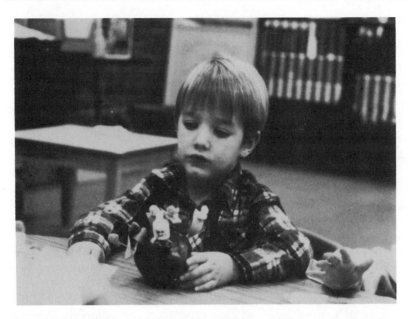

along with subject matter competencies. Children are given active experience through experimentation, exploration, and talking about their experiences. The instructional process encourages thinking and learning.

The classroom environment is designed to encourage children to make decisions, express opinions, work cooperatively with others, and exercise self-discipline. The teacher is seen as a facilitator and catalyst for children's learning.

The High/Scope model has produced impressive evidence of success using a true experimental design. Long-term follow-up of the program has corroborated its beneficial effects.

Engleman/Becker Model for Direct Instruction Operating from a different premise is the *Engleman/Becker Model for Direct Instruction* (DISTAR) that holds that disadvantaged and handicapped learners are slower than their peers, and in order to catch up, they must learn *basic skills* at a faster rate. Basic skills are task analyzed and presented via structured, carefully sequenced lessons.

The classroom environment is structured to provide small group sessions involving face-to-face, fast-paced drills between teacher and children. Children are required to remain on task and respond verbally in rapid-fire sequences. The teacher's role is to present programmed learning taks using preplanned and pretested materials.

The evidence of the effectiveness of this approach is impressive also, although no long-term effects are available. When High/Scope models and DISTAR models have been compared directly, the results have been inconclusive.

A variety of approaches ranging from waterbed stimulation in neonatal intensive care units, to attempts to stimulate cognitive development by improving parent/infant interaction, have been used to stimulate the cognitive development of infants. Infant stimulation programs have produced varying results. Bromwich and Parmalee (1979) devised a home-based stimulation program but only modest results were observed. More impressive scores were recorded for Field, et al. (1980), who combined home visits and parent training. Barrera, Rosenbaum, and Cunningham (1986) promoted parent/infant interaction and achieved modest results.

Several cognitive curriculum packages or approaches have been developed based on different conceptual frameworks. A list of these is presented in Table 11.2.

Table 11.2. Early intervention programs emphasizing cognitive development

Project name and location	Types of handicaps	Program component
Cognitive Early Education Project Carl Haywood Vanderbilt University Nashville, TN 37203	Mixed handicaps, ages 3–6	Seven curriculum units to enhance the development of specific cognition processes
Down Syndrome Project Rebecca Fewell, Director University of Washington Seattle, WA 98195	Down syndrome, ages 0–6	Cognitive curriculum
ERIN Project Peter & Marion Hainsworth 376 Bridge Street Dedham, MA 02026	Mild to severe mixed handicaps, ages 2–7	Academic readiness curriculum
High/Scope David Weikart High/Scope Educational Research Foundation Ypsilanti, MI 48197	Preschool, all abilities; ages 4–6	Cognitively oriented curriculum
MAPPS Project Glendon Casto, Director Utah State University Logan, UT 84322–6580	Mixed handicaps, ages 0–5	Preacademic curriculum
Portage Project George Jesien, Outreachages 626 East Slifer Street Portage, WI 53901	Mixed handicaps, ages 0–6	Preacademic curriculum
Rutland Center Project Karen R. Davis, Director 125 Minor Street Athens, GA 30606	Disturbed and autistic, ages 2–8	Behavior/socialization/ Preacademic curriculum

SUMMARY

Regardless of theories, models, and descriptions of cognitive development as seen in infants and young children, there is one major consideration that must be kept in mind. All cognitive development is based not only on inborn characteristic and potential, but also on the extent and quality of the experiences in infancy. Learning from experiences such as looking and listening is necessary in order for any child to take advantage of environmental events. Other learning experiences include mouthing, touching, and moving toward interesting objects. Piaget's observation of infants and young children, although much more detailed than that of most careproviders, describes the child's sensorimotor participation with people and objects that are familiar to the young child in his or her everyday life. For handicapped children to have these self-exploratory experiences, goals must be carefully selected (see Chapter 8), self-care routines must allow time for exploration (see Chapter 13), language activities must be supportive (see Chapter 9), and ample opportunity for motor experiences needs to be supplied (see Chapter 10).

STUDY QUESTIONS

1. Play "peek-a-boo" with a nonhandicapped infant and then with an infant who has a cognitive delay, both of the same chronological age. Compare and contrast the interaction.

2. Examine the items on the cognitive section of the Battelle Developmental Inventory. Try administrating them to some children.

3. Obtain parental permission and observe a cognitive assessment of an infant or young child.

4. Obtain parental permission and observe the interaction between a child with a cognitive deficit and a nonhandicapped child.

REFERENCES

Arbitman-Smith, R., Haywood, H. C., & Bransford, J. (1984). Assessing cognitive change. In P. H. Brooks, R. Sperber, & J. McCauley (Eds.), *Learning and cognition in the mentally retarded* (pp. 433–473). Hillsdale, NJ: Lawrence Erlbaum Associates.

Barrera, M. E., Rosenbaum, P. L., & Cunningham, C. E. (1986). Early home intervention with low birth weight infants and their parents. *Child Development, 57,* 20–33.

Baumeister, A. (1984). Some methodological and conceptual issues in the study of cognitive processes with retarded people. In P. H. Brooks, R. Sperber, & J. McCauley (Eds.), *Learning and cognition in the mentally retarded* (pp. 1–38). Hillsdale, NJ: Lawrence Erlbaum Associates.

Bray, N. W. (1979). Strategy production in the retarded. In N. R. Ellis (Ed.), *Handbook of mental deficiency, psychological theory, and research* (pp. 699–726). New York: McGraw-Hill.

Bromwich, R., & Parmalee, A. H. (1979). An intervention program for preterm infants. In T. M. Field, A. M. Sostek, S. Gokldberg, & H. H. Shuman (Eds.), *Infants born at risk* (pp. 389–411). Jamaica, NY: Spectrum Publications.

Brown, A. L., & Campione, J. C. (1977). Training strategic study time apportionment in educable retarded children. *Intelligence, 1*, 94–107.

Casto, G. (Ed.). (1979). *An early intervention program for the handicapped child.* New York: Walker & Co.

Detterman, D. (1986). Theoretical notions of intelligence and mental retardation. *American Journal of Mental Deficiency, 92*(1), 2–11.

Ellis, N. R. (1963). The stimulus trace and behavioral inadequacy. In N. R. Ellis (Ed.), *Handbook of mental deficiency, psychological theory, and research* (pp. 134–158). New York: McGraw-Hill.

Field, T. M., Widmayer, S. M., Stringer, S., & Ignatoff, E. (1980). Teenage, lower class, black mothers and their preterm infants: An intervention and developmental follow-up. *Child Development, 51*, 426–436.

Flavell, J. (1963). *The developmental psychology of Jean Piaget.* New York: Van-Nostrand Reinhold.

Fuerstein, R. (1980). *Instrumental enrichment: An intervention program for cognitive modifiability.* Baltimore: University Park Press.

Haywood, H. C. (1979). What happened to mild and moderate mental retardation? *American Journal of Mental Deficiency, 83*, 429–431.

Meeker, M. N. (1969). *The structure of intellect.* Columbus, OH: Charles E. Merrill.

Neisser, U. (1976). General, academic and artificial intelligence. In L. B. Resnick (Ed.), *The nature of intelligence* (pp. 118–130). Hillsdale, NJ: Lawrence Erlbaum Associates.

Peterson, N. (1987). *Early intervention for handicapped and at-risk children.* Denver: Love Publishing.

Sroufe, L. A., & Waters, E. (1977). Attachment as an organizational construct. *Child Development, 48*, 1194–1199.

Sternberg, R. J. (1984). Macrocomponents and microcomponents of intelligence: Some proposed loci of mental retardation. In P. H. Brooks, R. Sperber, & C. McCauley (Eds.), *Learning and cognition in the mentally retarded* (pp. 89–114). Hillsdale, NJ: Lawrence Erlbaum Associates.

Uzgirus, I., & Hunt, J. (1975). *Assessment in infancy: Ordinal scales of psychological development.* Urbana: University of Illinois Press.

Weisz, J. R., Yates, K. O., & Zigler, E. (1982). Piagetian evidence and the developmental difference controversy. In E. Zigler & D. Balla (Eds.), *Mental retardation: The developmental difference controversy* (pp. 213–276). Hillsdale, NJ: Lawrence Erlbaum Associates.

Wight, A. R., & Casto, G. (1979). *An instrumented self assessment laboratory.* Denver: Center for Research in Education.

Zeamon, D., & House, B. J. (1979). A review of attention theory. In N. R. Ellis (Ed.), *Handbook of mental deficiency, psychological theory, and research* (2nd ed., pp. 63–120). New York: McGraw-Hill.

Zigler, E. (1967). Mental retardation. *Science, 157*, 578–579.

Chapter **12**

Social Skills
in Early Intervention

Carol Tingey

———————— • ————————

Prerequisite to the effective use of all other skills is the ability to get along with others. One of the prime reasons for offering early services to families of handicapped children is to help avoid the isolation and expense of special schools and institutions. Although motor, language, and cognitive skills are useful in social settings, displaying these skills requires a degree of social/ emotional competence. Any child who is not well behaved is unwelcome almost everywhere. The development of adequate social/emotional skills in handicapped infants and children presents a challenge to both parents and professionals.

DEFINITION OF SOCIAL SKILLS

The exact description of social skills varies. Greshan's (1982) definition includes a description of social competence from an earlier definition (Foster & Ritchey, 1979), and identifies social skills as responses that "maximize the probability of producing, maintaining, or enhancing positive effects for the interactor." Greenspan's (1979) definition states that good social skills are those that make it possible to deal effectively with social and interpersonal objects and events. However, Reschly (1981) states that social competence is measured by the adaptive behavior concept and scales. A more simple definition of social skill competence might be "the ability to relate to other people who share the day-to-day activities of life" or enjoyment in being around others (Michaelis, 1979b, pp. 4; Tingey-Michaelis, 1983a). Mothers, grandmothers, and others who are experienced in child care, instinctively know when a child is *acting his age* or acting within the proper level of social skill competence.

In order to adequately plan for the opportunity to develop competent social skills, it is important to know the following:

1. What social and emotional skills are learned by normal children in the first 5 years?
2. What experiences do normal children have that help them learn the skills?
3. What specific procedures help handicapped children learn these skills?

SOCIAL SKILLS LEARNED BY NORMAL CHILDREN

It is important for staff of an early intervention program to be very familiar with social/emotional development of normal infants and children, in order to effectively understand skills and conditions their subjects need to learn. One experienced developmental psychologist who works in early intervention mentioned that her work in private practice with nonhandicapped children is almost identical to the work that she does with infants and children who have Down syndrome (Doret, 1987). Although handicapped infants and children may be ready to learn the skill at an older chronological age and need more learning trials, they need to learn the skills in the same sequence and with roughly the same learning experiences. "The handicapped child is similar to the normal child in many ways, especially in social skill development (Hewett & Forness, 1974).

Social/Emotional Skills of Infancy and Early Childhood

Social/emotional skills, like many others, are developed in a specific sequence from the most basic to the more complicated. In order to determine what skills are needed for handicapped children from infancy to early childhood, it is necessary to know what social/emotional skills normal children learn during that time. The following is a list of such skills:

Attachment to mother and other caregivers
Separation from caregiver for short and then longer times
Playing beside other children (parallel play)
Playing with other children (deciding rules/activities together)
Sharing objects of play or foods with other children
Taking turns in language and other action
Saying "Please" and "Thank you" to others without a reminder
Being quiet when waiting in line or for attention
Taking care of own toys/clothes
Respecting others' things/time
Obeying parents/adults instructions/directions

In addition to the direct skills of social development listed above, normal children also develop social habits to be used everyday. These habits allow others to help meet the child's needs, without totally sacrificing their own needs. Some of these habits include:

Sleeping and resting when tired in a comfortable place, even though it may not be a familiar place

Enduring illness and trips to the dentist and physician without creating a scene

Attending adult activities such as eating out, going to church, family dinners, holiday get-togethers, shopping trips, and picture taking sessions by cooperating with regular sleeping, eating, and playing routines

Attending child activities such as trips to the zoo; birthday parties; preschool; Sunday school class; and swimming, dancing, music, or gymnastic lessons when part of the family routine

Being comfortable with a baby sitter and with independent trips to the grandparents' homes

Wearing clothing appropriate for a specific occasion and changing clothing for various occasions without fussing

Dressing and undressing in private

Avoiding discussion of toilet behaviors in public

Playing safely by staying in own play area and using approved play objects

Enjoying walks, stories, and other activities with a familiar adult

Asking for help with items or activities that a child cannot do by him- or herself

Assisting with household chores

Using a loud voice when playing outside and a quiet one during indoor activities, with only minimal reminders

Assisting with the care of a pet (e.g., feed, walk dog); not squeezing a pet too tight or eating pet food

Performing short songs or games for familiar adults

Being polite to parents' friends and neighbors

During these years, children learn: 1) to have the spotlight alone, 2) to share the spotlight with the parent, 3) to share the spotlight with other children, then 4) to be able to give attention to others in order to receive attention in return. Children learn how to give by first learning the comfort of receiving. During the infancy and early childhood years, the child learns first that he or she is important, then that parents are important, and finally that other children and adults are important. The process of learning to value others begins with learning to value oneself.

Experiences that Develop Social Skills

Social/emotional skills are developed during regular day-to-day life activities of the child. These activities include the regular house work and daily care routines, and rely heavily on the adult/child interaction during such activities (e.g., feeding, dressing, washing, toileting, and play supervision). In addition to accomplishing the *task,* the adult also demonstrates appropriate social interaction during the project. In *freeplay,* children copy adult behavior while playing house, and make up things to do with toys, symbolic objects, or other children who are present. The child *copies* and adapts the mannerisms of significant adults and playmates.

Social/Emotional Skills Learned from the Environment

Although cognitive, sensorial, and motor deficits may exist that cannot be completely remediated, social skill attainment is largely the result of social interaction in the environment. Therefore, the social skills are determined not only by the child's condition, but by the sophistication of the adults who manage the surrounding environment. Emotional disturbance in children is largely due to a poor environment that results in an unhealthy climate for social development.

Young emotionally disturbed and behaviorally disordered children usually exhibit immature, rather than bizarre, behavior. Children labeled *autistic* can be described as lacking in social/emotional development, as well as being unable to understand gestures and the social aspects of communication (Rogers, Herbison, Lewis, Pantone, & Reis, 1986). In other words, the disorder stems from socially immature behavior rather than disordered behavior. Antisocial or socially destructive behaviors, it can be argued, are only exhibited when the individual has had enough experience to understand how disruptive behavior inhibits socially comfortable behaviors for others.

Social role valorization, a more current term for the *normalization principle,* suggests that the way a person is perceived determines how that person is treated and ultimately behaves (Wolfensberger, 1983). Siperstein and Bak (1985) found that normal children could accept mentally retarded schoolmates if negative social behaviors were not present. Benson, Reiss, and Smith (1985) discovered that poor social skills were correlated with psychosocial depression in mentally retarded adults.

SOCIAL SKILLS LEARNED BY HANDICAPPED CHILDREN

Procedures for the Development of Social Skills in Handicapped Children

The task of the adult trainers, whether they be parents or staff of an early intervention program, is to organize all caregiving activities in such a way that the demonstration and practice of socially appropriate interaction is possible. The adults must carefully demonstrate well-mannered behavior, personal caring, and respect during the daily interaction. The exact amount of adult direction needed to facilitate social development varies for each child and setting.

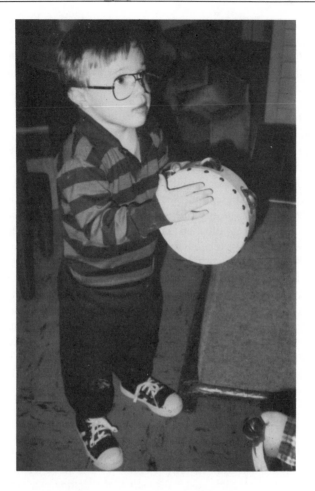

Social/Emotional Skills in Handicapped Children

For social skills to develop, it is necessary for the child to interact with other family members, as well as nonfamily children and adults. Social opportunities that are naturally available to other children are sometimes limited for handicapped children due to their special needs. Frequently, handicapped children require treatment that is delivered in settings where other young children are not present. Not only are the learning opportunities for the handicapped child limited, but, as a result of his or her learning problems, additional efforts and more practice may be needed to acquire these skills. Social/emotional skills are, therefore, doublely difficult to facilitate (see Chapter 7 for details on mainstreaming).

The special services provided to the handicapped child can potentially create a further handicap, the "poor little thing" attitude, by focusing on his or her special needs. Such specialized services can actually cause the child to become more demanding and dependent. Thus, the additional attention from the services themselves could possibly contribute to a delay in development of appropriate socially autonomous skills.

Assessment of Social Skills

Identification procedures to define deficits in infants and young children are unstable and problematic (see Chapter 2), especially in the social development area. Although standardized measures are available and most development scales include a section on social skills, the most important information can be measured on a "wide range of possible dimensions" (Strain & Kohler, 1988), gathered from both parents and others who know the child. However, it is not possible in a formal testing situation to have a sample of the child's interactional pattern in various social situations and with various people (Sexton, Hall, & Thomas, 1984). Most of the formal assessment instruments designed to evaluate social skills attempt to deal with the observational difficulties by including some or many interview questions for the caregiver in regards to the child's typical behavior (Bayley, 1969; Bensberg & Irons, 1986; Newborg, Stock, Wnek, Guidabaldi, & Svincki, 1984). Although these may be most appropriate for intial assessment and referral, direct observation of the child's behavior in an interactional setting is necessary in order to design appropriate individual goals and training procedures (Kohn & Rosman, 1972; Greshan, 1981; Schloss, Schloss, Wood, & Kiehl, 1986).

FORMAL AND INFORMAL INSTRUCTION

Instruction can take place in a planned, formal setting where the teacher and students perform predetermined activities that are measured against specific criteria in order to meet their goals. Teachers in this setting plan activities for students and *grade* the quality of their work on the specific task. Most of what we traditionally know as *school* is designed around this formal teaching and learning setting.

Informal instruction is quite different. Although there may be a *teacher* and a *learner,* there is not a rigid, formal role relationship, and the activity may not be designed to produce prespecified results. In fact, the activity may not be related to the learning that is taking place. For instance, one might *learn* not to be late by going to a party late and finding that all of the cake had been eaten. Or, one might *learn* to take turns because the other children in the group are sharing.

Formal instruction is, of course, the usual format for the school setting where teachers prepare lesson plans and students finish their *work.* Only during such times as field trips or perhaps physical education do the children learn incidently from the ongoing activity, at other times, for the most part, *lessons* are planned with a specific learning goal that needs to be accomplished.

A third term has been coined to include a formal setting with informal teaching. The term *incidental teaching* means that the structure of the learning setting is formal, and that the teacher has a set of goals that need to be learned by the students and plans activities to facilitate those goals. However, the learning activities in this setting are more spontaneous because the teacher alters the activities according to the flow of learning and the input of the students (Hart & Risley, 1975, 1978; Tingey-Michaelis, 1986). Experienced teachers have long used this technique to take advantage of unplanned opportunities (e.g., they have taught about how snowflakes are formed on the first day of snow, and discussed the bones in the arm on the day one student came to school with a broken arm).

Formal methods of teaching are important for academic skills such as reading and writing. Some formal instruction materials have been prepared for social skills training (Karnes, 1987) and direct instruction methods have been designed. However, for most children, social skills are learned in informal settings.

Adaptations of Daily Life Experience

Published curricula for the development of social/emotional skills suggest an interactive teaching setting. Experienced adults can make regular routines a teaching setting by understanding general guidelines and the sequence of development of social skills. In normal children, social skills are learned incidentally by the structure of the activity and the verbal input of the child's caregivers during the activity (Zahavi & Asher, 1978), rather than from a series of mini-lessons on how to behave. Although *mini-lessons* (direct instruction procedures) have been developed for children who have specific social skill deficits, most instructional material prepared for those deficits has been designed to be delivered in as natural a setting as possible. By using the natural setting, there is less the difference between direct instruction and incidental learning for social/emotional development (Michaelis, 1979b).

Teaching-Learning Interaction

Even in formal direct teaching settings, students not only learn what the instructor plans for them, but also what interests them or what they are ready to learn. Infants and young children learn from their primary caregivers not only the content of a *lesson,* but also various social responses (e.g., how an adult says "good morning," whether they look directly at the person they are speaking to, if they really pay attention when someone is talking to them) (Michaelis, 1978). In other words, children learn the pragmatics of social responsiveness by imitating the adults in their world. As social models, significant adults need to know how they appear to the children with whom they work.

Assessment of Teaching-Learning Instruction

Assessment of interactional strategies might begin with a videotape of the adult directing the child or children in a daily routine. The adult then watches and critiques his or her own behavior, noting particularly how much attention was paid to the child's actions. The adult must take special care to not be *directive,* since initiation and imitation are important for young children who are in the learning process. Although there are scales for careful mathmethical analysis of adult/child interaction (Ober, Bentley, & Miller, 1971), it is more important for personal feedback and training that the person get a *feel* for the interaction than to have an analytic score. To help make the process more objective, staff could be assigned to watch the tapes in pairs. The amount of directiveness that each adult naturally uses is determined by their attitudes toward children and sometimes these are difficult to change.

Facilitating Social Interaction Skills in Adult Caregivers

In order to change the interactional patterns in highly directive parents or teachers, it is important to show the adult exactly what is occurring by recording the activity. They can then watch the recording and count the specific behaviors that are exhibited in the interaction and code them (McCollum, 1986). Although most programs do not have the facilities to gather enough samples to be comfortable with the coding, it is important to have some type of self-monitoring procedure in order for the adult to become aware of his or her own behavior. If the adult is trying to be more positive during the interaction, a simple tally of positive and negative behaviors can be kept by marking on a piece of masking tape placed on the inside of the wrist.

SOCIAL SKILLS TAKE TIME

Social behavior cannot be rushed. Central to effective social behavior is providing ample time for each routine. This usually means limiting activities to daily routines. In doing so, the adult may feel that *enrichment* is lacking, but it is not. Children are not old enough to be bored with daily routines yet. To young children, eating, sleeping, dressing, and playing are still vital, exciting, and worth getting up for in the morning (Michaelis, 1979a).

Learning Setting

Social/emotional interaction occurs not only between people, but also in relation to ongoing activities. In addition to changing the behavior of adults to encourage better interaction, it is possible to change the setting where the interaction occurs. Space is important. Studies have determined that crowded laboratory animals' behavior deteriorates over time. The behavior of crowded children takes a similar course. Much of the learning of young children occurs in sensorimotor situations. It is difficult to learn in these situations unless there is ample room for each child to move around with ease. Since much of the social interaction is in relation to dressing, eating, toileting, and washing, space in these areas, in addition to the play areas, must not be cramped.

The setting includes not only the physical space, but the objects in the space. If there is only one attractive toy and three children, learning to share is difficult because there is nothing interesting to do while waiting for a turn. An ample number of similar toys helps children to be free of the strain of limited resources. They are assured of something at least somewhat interesting to do while they are waiting for what they think they really want to do.

Child-to-Child Interaction

One of the serious deficits of young handicapped children is the immature way that they interact with their peers. These interactions are difficult to measure, especially for children who cannot move freely due to sensory or motor impairments (Guralnick & Weinhouse, 1983). Mainstreaming questions revolve around concerns of whether or not the child can develop adequate interpersonal relationships with other children without an opportunity to interact in regular school settings, and whether it is possible to develop enough social skills in segregated settings to be ready to interact effectively in mainstreamed settings. Although there are strong opinions concerning the appropriate setting, little data exist about the impact of segregated and integrated settings.

Regardless of where the mainstreaming occurs, it is obvious that, in order to learn how to relate to other children, the handicapped child must first have extensive contact with nonhandicapped children (see Chapter 7). Unanswered questions concerning how such an interaction could best be accomplished place a tremendous responsibility on the early intervention program to find opportunities for the development of child-to-child skills that occur simultaneously with other developmental and remedial experiences. Handicapped children must be placed in regular settings from time to time and nonhandicapped children must be integrated into segregated settings. All experiences with other children in the family must be maximized. In order for this to happen, parents and families need assistance in understanding social learning at home in much the same way that early intervention staff do.

Although contact is necessary, it alone is not sufficient. Guralnick and Groom (1985) found that the observation of peer-related social interactions of 33 developmentally delayed preschool children showed that for a large part of the playtime, the children were either occupied with solitary play, unoccupied, or were onlookers. The data were collected in a play setting containing only delayed children. Such information indicates that the unstructured freeplay period for delayed children may not automatically give them the needed learning experiences. More active involvement of adults and normal children with handicapped children during that time may be necessary to facilitate development of interactional skills. In an analysis of effectiveness of early intervention, it was found that handicapped children need more structure and direction than nonhandicapped children (Tingey-Michaelis, 1986).

Play Setting

Adults who interact with normal children during playtime usually take a passive, cooperative role. Since most other children are not *cooperative* all of the time, it may be wiser for the adult to act like another child. This can be a difficult and rather unnatural role to play as shown in the following example:

Kallie, a two year old with Down syndrome, has developed a number of socially assertive skills as she interacts with her two triplet nonhandicapped sisters. They early on learned, however, that "Lally" as they called her (long

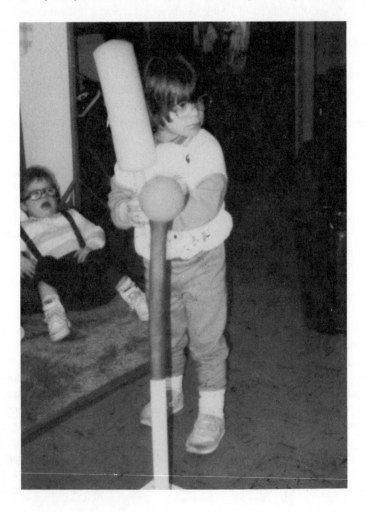

before they called each other by name), needed more assistance with eating, dressing and movement activities and they sometimes "help" mother care for their sister (Tingey, 1987). However, too much "help" can cause dependency.

Creating a more elaborate play setting (Anita, 1985) can provide the child with the opportunity to practice interactional skills in a creative drama-like situation (Warger, 1985). The teacher organizes a situation in which the child participates in playing "house," "school," or "bus," much in the same way that normal children create these experiences for themselves. The child plays the part of people who may be a part of his or her life. These people can be family members or people with whom the child interacts with publicly, such as teachers, doctors, dentists, or bus drivers (Michaelis, 1981). Role playing can be an event structured to be typical of the child's life-like situation (e.g., a birthday party, watching television, serving juice and cookies) (Michaelis, 1979b). Dress-up clothes can be an effective way to create the setting. Be certain that, although the clothes look authentic, they are not oversized for the child. Sometimes, just hats can create the effect without all the weight. Empty cereal boxes and other food packages can make grocery shopping appear more realistic. The adults or other children participate in the role-playing situation with movements and speech that is as natural as possible. However, the adults must make sure that the delayed child has ample time and opportunity to explore various actions and try out speech patterns.

SELF-MANAGEMENT SKILLS

As the child begins to develop comprehension skills, it is possible to help him or her learn self-control or self-management skills (Kelly et al., 1983; Wilson, 1984). Even though young delayed children may be deficient in verbal language skills, receptive language is usually much more developed. Most children can understand directions such as: "wait a minute," "you are doing fine," "it is your turn now," and "remember how we put things away." Through repeated occurrences of appropriate instruction, the child is able to develop self-monitoring skills. In order for this to happen, the adult must be patient enough to continue to give the child input in a calm manner. As soon as the adult becomes impatient, the input ceases to be an appropriate self-management model.

Teaching Appropriate Assertive Behavior

Although social behavior for young children frequently requires compliance with adult wishes, it is not completely submissive. During the preschool years, normal children learn to request repeatedly activities that are pleasurable (e.g., those that provide more food). The development of spontaneous requesting must be encouraged for the severely handicapped (Gobbi, Cipani, Hudson, & Lapenta-Neudeck, 1986). Sometimes, it is more effective when this is done in connection with food; therefore, snacktimes and mealtimes are particularly good times for the development of requesting for *more*. Many children also like movement activities (May, 1977; Tingey-Michaelis, 1983b) and can learn to request that the activities be repeated.

Tracking Social Behavior

The development of sophisticated social skills is a slowly developing process for anyone, and must be measured in fine increments. One of the best ways to track development is to observe frequently and systematically the emerging behavior of a child. Although a formal multiple baseline (Schloss, Schloss, & Harris, 1984) used for research purposes is probably too time consuming for teachers, a simple bridge tally record can show progress in such things as requesting more, taking turns, and saying "thank you" (see Figure 12.1). This kind of information can help show progress, even when it is slow. Fairchild (1987) suggests that a rather formal report card be sent home daily. Adaptations of the report to parents can be seen in the notebook that is sent home with the teacher's message and returned with the child after the parent writes a message. It is then sent back and forth between school and home for continued messages. (Michaelis, 1980) and in other frequent messages from school to home and home to school.

SOCIAL SKILLS IN THE IEP

Although the need for appropriate social skills is well documented in both professional literature and the personal experience of most professionals, the development of social skills as a primary goal of the educational program has not been a priority. Parents and teachers of young and teenage handicapped children still think of education as the development of academic-like skills and seldom realize the importance of social skills (Tingey, 1988).

A study of the IEPs of 40 mildly mentally retarded students (Down syndrome), ages 7 to 11, indicated that basic academics were part of the goal for 37, language for 37, motor for 36, and social skills for only 23 of the children (Weisenfield, 1986). This lack of emphasis on social skills at the elementary-school age is questionable. Lack of emphasis on social skill development in the infant and early childhood years could be disastrous.

For the implementation of the social/emotional skill to be effective, goals must be specific (see Table 12.1). A general desire to learn more socially acceptable behavior is not as effective as "This student will learn to share the blocks with children in the early intervention program and with his or her siblings at home." A specific plan that specifies who does what and when may also be helpful (see Figure 12.2). Social skill development requires continual attention and modeling by both adults and children.

Name if chart used for individual

Dates if chart used for group

Date if used for indiv. Name if used for group — Skill	Degree of Participation	Tally for Role Playing	Tally for Supervised Free Time	Tally for Spontaneous life
A.1 Thank You				
A.2 Please				
A.3 Sorry				
A.4 Excuse Me				
A.5 Knock				
A.6 Ans. Door				
A.7 Telephone				
A.8 Shake Hands				
C.1 Listen				
C.2 Stand in Line				
C.3 Quiet Time				
C.4 Ans. when called				
C.5 Look at speaker				
C.6 Take Turns				
C.7 Share				
C.8 Good-bye				

Figure 12.1. Social skills tally sheet. (Tally key—1 = skill produced; X = skill appropriate but not produced.) (From Michaelis, C. T. [1979b]. *Socialization skills adaptive behavior.* Long Branch, NJ: Kimbo Educational.)

237

Table 12.1. Sample long-term goals

Joe will say "thank you" when someone does something for him or gives him something.
Joe will say "please" when he wants help or to have or use something.
Joe will say he is sorry when he does something that makes someone feel bad or hurt.
Joe will say "excuse me" if he interrupts someone or disturbs him or her.
Joe will knock or otherwise ask before he enters a private or semi-private room.
Joe will answer the door when the bell rings or someone knocks.
Joe will answer the telephone when it rings.
Joe will shake hands when he meets people.
Joe will listen when someone is talking to him or giving instructions.
Joe will stand in line without disturbing others.
Joe will talk quietly and be quiet when the activity suggests it, or when he is asked to do so.
Joe will answer when he is spoken to or called.
Joe will look at the face of the person who is talking to him.
Joe will wait quietly while others are taking their turns.
Joe will share his things with others.
Joe will say "good-bye" when someone leaves.

From Michaelis, C. T. (1979). *Socialization skills.* Long Branch, NJ: Kimbo Educational; reprinted by permission.

INVESTMENT IN SOCIAL/EMOTIONAL SKILLS

Although it is generally known that children's physical development occurs in a predetermined sequence, it is sometimes not as commonly known that healthy social/emotional development also occurs in similar way. Early social/emotional skills are formed through participation in child and caregiver routines; therefore, it would only be possible to observe a lack of social/emotional competence in infants or young children who were severely deprived of care-provider attention and warmth. A child who is not able to relate warmly and naturally to adults and other children lacks not only the prerequisite skills for social/emotional health, but also the interactional skills that are the key to successful contact for other learning. Although transdisciplinary assessment of handicapped children may identify a multitude of skill deficits in the child, the primary need for the handicapped child, as for any child, is the development of the ability to live with and to relate to others in a warm, trusting way. With these skills, the handicapped child has access to a comfortable place in the community. Without these skills, any child is indeed a handicapped child.

SUMMARY

Social/emotional skills are prerequisite to the use of all other skills; therefore, the development of such skills is very important to the handicapped child as

Child name: Joey

Skill to develop: Sharing

Task: Play with blocks with another child

Dated started: 9-10-89   Date completed: 10-10-89

Who assists: Teacher aide—Volunteer

When: Freeplay time

Where: Carpet area of classroom

Materials: 30 multicolored 1-inch blocks

Methods: Children and blocks on floor. Teacher begins building a tower or a train.

Verbal cue: "Help make a tower, Joey."

Desired outcome: Joey hands blocks to other child—puts blocks on same tower.

Evaluation: Teacher observation

Reference: Social skills checklist

Figure 12.2. Specific plan for teaching: IEP summary sheet. (Adapted from Michaelis, C. T. [1980]. *Home and school partnerships in exceptional education.* Rockville, MD: Aspen Systems.)

well as other nonhandicapped children. Understanding which social/emotional skills are learned by nonhandicapped children during the first five years, and what experiences facilitate such learning, is basic to the understanding of how to organize the environment to assist the handicapped child in developing such skills. Procedures for enhancement include: adapting daily life experiences in order to implement informal instruction, and providing ample opportunity for the child to practice interaction with adults and other children. Children have the opportunity to recognize and practice social skills in play settings with both adults and children. The goal of skill development is for the child to gain the ability to manage his or her own behavior. Parents and teachers should include social skills attainment as part of the educational goals. This will ensure that it be an important investment in the child's present and future ability to live and interact with others.

STUDY QUESTIONS

1. Observe children during snack time at a day care center. Describe how children handle food and interaction during that time.

2. Observe children as they play together in the sand or other outdoor play activities. Describe how they relate to one another.

3. Observe an early intervention program as the teacher works with children in a group (circle) activity. Describe how various children relate to the teacher and to each other.

4. Observe and describe how children and parents say "goodbye" and "hello" during early intervention activities.

REFERENCES

Anita, K. F. Li. (1985). Toward more elaborate pretend play. *Mental Retardation, 23*(3), 131–136.

Bayley, N. (1969). *Bayley Scales of Infant Development.* New York: Psychological Corporation.

Bensberg, G. J., & Irons, T. (1986). A comparison of the AAMD Adaptive Behavior Scale and the Vineland Adaptive Behavior Scale within a sample of persons classified as moderately and severely mentally retarded. *Education and Training of the Mentally Retarded, 21*(3), 220–228.

Benson, B. A., Reiss, S., & Smith, D. C. (1985). Psychosocial correlates of depression in mentally retarded adults: II poor social skills. *American Journal of Mental Deficiency, 89*(6), 657–659.

Fairchild, T. N. (1987). The daily report card. *Teaching Exceptional Children, 19*(2), 72–73.

Foster, S. L., & Ritchey, W. L. (1979). Issues in assessment of social competence in children. *Journal of Applied Behavior Analysis, 12,* 625–638.

Gobbi, L., Cipani, E., Hudson, C., & Lapenta-Neudeck, R. (1986). Developing spontaneous requesting among children with severe mental retardation. *Mental Retardation, 24*(6), 357–363.

Greenspan, S. (1979). Social intelligence in the retarded. In N. R. Ellis (Ed.), *Handbook of mental deficiency, psychological theory, and research* (2nd ed., pp. 67–75). Hillsdale, NJ: Lawrence Erlbaum Associates.

Greshan, F. M. (1981). Assessment of children's social skills. *Journal of School Psychology, 9*(2), 120–133.

Greshan, F. M. (1982). Misguided mainstreaming: The case for social skills training with handicapped children. *Exceptional Children, 48*(5), 422–433.

Guralnick, M. J., & Groom, J. M. (1985). Correlates of peer-related social competence of developmentally delayed preschool children. *American Journal of Mental Deficiency, 90*(2), 140–150.

Guralnick, M. J., & Weinhouse, E. (1983). Child-child social interaction: An analysis of assessment instruments for young children. *Exceptional Children, 50*(3), 268–271.

Hart, B., & Risley, T. R. (1975). Incidental teaching of language in the preschool. *Journal of Applied Behavior Analysis, 8,* 411–420.

Hart, B., & Risley, T. R. (1978). Promoting productive language through incidental teaching. *Education and Urban Society, 10,* 407–429.

Hewett, F. M., & Forness, S. R. (1974). *Education of exceptional learners.* Newton, MA: Allyn & Bacon.

Karnes, M. (1987). *Know me, know you.* Allen, TX: DLM Teaching Resources.

Kelly, W. J., Salzberg, C. L., Levy, S. M., Warrenteltz, R. B., Adams, T. W., Crouse, T. R., & Beegle, G. P. (1983). The effects of role playing and self monitoring on the generalization of vocational social skills by behaviorally disordered adolescents. *Behavioral Disorders, 9*(1), 27–35.

Kohn, M., & Rosman, B. L. (1972). A social competence scale and symptom checklist for the preschool child. *Developmental Psychology, 6*(2), 430–444.

May, B. (1977). *Tickle snug kiss hug.* New York: Paulist Press.

McCollum, J. (1986). Charting different types of social interaction objectives in parent-infant dyads. *Journal of the Division of Early Childhood, 11*(1), 28–45.

Michaelis, C. T. (1978). Communication with the severely handicapped: A psycholinguistic approach. *Mental Retardation, 16*(5), 346–349.

Michaelis, C. T. (1979a). *Self care skills.* Long Branch, NJ: Kimbo Educational.

Michaelis, C. T. (1979b). *Socialization skills adaptive behavior.* Long Branch, NJ: Kimbo Educational.

Michaelis, C. T. (1980). *Home and school partnerships in exceptional education.* Rockville, MD: Aspen Systems.

Michaelis, C. T. (1981). *Housekeeping tasks.* Long Branch, NJ: Kimbo Educational.

Newborg, J., Stock, J. R., Wnek, L., Guidabaldi, J., & Svincki, J. (1984). *Battelle Developmental Inventory.* Allen, TX: DLM Teaching Resources.

Ober, R. L., Bentley, E. L., & Miller, E. (1971). *Systematic observation of teaching.* Englewood Cliffs, NJ: Prentice-Hall.

Odom, S. L., & Karnes, M. B. (1988). *Early intervention for infants & children with handicaps: An empirical base.* Baltimore: Paul H. Brookes Publishing Co.

Reschly, D. J. (1981). Assessing mild mental retardation: The influence of adaptive behavior, sociocultural status, and prospects for nonbiased assessment. In C. Reynolds & T. Gutkin (Eds.). *The handbook of school psychology* (pp. 132–147). New York: John Wiley & Sons.

Rogers, S. J., Herbison, J. M., Lewis, H. C., Pantone, J., & Reis, K. (1986). An approach to enhancing the symbolic communicative and interpersonal functioning of young children with autism or severe emotional handicaps. *Journal of the Division of Early Childhood, 10*(2), 135–145.

Schloss, P. J., Schloss, C. N., & Harris, L. (1984). A multiple baseline analysis of an interpersonal skills training program for depressed youth. *Behavioral Disorders, 9*(3), 182–188.

Schloss, P. J., Schloss, C. N., Wood, C. E., & Kiehl, W. S. (1986). A critical review of social skills research with behaviorally disordered students. *Behavioral Disorders, 12*(1), 1–14.

Sexton, D., Hall, J., & Thomas, P. J. (1984). Multisource assessment of young handicapped children: A comparison. *Exceptional Children, 50*(6), 556–558.

Siperstein, G. N., & Bak, J. J. (1985). Effects of social behavior on children's attitudes toward their mildly and moderately mentally retarded peers. *American Journal of Mental Deficiency, 90*(3), 319–327.

Strain, P. S., & Kohler, F. W. (1988). Social skill intervention with young children with handicaps: Some new conceptualizations and directions. In S. L. Odom & M. B. Karnes (Eds.), *Early intervention for infants & children with handicaps: An empirical base* (pp. 129–143). Baltimore: Paul H. Brookes Publishing Co.

Tingey, C. (1988). Cutting the umbilical cord: Parental perspectives. In S. Pueschel (Ed.), *The young person with Down syndrome: Transition from adolescence to adulthood* (pp. 5–22). Baltimore: Paul H. Brookes Publishing Co.

Tingey, C. (1987). Developmental study of triplets one of whom has Down syndrome. (Proposal sent to national Institute of handicapped Research) Logan: Developmental Center for Handicapped Persons, Utah State University.

Tingey-Michaelis, C. (1983a). *Handicapped infants and children handbook for parents and professionals.* Austin, TX: PRO-ED.

Tingey-Michaelis, C. (1983b). Make room for movement. *Early years, 13*(6), 26–29.

Tingey-Michaelis, C. (1986). The importance of structure in early education programs for disadvantaged and handicapped children. *Early Child Development and Care, 23*(10), 283–297.

Warger, C. L. (1985). Making creative drama accessible to handicapped children. *Teaching Exceptional Children, 17*(4), 288–293.

Weisenfield, R. B. (1986). The IEP's of Down syndrome children: A content analysis. *Education & Training of the Mentally Retarded, 21*(3), 211–219.

Wilson, R. (1984). A review of self control treatments for aggressive behavior. *Behavioral Disorders, 9*(2), 131–140.

Wolfensberger, W. (1983). Social role valorization: A proposed new turn for the principle of normalization. *Mental Retardation, 21*(6), 234–239.

Zahavi, S., & Asher, S. R. (1978). The effect of verbal instructions on preschool children's aggressive behavior. *Journal of School Psychology, 16*(2), 146–153.

Chapter **13**

Self-Care Skills

Adrienne L. Peterson and Kathryn Haring

————————— ● —————————

The development of self-care skills is an area of critical importance to serviceproviders and family members of infants and young children who are delayed or at-risk for delays. The ability to care for one's basic needs is a prerequisite for independent functioning. Teachers and parents of young children who are handicapped are primarily concerned with developing skills in the areas of eating, dressing, and toileting. Skill areas of secondary concern are washing and grooming (Lance & Koch, 1973).

THE DEVELOPMENT OF SELF-CARE SKILLS

The process of human development is frequently divided into several general categories including cognitive skills, communication skills, personal-social skills, motor skills, and self-care skills. For the sake of convenience, these areas are frequently dealt with as separate entities when attempting to describe them in detail. However, the use of the systems theory model provides a method of visualizing child development as a more unified, interactive process.

More than any of the other general areas of child development, the acquisition of specific self-care skills is culturally bound. All children normally learn to sit, walk, and then run; or, first babble, then speak in single utterances, and later form meaningful sentences. However, learning to feed oneself could have several different end products, such as learning to use conventional silverware, chopsticks, or even the fingers themselves. Likewise, types of clothing as well as clothing fasteners are quite simple in certain societies and more complex in others. Even within one society, parents usually expect children to acquire specific motor or language skills at a particular age, but in the area of self-care skills, these tasks and their appropriate ages of acquisition are not as firmly fixed in most parents' minds.

The normal acquisition of self-care skills for a young child is embedded from the start in the context of family expectations. Some parents want their children to gain proficiency in feeding, dressing, or toileting skills, then pride themselves and praise the child for their steps toward independence. Other parents gain satisfaction in helping their child to eat or to dress long after the child actually needs assistance, thereby prolonging the child's physical dependence on the parent.

Learning to do things for themselves, particularly to take care of their bodies, is part of the excitement of the day-to-day experiences of young children. They enjoy doing whatever they see people who are important to them doing (e.g., they imitate daddy shaving, mother putting on lipstick, Uncle Joe drinking a soft drink). Although daily routines change from time to time and from weekdays to weekends, self-care needs are constant and must be performed for the child by careproviders, whether they are the parents, grandparents, nursery school personnel, or other parents in a baby-sitting cooperative.

From the time of birth, the infant is directly involved as a participant rather than as an observer in each of the daily routines. Children do not watch themselves being fed, dressed, washed, and diapered; they learn by going through the motions. They feel the different textures of fabric, as well as the firmness of the grip of the adult. They experience the warmth of the bathwater and the flavor and texture of the applesauce, not just once but time and time again. It is no wonder that a very young infant grabs the bottle, pulls away from a wooly sweater, or cries when his or her nose is wiped.

It is not possible for the parent to do anything to the child without the child knowing it. The child also, to some extent, *gives permission* for the activity by allowing the adult to move the child from the high chair to the potty chair, or from the playroom to the crib. During each of these activities, the child may *cooperate* by going willingly, or *complain* by fussing and/or holding the body stiff.

Adults have learned ways to cajole the child into wanting to perform the next activity by using, for example, pajamas with stars on them, teddy bears that tell bedtime stories, and toothbrushes that have bells in the handle. Many of the toys created for children help them with the playtime goal of pretending to be like adults. Clothes, too, help accomplish this goal. Robes, slippers, T-shirts, small jeans, and ski parkas look almost identical to those worn by older children and adults. Even young children like to "dress up" in daddy's hat or mother's gloves.

The whole process of dressing and undressing for young children is an animated fashion show of "pretendland." Hooks to hang clothes on are shaped like ducks, bears, or even giraffes. The clothes hamper may look like a turtle or a Sesame Street garbage can. The feeding process is a similar one. Children practice feeding and eating skills with pastel-colored bottles, or those shaped like cartoon characters. They learn to use a spoon that has Mickey Mouse on the handle, and wear a bib decorated with the nearest university insignia or a bold print of "Yellowstone Park." The traditional "Tommy Tippy" cup may be blue, yellow, or covered with a bright design. Variety stores are filled with children's dishes that are unbreakable and come in all colors of the rainbow; some have spaces for hot water to keep foods warm while the baby plays with the food. High chairs have colorful decals and bright pads to make them more comfortable. Grocery stores are full of child-sized packages of anything from the traditional animal crackers to pudding, and rows of cereals that not only snap, crackle, and pop but have special prizes located somewhere inside. Baby food sections of the grocery store not only have ordinary things such as rice cereal and Zwieback® toast, but also exotic combinations of chopped, pureed, and cubed foods.

Each family has its own unique needs and preferences for the sequence of teaching self-care skills to their children. The reasons for these variations among families are too numerous to elaborate here, but the point is that even within average families, variety rather than uniformity is the rule for teaching and learning self-care skills.

For our purposes, self-care skills consist of eating skills, dressing skills, grooming skills, and toileting skills. By first discussing the so-called normal patterns of self-care skills, it is then easier to look at the differences and the problems facing infants and children with handicaps.

Eating Skills

Traditionally, the infant has been thought to be completely dependent upon his or her parents for feeding. Although the parent or another adult must be present to provide the breast or bottle, the normal infant is able to root, suck, and then discontinue nursing. Many of these behaviors are partially reflexive, but recent studies indicate that the infant has a greater degree of control than was previously thought. Table 13.1 is a chart of the major self-help skills developed from birth to 5 years of age.

During their first 6 months of life, the infant is able to let parents know when he or she is hungry, learns to open the mouth when the bottle or spoon is presented, and begins to actively move soft foods around in the mouth before swallowing. Tongue and mouth movements are at first less coordinated, gradually becoming more refined. Food preferences are also beginning to be established at this time.

The 6- to 12-month period and the acquisition of a few teeth bring greater variety in the types of food the baby eats as well as in his or her degree of control. The infant is now able to close his or her lips on a spoon to remove the food. He or she also increases head and trunk control, making mealtime a more interactive process, since the baby can now sit up during mealtime rather than be cradled in the parent's arm. In addition, the baby's hands become more involved in the feeding process by picking up small bits of food and placing them

Table 13.1. CAMS self-help developmental chart

Age range	Feeding skills	Dressing skills	Personal hygiene skills	Toileting skills
0–6 months	Closes lips on a nipple. Sucks on a nipple. Opens mouth on approach of a nipple. Brings hand to mouth.		Allows self to be bathed. Allows hair to be washed.	
7–12 months	Closes lips on spoonful of strained food. Moves food around mouth with tongue. Reachs for and holds bottle or breast. Drinks from a glass with help. Eats lumpy or *junior* food. Feeds self with fingers. Chews solid food.	Helps in dressing/un-dressing by holding out arms and legs.	Splashes hands in water. Allows teeth to be brushed.	
12–18 months	Begins to eat with spoon. Holds a glass in both hands and drinks. Feeds self using a spoon.	Pulls off socks.		
19–24 months	Unwraps food.	Takes off coat. Takes off pants. Puts on pants. Takes off and puts on a loose hat. Unzips a zipper. Removes shoe with laces loosened.	Allows nose to be wiped with a tissue.	

(continued)

Table 13.1. *(continued)*

Age range	Feeding skills	Dressing skills	Personal hygiene skills	Toileting skills
25–36 months	Eats with fork in fist. Drinks with a straw. Eats with a fork and spoon held under hand. Sits in a chair throughout a meal.	Loosens the laces and removes shoes. Opens snaps. Takes off a pullover shirt. Puts on coat (floor method). Puts on socks.	Dries face and hands. Washes hands with soap. Wipes nose. Obtains a tissue for use. Throws away the tissue after use. Blows nose with assistance.	Defecates in the potty. Indicates need to defecate. Urinates while on potty. Indicates need to urinate.
37–48 months	Drinks from glass held in one hand. Uses napkin at mealtime. Cleans up own spills. Serves self from a serving bowl. Clears place setting from table after meal. Chews with lips closed. Spreads food with a knife.	Puts on a pullover shirt. Unbuttons large buttons on front of clothing. Buttons large buttons on front of clothing. Hangs clothes on a hook. Puts on shoes with reminders. Folds own clothing. Ties a half-knot on shoelaces. Puts on boots.	Bathes self with assistance. Rinses mouth after having teeth brushed. Dries self with assistance. Brushes teeth with assistance. Washes face.	Stands to urinate in toilet (boys only). Flushes toilet after use. Obtains own toilet paper. Stays dry through night.
49–60 months	Cuts food with a fork. Passes a serving bowl. Helps to set table.	Laces shoes. Distinguishes the front from the back of clothing. Hangs clothes on a hanger in closet.	Keeps nose wiped and blown when reminded. Bathes and dries self. Brushes teeth. Uses toothpaste.	Wipes self with toilet paper. Wipes after urination (girls only).

(continued)

Table 13.1. (continued)

Age range	Feeding skills	Dressing skills	Personal hygiene skills	Toileting skills
		Closes a snap. Zips an open-ended zipper. Puts on coat (adult method). Puts dirty clothing in designated spot.	Combs hair with assistance. Adjusts water temperature.	Uses toilet independently.

into the mouth. Spoon- and cup-banging on high chair trays is a favorite pastime during this period. Many infants want to interact on a more cognitive level in the eating process, but their undeveloped fine motor skills limit it. Consequently, parents of these busy babies quickly learn that by allowing their baby to have a spoon or cup to bang while mother or father spoon feeds them, tends to make mealtime a smoother process.

By 18 months, most babies are able to drink from a cup, finger feed neatly, and use a spoon to eat foods from a bowl. However, family variation is quite apparent at this point. Although infants are capable of the degree of independence described, many toddlers may still be given a bottle because it is easier and not so messy. The same is often true for the baby-using-a-spoon versus parent-spoon-feeding-baby methods. Many parents knowingly or unwittingly continue to help a child with eating skills long after the child is capable of independence.

After 18 months of age, additional eating skills that a child learns are basically refinements of earlier skills. Improved eye-hand coordination and strength contributes largely to the ease with which a child eats and drinks. By 5 years of age, most children have learned to use a fork and knife, drink when holding a glass with one hand, pass a serving bowl, and use some basic table manners.

Dressing Skills

Whereas eating skills begin to develop shortly after birth, the infant's participation in dressing begins quite a bit later. The beginnings of control start to emerge when the infant attempts to make bodily adjustments to make it easier for the adult to put on and remove clothing. Putting a shirt on over an infant's head is much easier when the baby can hold his or her head up steadily. Between 7 and 12 months of age, babies are able to hold out their arms, then legs, when pulling clothes off and on. As stronger patterns of extension of the child's

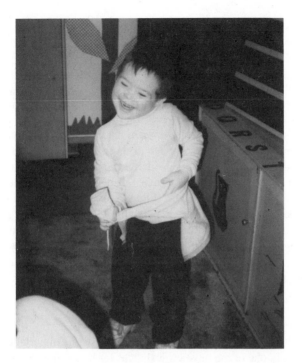

limbs develop, he or she is able to stand upright, walk, and stiffen and push arms and legs into the armholes and pantlegs. The ability to perform independent dressing skills closely parallels a child's gross and fine motor development.

Dressing independence usually follows a "take-it-off-first, put-it-on-later" pattern. Shoes and socks are pulled off somewhere after the first birthday. This may be accomplished in both a sitting position or a back-lying position with feet in the air, depending upon the child, the situation, and on whether the toddler is tired. In conjunction with toileting, pushing down soiled pants usually develops at the end of the second year.

Putting on clothes becomes more skilled during the third year as the child increases his or her need for independence with the "I'd rather do it myself!" attitude. This attitude varies quite a bit from child to child and family to family —some children demand that they are left alone while putting on a shirt and pants, even if they are upside down and backwards, while others melt into the parents arms, waiting for assistance. Patience and constant but gentle nudging are helpful concepts to remember when teaching dressing skills.

Skills that develop later include putting on various types of shirts, coats, and shoes, and then learning to manipulate the fasteners. In western cultures, a variety of closures is the rule (e.g., different buttons, zippers, snaps, ties, and Velcro®). Because of the greater variety of closures, children usually first gain competence with the types of fasteners that they typically have on their clothes.

Toileting Skills

Probably more than any other self-care skills, independence in toileting is prized by both child and parents. Most children are able to accomplish elimination into a potty chair or toilet between 18 and 36 months of age. However, several additional skills are necessary for toileting independence. These skills include going to the bathroom when necessary (and not having an accident), removing clothing, completing the elimination process, careful wiping, redressing, flushing, and hand washing and drying. When viewed this way, it is easy to see how a young child can get sidetracked somewhere along the way.

Although toilet training can be a frequent source of parent/child conflict, parents can apply the same useful rule of thumb for toilet training as for teaching dressing skills—patience and gentle nudging. A child usually acquires toileting independence, as described above, sometime before entry into kindergarten, although it is not unusual for a child to have an embarrassing accident during the first year of school. Suffice it to say that the social acceptability of a self-care mishap is heavily dependent upon the type of accident, that is, an open button or zipper is much less traumatic than soiled pants.

Grooming Skills

Personal grooming, although not at the top of the list of important self-care skills, is probably one of the most critical areas for handicapped children. Although a minor concern in the preschool years, a sloppy, disheveled appearance in later childhood and into adulthood heavily influences the perceptions of peers, teachers, and potential employers (Adams, 1975).

Personal grooming includes both personal cleanliness in regular bathing and hair washing, and neatness throughout the day, especially after eating, toileting, and physically active or messy activities. Very young children are rarely concerned about such things. Indeed, some families pay very little attention to personal grooming. Most children develop an awareness for personal grooming first through reminders by their parents, and later as they become aware of the expectations of their peers. The experience of being taunted because of sloppy or even unstylish hair or clothing is painful for any child.

In summary, the acquisition of self-care skills by preschoolers is a process that begins early in life and continues into adulthood. Parents are wise to use a little forethought when choosing clothing and equipment that encourage a child's independence, whether it be the size of a spoon or cup, a brightly colored potty chair, or Velcro®-fastened shoes.

TEACHING TECHNIQUES FOR HANDICAPPED CHILDREN

It is widely recognized that the use of behavioral procedures is effective in training self-care skills (Bailey & Wolery, 1984). Early research in training of self-care skills evaluated the use of operant conditioning techniques to train these skills (Westling & Minden, 1978). The proponents of the operant conditioning approach consider self-care skills as behavioral chains of varying complexity. This approach is based on the premise that a complex skill can be learned most effectively if the skill is broken down into simple, individual steps. This is commonly referred to as *task analysis*. Task analysis serves as a sequenced breakdown of behavior chains. Used properly, it identifies training steps and can serve as a checklist assessment of baseline skills (Snell, 1978). The following is an example of a task analysis of toileting behavior from Bailey and Wolery (1984):

1. Indicates need to use toilet (if necessary)
2. Moves to bathroom
3. Unfastens pants (if necessary)
4. Pushes pants and underwear down
5. Gets on the toilet
6. Maintains sitting balance on toilet
7. Eliminates urine or feces
8. Reaches and gets toilet tissue
9. Wipes self until clean
10. Disposes of toilet tissue
11. Gets off toilet
12. Flushes toilet
13. Pulls up underwear and pants
14. Washes and dries hands

Operant conditioning techniques generally involve the contingent delivery or withdrawal of reinforcement following the occurrence of targeted behaviors. These techniques also rely on various behavior antecedents used to cue, prompt, and shape desired self-care behaviors. Thirty-six studies of operant training of self-care skills in the areas of self-feeding, personal care behaviors, and a combination of the two were evaluated (Westling & Minden, 1978). The general results indicated that operant training is effective in helping individuals perform independent skills.

Traditionally in special education programs, a *multiple trials* format is utilized to train individuals who are severely and moderately disabled (Gaylord-Ross & Holvoet, 1985). Students are presented with a prespecified number of trials in order to practice a discrete movement or chain of movements. Many curricula developed for use with preschool-age handicapped children are based on a model that uses *massed trial training* or skills taught in isolation (Bricker, Casuso, Pearson, Mendoza, & Praeto, 1977; Mendelsohn, 1978; Shearer et al., 1970; Vincent, Dodd, & Henner, 1978). More recent curriculum models (Fiechtl et al., 1986; Guess et al., 1978; Holvoet, Guess, Mulligan, & Brown, 1980; McGreevy, Lacy, & Calkins, 1984; Rule et al., 1987) have concentrated on arranging tasks in functional sequences using naturally occurring opportunities for teaching self-care skills. In some cases, coincidental teaching sessions are presented (Rule et al., 1987) on occasions when a skill can be naturally applied. For example, dressing skills are taught in conjunction with recess, nap time, or toileting, while food preparation and self-feeding skills can be trained during snack- and mealtimes. Coincidental teaching sessions are short programs that include specified skills in sequence with specific numbers of repetitions and a measurement/recording system. This concept is based on Hart and Risley's (1975) work on incidental teaching (see Chapter 15 for a description of incidental teaching). However, coincidental teaching may be teacher-initiated and is used primarily to enhance the development of self-care skills (see Chapter 15).

There is support in the literature for training skills in the context in which they naturally occur, as opposed to training within a session which is called *multiple trial model* (Bronicki, Holvoet, & Guess, 1981; Neel, Billingsley, & Lambert, 1983; Neel, Billingsley, McCarthy, et al., 1983; Sailor & Guess, 1983).

A small number of studies have emerged that provide empirical evidence supporting the efficacy of total task training, as compared to the multiple trial format (Kayser, Billingsley, & Neel, 1986; Spooner, 1981, 1984; Zane, Walls, & Thvedt, 1981). Further research is clearly needed to support the intrinsically logical notion that self-care skills can be trained with graduated prompting in the natural environment during normally occurring opportunities in the home and the classroom.

One study (McGreevy, Lacy, & Calkins, 1984) compared a massed trial training format, in which 10 trials of a discreet task were taught at one time during one teaching session, with a model that taught clusters of skills in naturally occurring opportunities. The Individualized Curriculum Sequencing Model (ICS) (Guess et al., 1978; Holvoet et al., 1980) is a clustered skills model that focuses on skills that cut across domains. As can be seen in Figure 13.1, a student might be taught to sign for a cracker (communication skill), to crawl to the table (motor skill), and to pick up and eat the cracker (self-care skill) in one sequence. This approach was compared to the mass practice-isolated skill approach of giving a child 10 trials to manually sign for "crackers."

Both the massed trial and the ICS models of training occurred in functional environments, using age-appropriate and functional materials with varying instructional strategies. The results of this study that compared the massed trial and ICS methods indicated no practical or statistically significant differences in the subjects' skill acquisition between the models compared. However, the number of subjects in this study was small (16 parents of severely handicapped children were trained to apply the treatment, fewer completed every level of the study). Limited data available from this study indicated that

Name: Polly   Name of task: Sign for cracker

ANTECEDENT	CORRECT MOVEMENT	CONSEQUENCES
a) place crackers in front of Polly but out of reach b) stand by table and say "come here" c) allow Polly to grasp cracker	a) signs for cracker in count of 5 b) crawls to table in count of 10 c) holds cracker with one hand	Correct: Social praise Incorrect: a) show Polly correct sign b) help Polly crawl to table c) put your hands over her hand and help her pick up cracker

How to count:

+ =   Same as correct movement
- =   a) attempts to make a sign
       b) crawls part of the way
       c) picks up cracker with one hand and drops it
0 =   Does not attempt any movement, refuses, cries

Start Date

	Date													
1. a) Signs for cracker														
b) Crawls to table														
c) Picks up cracker with one hand														
2. a) Signs for cracker														
b) Crawls to table														
c) Picks up cracker with one hand														
3. a) Signs for cracker														
b) Crawls to table														
c) Picks up cracker with one hand														
4. a) Signs for cracker														
b) Crawls to table														
c) Picks up cracker with one hand														
5. a) Signs for cracker														
b) Crawls to table														
c) Picks up cracker with one hand														
Total minutes and seconds														

Figure 13.1. CAMS Self-help Curriculum's information obtaining tally sheet. (Adapted from McGreivy, P., Lacy, L., & Calkins, C.F. [1984].)

parents preferred mass trials of isolated skills, and that skills taught with massed trials were better maintained across new settings. Obviously, the differences between these two types of training require further examination.

The practitioner can conclude much from the literature surrounding the training of self-care skills. Research indicates that operant training, utilizing a task analysis of skills, and teaching in small steps is effective. However, some research indicates that the total task can be taught in an equally efficient manner. The prudent serviceprovider or parent should conclude that each child must be approached as an individual. Many possible models for self-care skills training are available, and all contain the fundamental component of training in a functional and age-appropriate way, which is critical to self-care training.

ADAPTIVE EQUIPMENT FOR CHILDREN WITH HANDICAPS

Feeding Equipment

Difficulties in teaching self-care skills to handicapped preschoolers result from a variety of obstacles such as physical deficits. They can be further influenced by cognitive delays, physical limitations, sensory impairments, and the child's temperament, as well as parental expectations, the physical environment of the house or preschool, and the choice of equipment. The use of appropriate or adaptive equipment can greatly enhance the acquisition of independent self-care skills for delayed individuals. Although adapted equipment has been in

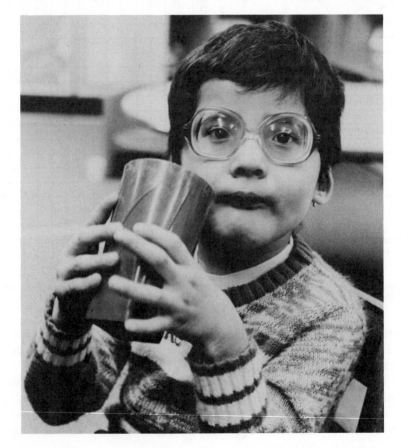

use for many years, an increase in national awareness of the rights of handicapped individuals has promoted the increased development of a wide variety of adaptations and devices. In general, regular equipment should be used and adapted prior to purchasing more expensive, ready-made adaptive equipment. Beginning with feeding skills, certain infants have difficulty using a standard nipple. Several different types are available to assist an infant in achieving better lip closure and suction on the nipple. Even normal infants may prefer using one of the variations of the standard bottle nipples. For at-risk infants and those with known delays, an occupational therapist or other infant specialist can assist a parent in choosing a nipple to assist the baby in nursing more efficiently.

As the infant approaches 1 year of age, self-feeding normally begins to emerge. Hand function is necessary for finger feeding and the use of utensils. Delayed infants may have a weak grip, fisted grip, or no functional grip at all, resulting from a variety of causes. By enlarging a spoon handle with lightweight foam padding and tape, a child is able to grasp the spoon more easily, and therefore, the child's independence is enhanced. The use of a Velcro® strap to hold a spoon in a child's hand aids an infant with poor hand function. Bowls and plates with steeper sides make it easier for a child to scoop. A nonskid surface on a high chair tray stabilizes cups and bowls. More specialized equipment should be acquired only after usefulness of the simpler methods is found to be inadequate.

Clothing

Learning to dress oneself is another area of self-care that can present a multitude of problems for delayed preschoolers, especially those with physical handicaps. Knit fabric is usually easier to take off and put on. Likewise, loose fitting clothes allow greater ease in dressing for both parent and child. The necessity to learn to button, snap, and zip has been lessened with the increased availability of garments with Velcro® closures. Similarly, shoe tying has been simplified since many children's shoes now have Velcro® fasteners. As with many things, however, trade-offs are involved when using adaptations. For example, easier clothing and fasteners should be used to facilitate a child's independence in dressing, but when the appropriate goal for a young child is learning to tie or snap, regular opportunities to learn these skills should be included in a child's program.

Personal Hygiene Equipment

A wide variety of adaptive equipment for personal hygiene is available for older children and adults. If the person's disability greatly interferes with his or her ability to take care of personal appearance and grooming, a large variety of products are available on the market to increase a person's independence in bathing, shaving, and toileting. However, for a young child, simplicity and persistence should be kept in mind.

Bathing Equipment Even if a child is moderately to severely delayed, parents need to begin self-care training by allowing him or her to be bathed and tidied up as they would with any child. Small children with motor delays may cry and be fearful when placed in a tub of water because the lack of physical control increases the child's sense of helplessness. Yet, as most parents realize, many young children may initially be fearful when bathing. Parents, especially those whose first child is delayed, should be reassured and instructed on how to make bathtime easier, as well as how to make it a learning experience for the baby. All too often, parents are embarrassed to admit that bathtime has become difficult, or do not even realize it. Often, for more severely involved children, bathing can be one of the more physically demanding responsibilities for parents. The infant specialist or the home visitor should routinely assess a child's and parents' needs in these areas.

Several simple techniques serve as a starting point for the child's bath before ordering more expensive equipment. A terry cloth hand towel placed on the bottom of the tub serves as a nonskid surface on which the baby is placed. Also available commercially is a contoured foam bath mat on which the baby can be placed. Two inches of water in the tub is sufficient for washing most infants and toddlers. The child can be made to feel more secure by placing a warm wet washcloth over the chest and stomach. A child with poor head control in this back-lying position may need an additional folded hand towel to cradle the back of the head and to raise it a bit more out of the water.

A small plastic innertube and a terry cloth towel underneath the child's bottom can be used while bathing infants who are just beginning to sit up but still unstable. The child with less control can be seated in the tube, bottom first, with the arms and legs bent over the sides. As the child gains more control, the tube can be placed around the chest and waist. This allows the arms to be free to splash and play with toys, and keeps the child from slipping through the tube. The water level is very important since it could increase the child's buoyancy in water, providing more stability. The optimal water level may vary from child to child, but a level somewhere between the waist and armpits provides a good deal of trunk support.

Lastly, but very importantly, parents should obtain a small stable stool to sit on at the side of the tub when bathing their child. Bending over the side of the tub can cause severe strain on the low back muscles. This is an important precaution to remember since parents of handicapped children are prone to back problems with the increased amount of lifting of their child and added equipment needs.

In addition to these simple techniques, several different types of bathing chairs and slings are available for children who need additional support. Again, occupational and physical therapists or other infant specialists are skilled in assisting a parent to choose the best type of equipment for a particular child and for the bathroom in which it will be used. A home visit is necessary to assess the arrangement of the bathroom. Expensive bathing equipment is quite useless if it cannot be maneuvered in a too small or unusually shaped bathroom.

Toileting Equipment As mentioned earlier in this chapter, independence in toileting is a highly valued area of self-care for parents of delayed children, as it is for parents with normal children. Some children prefer sitting on a child-sized potty chiar, while others prefer an adult-sized toilet fitted with a seat insert. Delayed children should be trained in the same trial and error manner as nondelayed children are before other equipment is ordered. In general, a child with poor balance achieves greater control if both feet are on the floor or a firm surface rather than dangling in the air.

Most parents do not regard their experiences with their children's toilet training as the most memorable and rewarding of their parenting years. Therefore, the parents of a handicapped child need a lot of reassurance as well as strategies and techniques that have been found to be useful for children with delays.

A child's opportunity for entry into and acceptance in less restrictive environments is greatly enhanced by his or her higher level of self-care skills. Therefore, a teacher or specialist who works with infants and young children is trusted and fondly remembered by parents for assisting with their child's acquisition of independent self-care skills.

CONSISTENCY BETWEEN HOME AND SCHOOL

Early intervention serviceproviders are frequently asked to develop and implement self-care programs. In order to ensure that self-care skills are acquired, maintained, and generalized, consistency between the school program and the home environment is necessary. Serviceproviders must elicit input from parents concerning which self-care skills are most important in the home. The meeting at which the Individualized Family Service Plan (IFSP) is developed provides a natural opportunity for this to take place (see Chapters 8 and 16). For assessment and programming purposes, it is useful to determine which self-help skills the child currently performs in the home.

Parents differ in what specific areas of self-care they value most. It is a responsibility of the serviceprovider to determine the self-care priorities for parents and to develop the child's program according to those priorities. As previously mentioned, the likelihood of a child's successful mastery of basic self-care skills is greatly enhanced if the school program and home environment are consistent.

Home-Based Programs

Many early intervention programs, particularly those for birth to 2-year-old children who are handicapped, utilize home-based models. Home-based programs offer serviceproviders excellent opportunities to assess parent needs and desires for their child's self-care development. Once the self-care goals and the program for meeting them are determined, the serviceprovider can offer concurrent intervention and parent training. The serviceprovider can model instructional strategies and reinforcement techniques (see Chapter 15). Parents vary in how much direct training they require. In some cases, serviceproviders may need to teach parents how to prompt, cue, and shape their child's behavior in a very direct manner. Some parents require assistance in how to provide reinforcement to their children. Such parents should be encouraged to supply social rewards such as smiling, hugging, clapping, and verbal praise for the child and specific desired child behavior. Parents are also trained to use naturally occurring consequences, such as, "If you put your shoes on, then you can go outside to play."

Providing parents with simple record keeping devices is helpful for documenting progress, and serves as a reminder to work with the child on a daily basis. Record keeping can be particularly beneficial in toileting programs, where it is essential that parents offer frequent opportunities for appropriate toilet usage and copious reinforcement. Progress on an objective from the CAMS Self-Help Program is documented by a simple record keeping system that is combined with a task-analysis (see Figure 13.2).

Center-Based Program

A primarily classroom-based intervention model is also responsible for home/ school consistency. However, if parent involvement is not stressed in the school program, serviceproviders have fewer opportunities to observe parent/child interactions and to intervene when necessary. The IFSP can still be instrumental in establishing what areas of self-care skill development are parental priorities. Classroom-based serviceproviders should be willing to assist parents in the extension of school-based self-care programs into the home environment. Parents must be encouraged to structure activities that promote self-care independence, and to take advantage of naturally occurring opportunities to train and reinforce self-care skills (see Chapter 15).

Serviceproviders should strive for cooperative and mutually respectful interactions with the families whom they serve. The coordination of programs between home and school enhances the development of independence in self-care skills for delayed preschoolers.

SUMMARY

Training self-care skills is absolutely essential in easing the transition of preschoolers who are handicapped into least restrictive environments. Children who experience a disability stand out as distinctly different from their peers; these differences are exacerbated if these children lack basic self-care skills (Fowler, 1982). In mainstreamed environments, the lack of self-care skills can

CAMS Self Help Program

Objective No. **F20 - THE CHILD FEEDS HIMSELF USING A SPOON**

Student's Name _____ Starting Date _____ Ending Date _____

Materials __A small spoon, a dish of favorite food__

		Date	Trials	%
Step 1:	THE CHILD FEEDS HIMSELF THREE SPOONSFUL OF FOOD.		1 2 3 4 5 6 7 8 9 10	correct
Method:	Seat the child at a table or in a high chair beside you. Place a bowl of food and a small spoon directly in front of the child. Encourage the child to pick up the spoon , and to eat without dropping the spoon between bites. The child may turn the spoon over just as it reachs the mouth.			
Criterion:	4 correct out of 5 trials.			

		Date	Trials	%
Step 2:	THE CHILD FEEDS HIMSELF THREE SPOONSFUL WITH THE SPOON HELD RIGHT SIDE UP WITH ASSISTANCE.		1 2 3 4 5 6 7 8 9 10	correct
Method:	Seat the child at a table or in a high chair beside you. Place a bowl of food and a small spoon directly in front of him. Encourage him to pick up the spoon , and to eat without dropping the spoon between bites. You may hold the child's hand to keep the spoon upright if the child begins to turn the spoon over .			
Criterion:	4 correct out of 5 trials.			

		Date	Trials	%
Step 3:	THE CHILD FEEDS HIMSELF THREE SPOONSFUL WITH THE SPOON HELD RIGHT SIDE UP.		1 2 3 4 5 6 7 8 9 10	correct
Method:	Seat the child at a table or in a high chair beside you. Place a bowl of food and a small spoon directly in front of him. Tell the child to pick up the spoon and to eat . The child may spill some of the food.			
Criterion:	4 correct out of 5 trials.			

		Date	Trials	%
Step 4:	THE CHILD FEEDS HIMSELF THREE SPOONSFUL OF FOOD WITH LITTLE SPILLING.		1 2 3 4 5 6 7 8 9 10	correct
Method:	Seat the child at a table or in a high chair beside you. Place a bowl of favorite food and a small spoon directly in front of him. Tell him to eat. Remind the child whenever the spoon is too full.			
Criterion:	4 correct out of 5 trials.			

Figure 13.2. CAMS self-help program's simple record keeping system.

be perceived as an additional inconvenience to the teacher and a cause for ridicule by peers.

The ultimate goal for all persons who are disabled is the achievement of independence. Serviceproviders and parents are expected to train preschoolers who are handicapped in basic self-feeding, dressing, and toileting skills. Fortunately, many opportunities to train these skills occur naturally in both the preschool classroom and home setting. Therefore, the training of self-care skills is a responsibility shared by persons in the child's home and school. It is advisable that a cooperative program be developed utilizing consistent instructional strategies and reinforcement in both settings. Classroom personnel may wish to help parents break down more complex behaviors, teach in small steps, and reinforce desired behaviors. Classroom personnel should definitely encourage parents to use naturally occurring opportunities to enhance coincidental learning in their homes. Parents may need encouragement to use guided practice or graduated prompting in assisting a child through a self-care task.

Allowing a child to self-feed or dress with appropriate assistance and prompting initially uses more parent time. Once the child masters these skills independently, the parent is awarded more time to devote to other tasks.

Self-care skills are necessary and may require direct teaching. It is best if the self-care skills are stressed across disciplines (e.g., teachers; careproviders; parents; and specialists in speech/language, occupational, and physical therapy), and settings (e.g., school, home, and community) for all young children who are disabled.

STUDY QUESTIONS

1. Observe equipment used for "pottie training" in the early intervention program in your community.

2. Observe as a child removes outer clothing and describe the movements involved.

3. Interview a parent of a young child concerning the clothing that the child prefers and which articles of clothing he or she is able to handle without assistance. Make diagrams of the favorite and most easily handled clothing.

4. Observe as a child eats finger food and describe the process.

REFERENCES

Adams, G. (1975). *Psychological attraction, personal characteristics and social behavior: Investigation of the effects of the psychological attractiveness stereotype.* Unpublished doctoral dissertation, Pennsylvania State University, University Park.

Bailey, B. B., & Wolery, M. (1984). Acquisition and use of self-help skills. In B. B. Bailey & M. Wolery (Eds.), *Teaching infants and pre-schoolers with handicaps* (pp. 333–360). Columbus, OH: Charles E. Merrill.

Bronicki, M. A., Holvoet, J., & Guess, D. (1981). The individualized curriculum sequence. In D. Guess, C. Jones, & S. Lyon (Eds.), *Combining a transdisciplinary team approach with an individualized curriculum sequencing model for severe/multiply handicapped children* (pp. 1–42). Lawrence: Department of Special Education, University of Kansas.

Bricker, D., Casuso, V., Pearson, E., Mendoza, B., & Praeto, M. (1977). *Family involvement*. Miami: Debbie School Institutue, Mailman Center for Child Development, University of Miami.

Fiechtl, B., Bonem, M., Morgan, J., Innocenti, M., Rule, S., & Stowitschek, J. (1986). *Coincidental teaching: A packet for trainers of preschool and daycare staff*. Unpublished manuscript from Utah State University, Social integration program, Logan.

Filler, J., & Kasari, C. (1981). Acquisition, maintenance, and generalization of parent-taught skills with two severely handicapped infants. *Journal of The Association for the Severely Handicapped, 6*, 30–38.

Fowler, S. A. (1982). Transition from preschool to kindergarten for children with special needs. In K. E. Allen & E. M. Goetz (Eds.), *Problems in early childhood education* (pp. 309–335). Rockville, MD: Aspen Systems.

Gaylord-Ross, R. J., & Holvoet, J. (1985). *Strategies for educating students with severe handicaps*. Boston: Little, Brown.

Guess, D., Horner, D., Utley, B., Holvoet, J., Maxon, D., Tucker, D., & Warren, S. (1978). A functional curriculum sequencing model for teaching the severely handicapped. *AAESPH Review, 3*, 202–215.

Hart, B., & Risley, T. R. (1975). Incidental teaching of language in the preschool. *Journal of Applied Behavior Analysis, 8*, 411–420.

Holvoet, J., Guess, D., Mulligan, M., & Brown, F. (1980). The individualized curriculum sequencing model (11): A teaching strategy for severely handicapped students. *Journal of The Association for the Severely Handicapped, 5*, 337–351.

Kayser, J. E., Billingsley, F. F., & Neel, R. S. (1986). A comparison of in-context and traditional instruction approaches: Total tasks, single trial versus backward chaining, multiple trials. *Journal of The Association for the Severely Handicapped, 11*(1), 28–38.

Lance, W. D., & Koch, A. C. (1973). Parents as teachers: Self-help skills for young handicapped children. *Mental Retardation, 11*, 3–4.

Mendelsohn, M. B. (1978). Behavioral training by paraprofessionals for families of developmentally disabled persons. *AAESPH Review, 3*, 216–221.

McGreevy, P., Lacy, L., & Calisius, C. F. (1984). *A comparison of two approaches to home-based training for parents of severely handicapped preschool children*. A final report submitted to U.S. Department of Education: Special Education Program. (Grant No. G 008300195).

Neel, R. S., Billingsley, F. F., & Lambert, C. (1983). IMPACT: A functional curriculum for educating autistic youth in natural environments. In R. B. Rutherford, Jr. (Ed.), *Monograph in behavioral disorders: Severe behavior problems of children and youth* (Series No. 6) (pp. 40–50). Reston, VA: Council for Children with Behavioral Disorders.

Neel, R. S., Billingsley, F. F., McCarty, F., Symonds, D., Lambert, C., Lewis-Smith, N., & Hanashito, R. (1983). *Teaching autistic children: A functional curriculum approach*. Seattle: University of Washington.

Rule, S., Stowitschek, J. J., Innocenti, M., Striefel, S., Killoran, J., & Swezey, K. (1987). The social integration program: An analysis of the effects of mainstreaming handicapped children into day care centers. *Education and Treatment of Children, 10*(2), 175–192.

Sailor, W., & Guess, D. (1983). *Severely handicapped students: An instructional design*. Boston: Houghton Mifflin.

Sedjo, K., & Peterson, A. (1987). *The CAMS self-help program*. Logan: Utah State University.

Shearer, D., Billingsley, J., Frohman, A., Hilliard, J., Johnson, F., & Shearer, M.

(1970). *The Portage guide to early education: Instructions and checklist.* Portage, WI: Cooperative Educational Service Agency #12.

Snell, M. (1978). *Systematic instruction of the moderately and severely handicapped.* Columbus, OH: Charles E. Merrill.

Spooner, F. (1981). An operant analysis of the effects of backward chaining and total task presentation. *Dissertation Abstracts International, 41,* 3992A. (University Microfilms No. 81–05,615).

Spooner, F. (1984). Comparisons of backward chaining and total task presentation in training severely handicapped persons. *Education and Training of the Mentally Retarded, 19,* 15–22.

Vincent, L., Dodd, N., & Henner, P. (1978). Planning and implementing a program of parent involvement. In N. Haring & D. Bricker (Eds.), *Teaching the severely handicapped* (Vol. 3, pp. 282–297). Columbus, OH: Special Press.

Westling, D. L., & Minden, L. (1978). Self-help skills training: A review of operant studies. *Journal of Special Education, 12,* 253–283.

Zane, T., Walls, R. T., & Thvedt, J. E. (1981). Prompting and fading guidance procedures: Their effect on chaining and whole task teaching strategies. *Education and Training of the Mentally Retarded, 16,* 125–135.

RELATED CONCERNS

———————————— • ————————————

All children, handicapped and nonhandicapped, are susceptible to childhood diseases and have need for sanitary environments in which to live, play, and learn. When children are grouped together, it is even more important to deal with issues concerning communicable diseases and for staff to learn appropriate health management techniques. It is also important to be able to manage learning environment efficiently and to allow for goal directed individualized teaching activities. This teaching must occur in the most natural interaction patterns possible and during the regular routines of the day. And, of course, first, last and always. In order to even have access to the child, it is necessary to understand and to relate to the family. Although each family is unique and therefore has unique needs, there are some guidelines.

Chapter 14

Health Concerns

James A. Blackman

———————— • ————————

Many states have regulations regarding the health and safety of children enrolled in day care or preschool programs. However, these regulations are usually minimal and do not address the wide range of health concerns that administrators, practicing professionals, parents, and children face in early intervention programs. Besides the basic obvious requirements for sanitation and management of communicable diseases, there exists an opportunity to create a healthful environment and promote concepts of health among children, their parents, and the program staff. Such an effort for an early childhood program must be well planned and carefully followed to be effective, as well as coordinated with other community resources such as health departments and private health care providers.

The purpose of this chapter is to review effective approaches in creating a healthful environment for children, staff, and parents involved with early intervention programs. The focus is on center-based programs, however, the concepts are equally applicable to home-based services. The generic health issues discussed are germane to all group care settings including day care, early intervention, or other types of preschool programs. They include the prevention of illness and injury through immunization and environmental controls to halt disease transmission and avoid accidents; the management of illness, including recognition of illness and developing policies for working with sick children; and consideration of precautions for children with special needs, such as those with developmental disabilities and chronic illnesses. Health promotion through diet, good dental care, and family support are also discussed. It is beyond the scope of the chapter to discuss in detail specific diseases or health problems of children. However, additional resources are suggested at the end of this chapter for such details.

PREVENTION OF ILLNESS AND INJURIES

Immunizations

The most obvious means of preventing illness is through immunizations. The rate of full immunization achieved by school-age children is very good since most states require completion of the immunization schedules prior to school entry. However, due to illness or parental noncompliance, there are frequently interruptions and delays of immunizations during infancy and early childhood, when vulnerability to certain diseases such as whooping cough (pertussis) is at its peak. Thus, early childhood programs should adopt requirements of their own stating that children must maintain the appropriate immunization schedule in order to qualify for participation. Table 14.1 contains the most recent recommendations of the American Academy of Pediatrics.

Vaccine against *Haemophilus influenzae,* a bacterium that is a major cause of meningitis, otitis media, and other serious illnesses, is recommended for all children at 18 months of age. It is likely that a vaccine will be available for very young infants who are highly susceptible to this organism.

Approximately 12% of Indo-Chinese refugees are estimated to be carriers of the hepatitis B virus. Most of these individuals do not have symptoms, and the likelihood of transmission is very low with good hygienic practices. Local health authorities should be consulted regarding the risk to staff in these situations. If rates of virus carriage are high in a particular setting, a vaccine is available for susceptible individuals.

A Safe Environment

There are many precautions that can be taken to ensure a safe environment in an early intervention program. Three such precautions include: 1) keeping the pro-

Table 14.1. Recommended immunization schedules

Recommended age	Immunization(s)
2 months	DTP,[a] OPV[b]
4 months	DTP, OPV
6 months	DTP (OPV)
15 months	MMR[c]
18 months	DTP,[d,e] OPV,[e] PRP-D[f]
4–6 years[g]	DTP, OPV
14–16 years	Td[h]

[a]Diphtheria and tetanus toxoids with pertussis vaccine.
[b]Oral poliovirus vaccine.
[c]Live measles, mumps, and rubella viruses.
[d]Should be given 6–12 months after the third dose.
[e]May be given simultaneously with MMR at 15 months of age.
[f]*Haemophilus* b conjugate vaccine.
[g]Up to the seventh birthday.
[h]Adult tetanus toxoid (full dose) and diphtheria toxoid (reduced dose) in combination.

gram free of potential accident-causing materials or events, 2) providing adequate air and water management, and 3) conducting proper sanitation practices.

Accidents The term *accident* implies that an event is beyond one's control. However, prevention programs have demonstrated that death and injury due to accidents can be averted. The preschool child is particularly vulnerable to accidents because of the potentially lethal combination of increased mobility and independence with relatively immature judgment. Most of the younger child's learning during this period is through experience, and minor accidents are inevitable. The risk of serious injury, however, can be lowered. The following is a list of suggestions for accident prevention:

1. Modify facility design; tables should have rounded edges, windows should be made of safety glass, and stairs should be carpeted and should have frequent landings.
2. Examine toys each day to determine potential for injury. Small toys or broken parts of toys should be eliminated to prevent choking, and balloons, peanuts, and other small objects should be avoided.
3. Use protective covers on electrical outlets and check for frayed or worn electric cords.
4. Outdoor play areas should be enclosed and equipment inspected for potential hazards such as projections, sharp edges, loose parts, entrapment spaces, hard swings, and moving parts that can pinch. Equipment should be placed to prevent tipping, and positioned so there are soft landing places and other objects in children's pathways are avoided.
5. Establish a fire escape plan.
6. Use smoke detectors.
7. Use appropriately textured food for infants and young children.
8. Poisons (e.g., cleaning materials, rodent poisons) should be kept out of reach or placed in a secured area. Medications used by staff or children should be kept in a locked cabinet. Serum of ipecac, used to induce vomiting, should be on hand, but used only if advised by a poison control center or a physician.
9. Maintain settings on hot water heaters at a maximum of 120°–125° F.
10. Child auto restraints should be used for transporting children. Their use by parents should be encouraged. Many states now have motor vehicle child restraint laws in effect.
11. Instill a sense of safety consciousness among staff.

An actual emergency is not the time to train staff in appropriate procedures. When an accident or a poisoning occurs, staff should be familiar with a plan of action. The telephone numbers of the poison control center, the emergency care system (e.g., 911), and a medical consultant (physician or nurse) should be prominently displayed on each phone. Staff working directly with children should take a basic CPR (cardiopulmonary resuscitation) course and have updated training annually. Choking is the most frequently encountered emergency and staff should be particularly competent in dealing with this problem. An individual trained in basic first aid should be present at all times as well.

Air and Water Management   Adequate ventilation, especially in enclosed spaces during the winter months, contributes to the comfort of the inhabitants and possibly decreases the incidence of respiratory illness. Hot air heating systems may need to be accompanied by some method of air humidification.

Passive smoking, the inhalation of cigarette smoke by nonsmokers, is now recognized to be harmful, particularly to those individuals with respiratory problems (children with asthma or a history of bronchopulmonary dysplasia). Therefore, smoking should be prohibited in areas utilized by nonsmokers. Restriction of smoking entirely or to designated areas may encourage smokers to quit or reduce the habit.

When drinking water is not obtained from a purified source, it should be tested for chemical, organic, and infectious contaminants. Fluoride is now recognized as an important means of tooth decay prevention. If fluoride is not added to the school or home water supply, an early intervention program could play an important preventive health care role by establishing a fluoride supplementation program. This may be particularly important for children with significant disabilities whose oral and dental hygiene may be suboptimal.

Sanitation   Diarrheal diseases are common in group care settings but, if staff employ basic hygienic practices, it is easier to control the spread of diarrheal disease than it is to control respiratory diseases. There are three important steps to take. First, hands should be washed after diapering or helping with toileting. If children do their own toileting, they should be taught proper handwashing. Handwashing is the single most effective means of preventing spread of diarrhea. Second, potty chairs should be kept clean and have a removable container. Third, diapers should be changed in a specially designated area. The Centers for Disease Control have issued the following guidelines for maintaining a sanitary environment:

Diapering   Change diapers directly on paper towels, roll paper, or other disposable covering. Place this disposable covering on a surface that is:

Smooth, not absorbent, and easily cleaned
Out of children's reach
Separate from the food preparation area
Within reach of a sink not used for food preparation

Store diapers and supplies together in a location that is easily accessible to caregivers and out of children's reach.

Potty Chairs   Keep potty chairs in bathrooms, not in classrooms or hallways. After the child uses the potty chair:

Wash the child's hands
Empty the potty contents into the toilet
Rinse the potty in a sink used only for this purpose, not for washing hands
Clean and disinfect the sink
Wash your hands

Cleaning and Disinfecting Environmental Surfaces Cleaning and disinfecting all surfaces is as important as washing your hands. The following are a few important tips on cleaning and disinfecting:

Wash all surfaces with soap and water, then, disinfect them with a bleach solution or a commercial disinfectant. An effective bleach solution can be made by mixing one part bleach with 10 parts water. A spray bottle is easy to use and handy for storage. Prepare a fresh bleach solution daily and keep it out of children's reach.

Bathroom surfaces, like faucet handles and toilet seats, should be washed and disinfected more than once a day if possible. Floors, low shelves, doorknobs, and other surfaces often touched by diapered children should be washed and disinfected weekly. Mattress covers and linens should be washed daily unless each child uses the same mattress cover every day.

Do not wash clothing that is soiled with stool. Instead, empty the stool into the toilet, being careful not to touch toilet water with your hands. Then, place the clothing in sealed plastic bags to be picked up by the child's parent or guardian at the end of the day. Always wash your hands after handling soiled clothing.

Allow children who wear diapers to play only with washable toys. Provide toys for each group so that toys are not shared among groups. Ideally, hard-surfaced toys should be washed daily, and stuffed toys should be washed weekly (more often if they are heavily soiled). Whenever possible, a toy that is mouthed by a child should be washed before other children handle it. Some programs keep an empty container out of the children's reach for storing heavily soiled toys. When time allows, these toys can be washed, disinfected, dried, and safely reused.

Keep on hand sufficient quantities of facial tissues, paper towels, and supplies for handwashing, diapering, and cleaning. Stock extra linens and mattress covers in case of accidents. Because handwashing is the most important deterrent to the spread of infection, signs to remind staff to wash hands would be very useful (see Figure 14.1).

MANAGEMENT OF ILLNESS

Most illness in young children is due to infectious diseases that are usually minor and transient. However, in a group setting, the result of minor illnesses can be magnified because of the inconvenience to parents who may have to

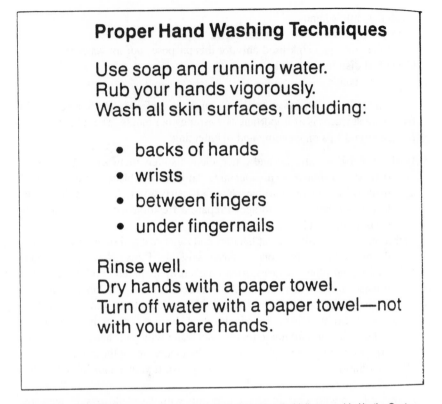

Proper Hand Washing Techniques

Use soap and running water.
Rub your hands vigorously.
Wash all skin surfaces, including:

- backs of hands
- wrists
- between fingers
- under fingernails

Rinse well.
Dry hands with a paper towel.
Turn off water with a paper towel—not
with your bare hands.

Figure 14.1. Hand washing reminder sign for staff. (Adapted from guidelines provided by the Centers for Disease Control, Atlanta, GA.)

rearrange schedules, because of lost educational time due to absence or discomfort of the child, and because of the potential for the spread of disease to other children and staff. Diarrhea caused by rotavirus, for example, can quickly spread from one child to the majority of children and staff in a program, and beyond that to their families. In this instance, the chain of transmission could be prevented by a simple hygienic practice: handwashing.

A useful way of understanding the transmission of infectious diseases is to consider the agent-vector (or vehicle) -host relationship. The *agent* is an infectious organism such as the hepatitis A virus. A *vector* (a living organism such as a rodent or fly) or *vehicle* (nonliving material such as air or water) carries the infectious agent to the *host,* the individual who potentially becomes infected and ill. Depending upon general health and previous experience with the disease, the host may repel the infectious agent, have only mild symptoms, or become severely ill. Infection control must be aimed at all three factors. Disinfection of toys kills the infectious agents, chlorination ensures that water does

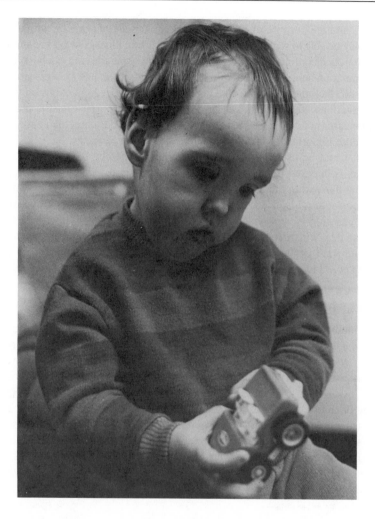

not become a vehicle of transmission for diarrhea-producing organisms, and a proper diet strengthens the host's ability to resist infecting organisms. It is easy to think of many ways that communicable diseases can be controlled by attending to the agent-vehicle-host relationship. The resources listed at the end of this chapter provide information on specific diseases and their management.

It is important that a program develop a clear policy for managing infections. Staff should learn to recognize signs of illness, especially when they indicate a serious problem that requires evaluation by a physician or possible quarantine. Policy must be consistent with local and state guidelines for management of infections.

In part, the policy depends upon the facility size and staff, the population served, and the purpose of the program. For example, a program with a large staff may be able to segregate children with a certain illness, such as respiratory infection, and continue to serve them without exposing the entire population. If the population being served includes children whose immune systems are compromised, then measures must be taken to protect them from exposure to certain infections, such as chicken pox. Finally, if the purpose of the program encompasses not only education and therapy, but also day care, then it would be even more important to exclude children with minor illnesses.

It would be useful to have a daily routine whereby the health status of children is checked upon their arrival at the program. Although it is neither practical nor within the purview of teachers to conduct health examinations, a brief look at the child to see whether he or she appears well, and a few questions to the parent or careprovider about health status are appropriate. It is much easier to deal with management plans for illness at the time of arrival than later when a parent would have to be called back and other children and staff have been exposed to an illness that would be best left outside the program.

Signs of Illness

The following are important signs of illness: fever (rectal temperature of approximately 100.4° F, oral temperature of approximately 100.0° F, or axillary temperature of 99.0° F), irritability, skin rash, pulling at ears, food and/or fluid refusal, excessive crying, difficulty breathing, and persistent vomiting or diarrhea. If these signs of illness are present, they should be reported to the child's parent or careprovider, and the child should be evaluated by a physician. They are particularly worrisome in a very young child because they may represent a very serious illness, such as meningitis. Cold symptoms, unaccompanied by any of the other problems listed, are generally of little concern, although it must be recognized that the organisms that cause them, usually viruses, are readily transmissible.

Excluding Sick Children from Programs

Sick children may need to be excluded, isolated, or cohorted (i.e., grouped together with other children with the same symptoms). Depending upon the nature of the disease and upon the availability of staff and special facilities, it may be possible to cohort all ill children apart from well children, particularly if it appears that they have the same illness, such as diarrhea. However, most programs must have some type of exclusion policy in order to prevent the spread of disease. Exclusion criteria should meet the needs of both the early intervention program and the parents, as closely as possible. They also must meet state health department standards. The Centers for Disease Control have developed some exclusion guidelines for day care centers. These guidelines are presented in Table 14.2.

Table 14.2. Exclusion guidelines for day care centers

Some important symptoms of illness to look for:

Diarrhea (more than one abnormally loose stool)   If a child has only one loose stool, observe the child for additional loose stools or other symptoms. Be sure that the child and careproviders wash their hands at all recommended times.*
Severe coughing   The child gets red or blue in the face or makes high-pitched, "croupy," or "whooping" sounds after coughing.*
Labored or rapid breathing   This is especially significant in infants less than 6 months old.*
Yellowish tint to the skin or eyes (jaundice)*
Tearing, irritation, and redness of eyelid lining, followed by swelling and discharge of pus (conjunctivitis, also called "pink eye")*
Unusual spots or rashes
Sore throat or difficulty in swallowing
Infected areas of skin with crusty, bright yellow, dry, or gummy areas
Unusually dark, tea-colored urine
Grey or white stools
Headache and stiff neck
Vomiting
Unusual behavior (crankiness, listlessness, crying more than usual, obvious general discomfort)
Loss of appetite
Severe itching of body or scalp or constant scratching of the scalp.

What to do if a child at your center develops symptoms of disease:

Symptoms	*Action*
Any of the signs or symptoms listed	Isolate the child from other children and watch for other symptoms.
Feverish appearance	Take the child's temperature Fever = 100° F (37.8° C) by oral thermometer and 101° F (38.3° C) by rectal thermometer. Take a rectal reading when the child is too young to use an oral thermometer without risk of injury.
Any of the signs or symptoms marked with an asterisk(*)	Contact the parents and ask them to take the child home.
A fever and any of the signs or symptoms (with or without asterisks)	Contact the parents and ask them to take the child home.
Any of the symptoms not marked by asterisks; no fever	Contact the parents to ask if they are aware of the symptoms and to obtain any information they may have about the child's condition.

Adapted from Centers for Disease Control (1984). *What you can do to stop disease in the child day care center.* Washington, DC: Department of Health and Human Services.

PRECAUTIONS IN SPECIAL POPULATIONS

Three groups of children warrant special consideration, either because they are unusually susceptible to infection or because they may infect other children. They are children with developmental disabilities, chronic illnesses, or impaired immunity.

Children with Developmental Disabilities

In general, children with developmental disabilities are not particularly susceptible to infection and require no special precautions or procedures. A few categories of disabilities are associated with higher rates of infection, however.
Children with spina bifida (meningomyelocele), for example, are particularly
prone to urinary tract infections (UTIs). While these infections pose no risk to
other children or careproviders, the staff in day care and preschool settings may
be called upon to participate in special preventive procedures, such as intermit-
tent catheterizations of the bladder. Staff should also be alert to signs and symptoms of UTIs, such as fever or foul-smelling urine, and bring these to the attention of the child's doctor.

Children with certain disabilities may be especially susceptible to respiratory and ear infections. For example, children with severe neuromuscular involvement (cerebral palsy) may not have an effective cough or may be unable to
swallow oral secretions well, which can lead to frequent bouts of pneumonia.
Children with Down syndrome seem to have a higher than normal number of
respiratory infections, and children with cleft palates have frequent ear infections, which can lead to chronic serous otitis media. While these children may
have a high incidence of infection, their symptoms are often no different from
those of other children.

Many careproviders are concerned that certain infections acquired before
or around the time of birth (e.g., rubella, cytomegalovirus, herpes simplex,
hepatitis, AIDS) may persist and be spread to other children or staff members.
In most cases, these congenital infections pose a very small risk to others, and
with proper precautions, affected children may safely participate in most day
care or educational programs. However, in some cases, special precautions are
warranted.

Since AIDS was first reported in 1981, there has been growing concern
about the potential for the transmission of this disease to uninfected persons.
Can young children with AIDS be safely integrated into group care activities?
To date there is no evidence that the AIDS virus is transmitted by normal, ca-
sual, and nonsexual contact in home, school, day care, or foster care settings.
Therefore, it appears that infected children can participate in group care without significant risk through contact. Consistent appropriate hygienic practices,
such as handwashing, should protect caregivers from the remote risk of becoming infected with the AIDS virus. Such practices will serve to prevent the spread
of all infectious agents, most of which are much more likely to cause disease
among those who work with young children. Because the immune system of
children with AIDS is weakened, they are at increased risk of acquiring both
common and unusual infections which can, themselves, be life-threatening.
The child's physician should be involved in guiding early intervention program
personnel in minimizing risk to staff and other children where there are special

circumstances, such as an excessive biting behavior, and providing guidelines for protecting the child with AIDS from other infections. The local health department is an excellent and definitive source of up-to-date information regarding the latest recommendations from the National Centers for Disease Control.

Children with Chronic Illnesses

Children with chronic illnesses, prolonged states of debilitation, or malnutrition are particularly susceptible to infection. For example, infants with a history of prematurity who have chronic lung disease (bronchopulmonary dysplasia), and children with cystic fibrosis, frequently have a higher than average incidence of respiratory infections. Similarly, children with congenital heart disease may have unusual difficulty with some respiratory viruses. Children with diseases or structural abnormalities of the urinary tract are highly susceptible to infections of the bladder and kidneys. Although it is not always possible to prevent these diseases, careproviders should be alert to the symptoms of infections and notify the child's parents and/or physician if they occur. Once treatment is initiated, these children should be able to participate in regular group care activities.

Children with Impaired Immunity

Certain diseases or treatments can lower the body's natural defenses against infection. AIDS, cancer of the blood or lymphatics, and some other diseases of the immune system significantly alter the body's ability to fight infection, allowing even common organisms to quickly become life threatening. In children with previously normal immune systems, some drugs that are used to treat chronic conditions (e.g., steroids for nephrotic syndrome) suppress the body's ability to fight infection. Drugs used to prevent rejection of organ transplants or to temper the body's attack on its own organs can also interfere with the normal immune response. In a child with cancer, both the disease itself and the drugs used to treat it inhibit the body's defense mechanisms.

Children with diseases or treatments that affect the immune system may need to be isolated from other children during periods of particular susceptibility. Their physicians may prescribe special precautions to limit exposure to infection, particularly to chicken pox, since this disease can be fatal in individuals with suppressed immunity.

Despite the risks of spreading or acquiring infections, children in these special population groups need to socialize as normally as possible. With care and planning, the majority of these children can be safely integrated into day care and school settings. Administrators, teachers, and careproviders should work closely with parents and health care providers to establish a safe environment for these children, their peers, and staff members who care for them.

HEALTH PROMOTION

It has been estimated that as much as 70% of chronic illness (including such diseases as heart attack, stroke, and cancer) could be prevented by alterations in people's lifestyles. Since disease prevention measures must be instituted in childhood, programs for young children, including early intervention programs, provide an opportunity to develop patterns of behavior that will reduce the risk of serious disease later. Furthermore, disease prevention activities are consistent with the philosophy of providing comprehensive services to children with disabilities and their families.

Diet

The importance of good nutrition in young children cannot be overemphasized. A high percentage of children with developmental disabilities have feeding and nutritional problems. A child with cerebral palsy or severe mental retardation is at-risk for malnutrition; the child with spina bifida or one who is receiving gastrostomy feedings may become obese. A child with a disability who is receiving inadequate caloric or nutrient intake may become further impaired as a result. Thus, attention to feeding techniques and appropriate intake is an essential part of an early intervention program. In general, helping children and families get used to a high quality diet (e.g., low saturated fat content, adequate fiber, sodium limitations) establishes behaviors that have been shown to reduce the risk of cardiovascular disease and cancer.

Dental Health

Dental care should begin early with the eruption of the primary teeth. Teeth should be brushed as soon as they begin to erupt. A convenient method is to place the young child in a cradle developed by two adults sitting in a knee-to-knee position: one stabilizes and keeps the child involved while the other wields a small multitufted soft brush that effectively cleans the teeth and massages the gums. Toothpaste is not necessary for cleaning and may in fact cause gagging. Toothpaste can be used when the child can spit it out after brushing. The cleaning should take place at least once a day. As the child grows and becomes more involved in the cleaning process, adults should continue to evaluate and reinforce the efforts.

Prevention efforts, such as the use of fluoride, have dramatically reduced the incidence of cavities and gum disease. However, such progress can be negated by other practices. For example, overuse of bottles with liquids high in sugar must be avoided to prevent destruction of the incisors.

Family Support

It has been suggested, although not without controversy, that a child with a disability brings increased stress to a family, a higher incidence of family break-up, and increased risk for child abuse. Although these risks may be overestimated, the psychological and social needs of special needs family members should not be overlooked. Early intervention programs should be able to suggest appropriate resources. Staff can help parents adjust and cope with the special needs child by encouraging questions, by asking for the parents' expertise in learning how to work with a child, and by being attentive and nonjudgmental listeners. Such resources as parent support groups and respite care programs can be very helpful as well, and all staff should be knowledgeable about such community resources.

Whether or not there is a higher than normal rate of child abuse among special needs families, statistics show that, in general, child abuse is a major cause of death for very young children. For this reason, any staff working with children in this age group should be knowledgeable about the signs of abuse. Half of all abused children are beaten on repeated occasions. Ten percent of children whose abuse is not detected when they are first examined by a physician die of subsequent abuse. Two-thirds of all abused children are less than 3 years old. Young children are the most frequent abuse victims because they are at the most demanding and most defenseless stage of development.

All professionals involved in services to children should be alert to the signs of abuse and neglect. Child abuse should be suspected when the size, shape, and color of the child's bruises or burns are inconsistent with how the injury is said to have occurred. Ninety percent of mistreatment leaves signs on the skin. Neglect might be considered if the child is consistently dirty or malnourished. It is sometimes difficult to determine whether a child's poor nutrition is due to neglect or feeding difficulties as a result of the child's disability. Sometimes it is due to a combination of both factors. Neglect may be manifested by failure to keep a child's health care appointments and to maintain the recommended immunization schedule. Some parents may be overwhelmed by the needs of a disabled child and be particularly at-risk for abusive activity. Parent support efforts may serve an important function in preventing child abuse.

SUMMARY

An early intervention program must view itself as having more than just educational goals. Successful intervention requires attention to all aspects of the child's and family's needs. Health care is one important component of comprehensive services. Directors of programs and their staff should consider each of the points discussed in this chapter and ensure that they become integral parts of the overall intervention program.

STUDY QUESTIONS

1. Wash own hands according to diagram on page 270. Compare this to the first 15 handwashes you observe in a public restroom.

2. Interview parents of young handicapped children concerning their attitudes about immunization.
3. Observe an early intervention program to see how staff handles washing hands after diapering and before food service.
4. Look at the attendance data to determine the absentee rate for children in early intervention programs. Determine which of these absences are for illness.

SUGGESTED READINGS

Health and Developmentally Disabled Children

Batshaw, M. L., & Perret, Y. M. (1986). *Children with handicaps: A medical primer* (2nd ed.). Baltimore: Paul H. Brookes Publishing Co.

Blackman, J. A. (Ed.). (1984). *Medical aspects of developmental disabilities in children birth to three*. Rockville, MD: Aspen Systems.

Bleck, E. E., & Nagel, D. A. (Eds.). (1982). *Physically handicapped children: A medical atlas for teachers*. New York: Grune & Stratton.

Health in Group Care Settings:

Andersen, R. D., Bale, J. F., Jr., Blackman, J. A., & Murph, J. R. (1986). *Infections in children: A sourcebook for educators and child care providers*. Rockville, MD: Aspen Systems.

Health in day care: A manual for day care providers. (1986). Washington, DC: Georgetown University Child Developmental Center.

Health in day care: A manual for health professionals. (1987). Elk Grove Village, IL: American Academy of Pediatrics.

Chapter **15**

Managing Learning Time
Structured Teaching
during Unstructured Times

Norris G. Haring and Mark S. Innocenti

●

This chapter is about managing learning time, or more accurately, structured (formal) teaching during unstructured (informal) times. This chapter includes the rationale for teaching during unstructured times, types of skills that can be taught, and techniques for teaching during unstructured times. Examples include a variety of skill areas. The chapter concludes with a discussion of procedures for training parents to teach at unstructured times.

WHAT IS MEANT BY STRUCTURE

The term *structure* has been used to refer to many different teaching strategies, most of which are thought of in terms of a formal learning enviroment (Lehane & Goldman, 1976). These strategies are characterized by planned lectures with questions and recitations used to achieve specific learning objectives. Structure can also mean the sum total of modifications in the classroom environment, including a reduction in the number of environmental stimuli and the size of the learning space (e.g., cubicles), the imposition of an organized school program with planned daily routines, and an increase in the amount of stimulus value contained in teaching materials (Cruickshank, Bentzen, Ratzeborg, & Tannhauser, 1961). Another way to achieve structure involves clarifying classroom objectives, arranging tasks to provide successful experiences, providing concrete instructional presentations, using immediate feedback to responses, and providing positive consequences for correct responses (Haring & Phillips, 1962). Finally, a structured intervention program for a child can be based on a detailed set of outcomes that are supported by a task analysis with a scripted presentation of activities, as well as procedures and criteria for progressing to new material (Casto & Mastropieri, 1986; Casto & White, 1985).

Using structure to refer to all of these ideas or procedures may be confusing. It is possible, however, to categorize these various meanings into two general headings: 1) *environmental structure* (organization of the physical setting) and 2) *learning structure* (organization of the activities or responses expected of the learner). Environmental and learning structures are not mutually exclusive. For example, Hoyson, Jamieson, and Strain (1984) combine the two in a curriculum design in which children are in a group situation (high environmental structure), but the subject matter taught is individualized for each child (high learning structure). This can be contrasted with coincidental teaching (high learning structure) where a social skill is taught during freeplay (low environmental structure) (Rule et al., 1987).

Research that has focused on early intervention for disadvantaged and handicapped children concludes that high environmental structure alone is not sufficient for learning (Blank & Solomon, 1968). In contrast, high learning structure appears to be an effective component of successful early intervention programs for environmentally at-risk children (Casto & White, 1985) and, to a lesser degree, for developmentally delayed children (Casto & Mastropieri, 1986; Tingey-Michaelis, 1986).

The knowledge of different kinds of structure can affect the way young children who are developmentally delayed are taught. Preschool children are not just younger third-graders. They cannot be expected to sit in large groups for long periods or to work independently for 20 minutes at a time. Thus, environmental structure of early intervention classes must be low. This is not necessarily bad. Children can learn many functional skills in environments that have low environmental structure (e.g., snack, freeplay). Children can also be taught skills during brief, highly environmentally structured times, as in individualized programs or microsessions (Rule, Killoran, Stowitschek, Innocenti, & Striefel, 1985). Both types of teaching can be beneficial.

Instead of categorizing environmental structure as only high or low, the term *natural environment* can be used to refer to environments where formal teaching is not occurring, and the term *naturalistic training techniques* to describe structured teaching techniques that might be used in natural settings.

WHY TEACH IN THE NATURAL ENVIRONMENT?

The ability to demonstrate general use of skills taught during formal training settings in other settings (i.e., generalization) has long been a concern of those attempting to teach new skills to delayed populations (Stokes & Baer, 1977).

This problem has received emphasis from clinicians and researchers interested in the development of language skills (Guess, Keogh, & Sailor, 1978; Warren & Rogers-Warren, 1980). The concerns expressed for training language skills also exist for other functional skills such as social skills (Berler, Gross, & Drabman, 1982; Gresham, 1981) and, to some degree, self-help skills (Kayser, Billingsley, & Neel, 1986).

The concern when training these functional skills is that they be used in the natural environment, not just in a training environment. Generalization problems occur, at least in part, because of the differences between the training environment and natural environments (Haring, in press). Training groups are often artificial; the trainer controls the material presented and prevents distraction. The stimuli (setting events or discriminative stimuli) in the training environment are frequently different from those in the natural environment. The consequences in the training environment (e.g., praise, token) are different than those in the natural environment (e.g., continued interaction, getting a desired item). Differences in these and other features of various environments require the use of techniques that are appropriate for the natural environment.

Halle (1982, p. 29) has provided the following reasons for using natural training techniques for language training and facilitation. These apply to all functional skills:

1. The problem of transferring stimulus control from the training setting to the natural environment is reduced.
2. Persons indigenous to the target children's environment are exposed to, and perhaps involved in, training; thus increasing the likelihood of facilitative interactions even when formal training is not in effect.
3. When training and facilitation occur in natural settings, they are more likely to be functional.

Most Common Natural Training Techniques

The three primary naturalistic training strategies are: 1) *incidental teaching,* 2) *mand-model procedure,* and 3) *naturalistic time-delay.* All naturalistic training strategies involve embedding instructional trials within the content of routines or activities that are already occurring in a natural environment (Halle, Alpert, & Anderson, 1984), although some environmental modifications are usually required. The naturalistic training strategies are all teacher-directed. These strategies all focus on transferring stimulus control from the teacher to novel stimuli in the environment.

Incidental Teaching   Incidental teaching (Hart & Risley, 1968, 1974, 1975) is a naturalistic training technique that consists of an interaction between an adult and child, used by the adult to teach information or to give the child practice in developing a skill. The interaction is child-initiated and occurs naturally during an unstructured time.

The incorporation of incidental teaching into the daily routine begins with an assessment to determine what skills will be the focus of attention. Then, the environment is arranged to increase the probability of an incidental teaching interaction. For example, if the goal is to have the child request toys using adjective-noun combinations during freeplay, toys are placed where the child cannot obtain them without assistance (e.g., on a high shelf). During freeplay, the teacher waits until the child initiates a request or begins an interaction. If there are no emergencies to attend to or other distracting events occurring, the teacher can begin an instructional trial. The teacher focuses attention on the child and determines what level of response is desired and what level of prompt may be necessary. If the child responds incorrectly (e.g., only points to the toys or uses a single word), the teacher provides a prompt. The level of prompt varies for each child, but generally the least intrusive prompt is provided. If the response continues to be incorrect, the teacher provides a more intrusive prompt. If the child responds correctly, he or she is praised and is given the toys.

Mand-Model Strategy The mand-model strategy (Rogers-Warren & Warren, 1980) is the second naturalistic training approach. This approach differs from incidental teaching in that a child initiation is not required to begin the teaching interaction. A trial begins with the teacher initiating a *mand* (a task question or direction) related to the child's focus of attention. The teaching interaction then follows.

Preparation for using the mand-model strategy begins with the teacher altering the environment to provide a variety of materials that attract the child's attention. As in incidental teaching, the child must be assessed to determine what skills are going to be taught and what levels of prompting are required prior to using this strategy. When the child approaches the materials, the teacher mands (e.g., "Tell me what that is."). If the child does not respond or gives a minimal response, the teacher provides a prompt (model). Again, the least intrusive level of prompt for that child is the better prompt. If the child responds appropriately to the mand or to the prompt, the teacher praises the child and provides the materials.

Naturalistic Time-Delay Procedure The third naturalistic training strategy is the naturalistic time-delay (Halle, Marshall, & Spradlin, 1979). The time-delay strategy is designed to provide more opportunities or reasons for children to respond, and to teach them to respond to physical or visual cues rather than adult verbalizations. This strategy is more of an environmental modification, but it is mediated by the teacher.

The time-delay strategy begins with the teacher identifying regularly occurring routines in the environment. Next, the teacher analyzes the routines in order to pinpoint steps where instruction can be provided. Such steps are usually those points where the teacher is currently providing assistance to the child or not promoting independence. Again, the child must be assessed to determine what skills are appropriate during the trial. A trial begins when the child comes to the identified step in a routine. The teacher does not speak and delays assistance for a predetermined number of seconds. The teacher provides a visual prompt, such as looking at what the child needs or holding out the item. At this point, the teacher faces the child with an expectant look and checks to see if he or she is paying attention, at least intermittently, to what is happening in the environment. If the child is not intermittently oriented, then the teacher moves closer to the child or provides a visual prompt. If the child responds correctly before the delay period ends, he or she is praised and provided the item. If the child responds incorrectly or not at all, the teacher provides the designated prompt. Correct responses to the prompt are followed by the child receiving the item. The rules for prompting remain the same for this strategy.

In short, incidental teaching, the mand-model procedure, and naturalistic time-delay are teaching strategies that take advantage of natural environments where children actually use the skills they are taught. All three naturalistic training strategies have been found effective with a variety of populations. Research has demonstrated the role of naturalistic training in facilitating generalization of skills trained and in skill maintenance. Results of selected studies are summarized in Table 15.1.

Commonalities between Naturalistic Training Techniques

Naturalistic training techniques share several common features, the first being that they all take place in the natural environment. For this reason, naturalistic training techniques are sometimes referred to as *milieu training* techniques (Halle, 1987). This environment is not restricted to freeplay or snack times, but can also include planned academic activities (Campbell & Stremel-Campbell, 1982; Halle et al., 1981; Neef et al., 1984; Peck, 1985; Stowitschek et al., 1985) or daily routines (Halle et al., 1979; Schepis et al., 1982).

The second common feature is that all of these training techniques involve some arrangement of the environment. This arrangement is oriented toward facilitating the natural occurrence of the target behavior. Arrangement of the environment also includes training staff to facilitate target behaviors.

A third common feature of these techniques is that they all involve programmed natural consequences. The use of natural consequences in a training program is considered to be a feature that aids generalization (Stokes & Baer, 1977). In many research studies, receiving a desired item is the natural consequence (e.g., Cavallaro & Poulson, 1985; Halle et al., 1979, 1981; Hart & Risley, 1974). Other natural consequences include positive teacher/child interactions (Peck, 1985) or positive child/child interactions (Stowitschek et al., 1985). Desirable activities can also become natural consequences. For example, in the Social Integration Program (Rule et al., 1987), the natural consequence for learning how to zip a jacket was getting to go outside to play.

The use of a continuum of prompts is the fourth feature that is common to

Table 15.1. Selected studies in natural environment

Study	Strategies	Population	Goals	Effect
Hart and Risley (1968, 1974, 1975)	Incidental teaching	Disadvantaged preschoolers	Verbal adjective/noun requests to compound sentences	Prompted and unprompted language increased
Cavallaro and Poulson (1985)	Incidental teaching	Developmentally delayed, language-delayed children	Verbal response to pictures	Increased spontaneous speech
Rogers-Warren and Warren (1980)	Mand-model strategy and one-to-one language training	Moderate to severe language-delayed children	Increase vocabulary and utterance complexity	Verbalization rates at least doubled, increase in newly trained words and grammatical forms
McGee, Krantz, Mason, and McClannahan (1983)	Mand-model strategy (modified incidental teaching)	Autistic children	Teach receptive labeling skills	Unprompted object identification
Warren, McQuarter, and Rogers-Warren (1984)	Mand-model strategy in a natural environment	Speech and language impaired preschoolers	Increase verbal initiations, verbalizations, and two-word utterances	Generalized skills to other settings; maintained skills
Fabry, Mayhew, and Hanson (1984)	Mand-model strategy; incidental teaching	Mentally retarded children	Teach sight-word vocabularies	Acquired sight-word vocabularies
Halle, Marshall, and Spradlin (1979)	Naturalistic time-delay procedure	Mentally retarded adolescents	Teach subjects to request meal trays	Requested their trays; generalized skill to another meal
Halle, Baer, and Spradlin (1981)	Naturalistic time-delay procedure	Moderately handicapped children	Ask for worksheets during academic activity, helpings during snack, toys during freeplay, toys to be handled during sharing period	Vocalization increased in each setting

Oliver and Halle (1982)	Naturalistic time-delay procedure and incidental teaching	Mentally retarded child	Teach functional sign use	Increased use of sign initiations
Schepis, Reid, Fitzgerald, Faw, van den Pol, and Welty (1982)	Modified incidental teaching	Profoundly retarded and autistic children	Increase manual signing using direct-care personnel in a ward setting	Significant increase in signing
Campbell and Stremel-Campbell (1982)	Incidental teaching and mand-model strategy	Moderately mentally retarded children	Teach the use of three syntactic structures (language behavior)	Increased use of syntactic structures; generalized effects in freeplay setting
Neef, Walters, and Egel (1984)	Mand-model strategy and embedded instruction	Developmentally delayed children	Train appropriate yes/no responses	Generalization to action, possession, and spatial relation questions
Peck (1985)	Naturalistic time-delay procedure and mand-model strategy	Autistic and/or mentally retarded children	Increase social/communication behavior	Produced small increases that were generalized to other tasks
Stowitschek, Czajkowski, Rule, Striefel, Innocenti, and Boswell (1985)	Coincidental teaching	Developmentally delayed children	Teach social interaction skills	Social interaction increased; generalized to a freeplay setting

all of these techniques. All procedures use prompts when incorrect responses are given. The goal of prompting is to obtain a correct response while giving the least amount of assistance possible. Many of the most recent studies using these naturalistic training techniques make use of the time-delay procedure, to some degree, because a delay is a nonintrusive prompt and many handicapped children need a longer time to respond (e.g., Campbell & Stremel-Campbell, 1982; Cavallaro & Poulson, 1985; Peck, 1985). If the target behavior does not occur in response to the delay, then more intrusive prompts are required. Halle (1987) discusses this continuum of prompts as it relates to spontaneous language production. Halle (1987) states that the final goal is for the child to exhibit the target behavior without cues from the teacher but in the presence of natural interceptive and contextual stimuli (e.g., the desire to talk and the presence of a listener). The prompts that are used must be consistent with the goals for any child.

Trends in Naturalistic Training

Naturalistic training tends to combine the three strategies. By combining them, it is possible to make use of the best aspects of all three. The mand-model strategy, according to research results, has the strongest generalization effects and the best maintenance capacity of all three techniques (Wolery, Ault, Doyle, & Gast, 1987). Another advantage of the mand-model strategy is that the training trial can be initiated by the teacher. In the time-delay procedure and incidental teaching strategies, the child initiates the trial. This may be a possible drawback as many handicapped children initiate infrequently. The teacher can combine these procedures (taking advantage of their strong features) to overcome drawbacks.

The following example describes how the combined techniques can be used. Begin by evaluating the environment and arranging it to promote the target behavior (e.g., requesting objects). The environment is arranged so that the child must ask the teacher for the desired objects. During freeplay, the child approaches the teacher. Along with making eye contact with the child, the teacher delays vocalizing—a first level of prompting. If the child initiates and responds inappropriately, the correct responses can be prompted (incidental teaching). If the child does not initiate, the teacher can provide a mand and then a prompt for a correct response. In all cases, once the child responds correctly, the child receives the desired object.

Language behaviors have been the most frequent target of intervention when using naturalistic training techniques. However, other behaviors can also be promoted. For example, interventions with manual signing (Oliver & Halle, 1982; Schepis et al., 1982), sight-word vocabulary (Fabry et al., 1984), and social/communicative behaviors (Peck, 1985) have been successful. In addi-

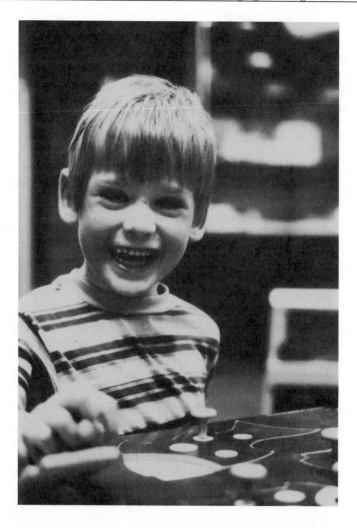

tion, social skills have been successfully facilitated in the natural environment (Stowitschek et al., 1985). A curriculum to teach social skills exists that focuses on using naturalistic training techniques in the environment (Rule, Killoran, Stowitschek, & Innocenti, in press). Self-help skills such as zipping a coat and brushing teeth have been targeted using naturalistic training techniques (Kayser et al., 1986; Rule et al., 1987). Research has demonstrated that intervention can be focused on training new responses and not on facilitating the use of trained responses in new environments (e.g., Cavallaro & Poulson, 1985). Clearly, there are a variety of skills that can be developed by means of naturalistic training techniques.

Facilitating Generalization

Research findings support the usefulness of naturalistic training strategies for promoting the generalization of skills trained. Receiving training in a natural environment makes it easier for the child to apply new skills to other natural settings. Even so, the child does not always spontaneously use the skill in untrained situations. Educators using naturalistic training techniques must actively plan to help the child generalize by taking into account those factors that are essential for success.

First, teachers must examine the types of skills targeted for instruction. Are they skills that a child uses over and over again in a variety of situations? Is the child being reinforced for displaying these skills? If a skill is not reinforced when it occurs, the child is not likely to use it again. In other words, teachers must select those skills that can be naturally reinforced and that are useful to the child rather than merely convenient or functional for others in the child's environment. (See Chapter 8 for a discussion of appropriate goal selection.) Skills that attract appropriate attention from parents, other adults, and other children are more likely to generalize than skills that do not.

In addition, skills should be useful in more than one situation and in settings that offer frequent opportunities for use. The greater the opportunities, the more likely that generalization will occur and maintain itself because the child will have more chances to recognize appropriate cues for the skill and receive more frequent reinforcement for performing it. This is especially the case with communication or language skills (see Chapter 9).

During the process of goal selection, it must be determined whether the child may already know how to perform a skill in some, but not all, settings. In such an instance, the child's IEP should specify the natural environments in which training and generalization will take place. For example, if the goal is independent hand washing, the child may be able to do this after toileting but not before eating. In such a case, additional training is necessary. Any differences in the targeted environments (and they should be minimal with regard to stimuli and natural consequences) must also be identified prior to instruction in the skill.

Finally, teachers must closely observe and measure the child's progress to determine that generalization has occurred following instruction. If it hasn't, then the reasons must be identified and procedures changed. The data on child performance in the generalization situation should provide clues for making decisions about what strategy to use in solving the problem (data collection during naturalistic training is discussed in a later section in this chapter).

In short, naturalistic training techniques contain the elements of a technology of generalization (Haring, in press) that increases the probability of children learning skills and using them successfully in a variety of settings. This technology emphasizes the selection of appropriate skills (those that are useful and naturally reinforcing); the development of instructional objectives that include generalization; and careful attention to generalization probes, data collection, and the identification of problems that may impede generalization.

Facilitating Peer Interaction

Children with developmental delays must be able to perform new skills in different settings as well as with a variety of people, especially nonhandicapped children. All three naturalistic training techniques (incidental teaching, mandmodel procedure, and naturalistic time-delay) are useful for developing important social skills such as negotiating (e.g., settling differences) or sharing. There are several appropriate intervention strategies that incorporate these techniques for encouraging desirable social interaction between children with handicaps and their nonhandicapped peers (Simpson, 1987).

Teachers may take responsibility for prompting and reinforcing appropriate social behavior. Nevertheless, on the basis of a review of research, McEvoy and Odom (1987) identified as two problems with teacher-mediated interventions the length of training time needed to reduce teacher prompts, and the continued need for highly structured (hence "unnatural") training environments. Other research has demonstrated that the teachers' presence hinders peer interaction (Innocenti et al., 1986). Because most children like to spend time with peers, researchers have investigated the feasibility of peer-mediated interventions as an alternative. The most frequently used strategy calls for peers to act as intervenors (Strain & Odom, 1986). The educator or researcher teaches socially competent peers to direct social initiations to children with developmental delays. When necessary, the teacher may provide verbal prompts or reinforcement to the peer at the end of the interaction session if he or she reaches an established criterion. Alternately, the teacher may show peers how to prompt the desired responses from the child with developmental delays, and then provide the reinforcement themselves. The same techniques can be used with less severely handicapped children acting as mediators (e.g., they are taught to initiate interactions with peers).

To ensure the successful facilitation of peer interaction, educators must take into account certain contextual factors that affect social skill training (McEvoy & Odom, 1987). The type of activity in which children engage determines to a large degree whether they interact with other children or play by themselves. Moreover, nonhandicapped peers in the environment must also be socially competent and responsive to the presence of handicapped classmates in order for social interactions to be naturally rewarding. In addition, social skills training must take place under naturally occurring conditions. Even certain kinds of social interactions among children in the classroom may appear to be contrived when compared to events in other environments. Peer tutoring, for example, is a popular practice in mainstreamed classroom settings. Nevertheless, since the relationship between the peer tutor and the child with developmental delays is not based on the equal role status that normally exists among peers, it is doubtful whether any interactional skills learned in the classroom can be generalized to the natural settings of home and community (Simpson, 1987).

Recent research on elementary school students with behavioral disorders emphasized the importance of a natural physical environment and the natural reinforcement of behavior by peers, a process called *entrapment* (McConnell, 1987). When the social behaviors of the handicapped child change positively, they require reinforcement from nonhandicapped peers during interventions in naturalistic settings in order to become entrapped or embedded in the child's behavioral repertoire. If such behaviors are thoroughly learned, they are likely to generalize to new settings and circumstances long after intervention is complete.

In the process of entrapment, as in facilitating generalization, the teacher who wants to promote skill development through social interaction must: 1) focus on behaviors that will be maintained after intervention, 2) select skills that will generalize across settings or other behaviors (e.g., sharing), and 3) choose target behaviors that either reliably follow specific peer initiations or precede positive peer responses (McConnell, 1987).

The application of naturalistic training procedures in unstructured settings with nonhandicapped peers taking the lead is one way to ensure that children with developmental delays acquire and maintain the social skills they need to function in everyday life.

COINCIDENTAL TEACHING

The term *coincidental teaching* is used to describe teaching that coincides with other activities that occur on a daily basis (Stowitschek et al., 1985). It is a naturalistic training technique that incorporates aspects of incidental teaching, the mand-model technique, and the time-delayed procedure. It has been used to teach language skills, social skills, and self-help skills. It may be the primary strategy for teaching a skill, or it may be used in conjunction with individualized training programs. A model/demonstration early intervention project, the Social Integration Program (Rule et al., 1987), has frequently used this procedure with success (Fiechtl et al., 1986; Rule et al., 1987; Stowitschek et al., 1985).

Coincidental teaching contains those elements common to all naturalistic training techniques: 1) training occurs in the context of using a skill when it would naturally be expected to occur; 2) the environment is arranged to facilitate the natural occurrence of the target behavior; 3) there is a continuum of prompts, with the least restrictive prompt being the most preferred; and 4) natural consequences, along with social reinforcement, result from engaging in the desired behavior. It is important to remember that coincidental teaching is a *planned procedure* that *focuses on a specific skill* that has been targeted because the child needs to master that skill.

Procedures for using coincidental teaching follow a specific format. First, the child is assessed to determine skills that need to be targeted for intervention. Second, a selection is made for those skills that can be taught in the natural environment. Generally, language, self-help, and social skills are appropriate for coincidental teaching. Third, assessment of the classroom environment is made to determine possible times for teaching these skills. In order to perform step three, it may be helpful to task analyze the school day. This can be done by dividing a sheet of paper into three columns. Record in the first column the schedule for an entire school day, including transition times, freeplay activities, and mealtimes. It is beneficial to break larger activities into their smaller components. For example, the breakdown of snack time activity may be as follows: 1) utensils and plates placed on table, 2) children come to table, 3) children sit, 4) teacher passes out snack, 5) children eat, and 6) children clean up on their own when finished.

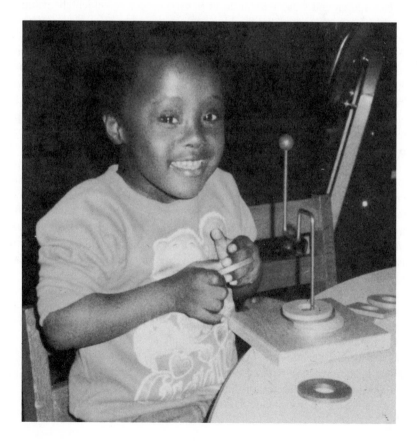

After completing this classroom task analysis, the second column can be used for writing (next to each activity) the skills that can be taught during the various components of the activity. By examining each activity, the best method for facilitating the occurrence of targeted skills can be determined. Procedures for each task can be written in the third column. Using the above example, the following teaching activities may be possible: 1) have two children work together to set out utensils, but they need to ask the teacher for utensils; 2) instead of the teacher passing out food to quiet children, each child must ask for the snack using a request appropriate to his or her language skills; and 3) when children leave the table, they must say "excuse me" and/or state what they are going to do next.

After completing the assessment of the environment for appropriate activities and possible skills that can be taught using coincidental teaching, the classroom activities can be altered to facilitate the natural occurrence of these skills. Procedures should be taken directly from the third column of the environmental assessment. Child assessment data can then be used to determine which children and what skills need to be targeted for coincidental teaching, and during what activities the teaching can occur.

In some activities, such as asking for a snack, coincidental teaching may occur for all children in the class. The teacher's behavior would not differ dramatically from child to child, except in regard to prompts for each individual child. Each child, however, would have to respond using language skills appropriate to the developmental goals. At other times, only one or two children may be targeted for coincidental teaching. For example, two children may frequently fight over table items. Coincidentally teaching these two children how to settle differences would be appropriate.

The third step in implementing coincidental teaching is to determine the specific teaching strategy to be used for each skill and/or child. The specific strategy will identify the type of mand, if any, that will be used by the teacher, and the length of the delay, if one is to be used. Also defined are the specific prompting strategies to be used. These can be child or skill specific. A general prompting strategy can be established for many skills. A general strategy, if used, should progress from the least intrusive prompt (delay or mand) to more intrusive prompts (model or physical guidance).

When conducting a coincidental teaching episode, it is important to remember that the spontaneous (unprompted) occurrence of a behavior is as important as a prompted one. Appropriate responses, prompted or unprompted, are considered part of the coincidental teaching episode. The unprompted responses are the desired outcome (cf. Halle, 1987). If the child continuously responds appropriately without prompting, then the goal has been achieved, and new goals should be set for him or her.

The final step in coincidental teaching is providing the consequences for the child's response. The primary consequence should be the one that is naturally occurring. This could be the child getting what he asked for, engaging in a social interaction, or moving on to another activity. Praise should be a secondary consequence from the teacher. Praise can be provided after a child-initiated or a prompted response.

Data Collection

Data collection is sometimes difficult when using naturalistic training techniques on a daily basis. Unlike discrete trial programs where a data sheet is available and scoring the responses is part of the teaching sequence, coincidental teaching occurs in the natural environment and data sheets are not usually at hand. Yet, two methods are available for overcoming this obstacle. The first method involves placing data sheets on the walls of the classrooms in areas where coincidental teaching will most likely occur (e.g., near the snack table, on the wall of the freeplay area, near the sink where children brush their teeth, by the door where they zip up their coats). If coincidental teaching occurs in the context of some other teaching activity, the data sheets can be added to the bottom of the already existing data records.

These data sheets should be simple, listing the name of the targeted skill and the children who will be learning that skill. There should also be a code describing the level of prompting needed to elicit the desired response (including spontaneous initiations). The teacher records the date on the data sheet prior to beginning the activity. After a coincidental teaching opportunity occurs, the teacher merely reviews the data sheet and enters the appropriate code.

Although this method of data collection is simple, a teacher can easily forget to enter the data while supervising an activity. This can lead to post activity estimates of what actually occurred. The second method of data collection avoids this problem. Instead of recording data on a daily basis, the teacher selects children and/or skills for observation on a regular basis, approximately once a week. Although this method does not provide daily data, it can generate more accurate data.

Using this method, the teacher observes a few children each day (or in each activity), and uses data sheets to record coincidental teaching episodes as they occur. The teacher does not ignore other children on these days (other children still receive coincidental teaching), but collects data for the designated children only. Using this data collection method for all the children in turn provides a good estimate of each child's skills.

The method used by any teacher to collect data varies based on a number of factors. However, teachers should collect data on a regular basis in order to evaluate the child's skills in relation to the achievement of specific goals. It might also be possible to recruit and train volunteers to collect data (see Chapter 4).

Coincidental Teaching Examples

Planning a lesson requires knowing the goals for each child in the group. Sharing is a social skill that can be taught through coincidental teaching during naturally occurring activities such as freeplay, lunch, and art. To facilitate the occurrence of sharing during art activities, the teacher can modify the environment by limiting the art supplies. The teacher's instructions to the children can stress the fact that they will need to share these supplies. Then, the sequence of prompts that will be used is identified. These environmental modifications, teacher behaviors, and child prompts should be written down on a teaching program plan (cf. Stowitschek, Stowitschek, Hendrickson, & Day, 1984) or other form. The teacher must then determine how many instances of sharing are appropriate for this activity and, once the activity begins, focus on implementing the prescribed number of teaching episodes.

Self-help skills require a slight modification of the coincidental teaching technique used for language or social skills. The need for self-help skills is evident when the child participates in activities in the natural environment. Therefore, it is better to teach self-help skills coincidentally rather than by using a discrete trial method. Coincidental teaching focuses on teaching skills at the times that they should occur. A child learns how to zip his or her coat before going home or out to play, as opposed to learning the same skill in a 10-trial session in the middle of the day. The consequences for the same behavior (going out to play versus a star on a chart) are very different, the first being much more natural.

When teaching self-help skills, the teacher must identify the activities where the skills fit naturally, then task analyze the skills and develop prompts to be used with each step. All of this should be written down. The teacher then sets the context for engaging in a skill by saying, for example, "No one can go out until he or she has his or her jacket zipped." The teacher would then focus on the child targeted to learn this skill. With self-help skills, the first step should always be a planned delay to see what the child does on his or her own. As the child completes the steps of the task, the teacher checks off on the task analysis sheet those steps done independently. When the child makes an incorrect response, the teacher intervenes and prompts, as needed, through the final steps of the task. When the child completes the task, the teacher praises the child, allowing him or her to move to the next activity (e.g., freeplay).

Training Staff to use Naturalistic Methods

Staff training does not appear to be a major issue when using naturalistic training techniques. Studies in which researchers have trained others in using these techniques have not reported problems (Cavallaro & Poulson, 1985; Halle et al., 1981; Neef et al., 1984; Peck, 1985; Schepis et al., 1982). In fact, there have been reports of the staff generalizing the use of these techniques to other activities (Halle et al., 1981). In addition, the social validation of naturalistic training techniques has made the staff willing to implement them (Schepis et al., 1982). Also, naturalistic training techniques have a positive effect on the training environment (Peck, 1985).

Mudd and Wolery (1987) conducted a systematic evaluation of teachers trained to use incidental teaching. In-service training was sufficient for two of the four teachers, whereas the other two teachers needed written and verbal feedback on their use of incidental teaching in the classroom before they were able to use it on a regular basis. Mudd and Wolery (1987) observed concurrent increases in child target behaviors after the teachers had learned incidental teaching.

These results from the research literature suggest that one would expect few difficulties when training staff in how to use these techniques. However, trainers should use organized preservice or in-service training procedures (cf. Mudd & Wolery, 1987) or programs with explicit directions on how to teach these techniques (e.g., Fiechtl et al., 1986).

Training procedures must be clearly outlined, and data on the accomplishment of program objectives must be available. Naturalistic training does not mean unstructured training. Nor does it mean that activities are not based on specific child goals. Components of naturalistic teaching are based on normal modes of interaction with developing children (Hart, 1985) and, as such, occur to some degree in interactions with all developmentally young learners. Therefore, this form of teaching is familiar to adults who have had experience with young children. When educators use naturalistic training techniques for specific goals, rather than as a general interaction strategy, training for teachers must maintain the best practices of special education programming (cf. Stowitschek et al., 1984), including accurate data collection procedures (see later section in this chapter).

PARENTS AS INTERVENORS
IN THE NATURAL ENVIRONMENT

Parental involvement in the education of a handicapped child has received renewed interest with the passage of Public Law 99-457. What is the best way to involve parents? In many programs, the most effective techniques (e.g., discrete trial training) have been taken from the classroom and taught to parents for use at home (Baker, 1976), but not without problems. Parents report difficulty in implementing this type of training (Culatta & Horn, 1981; MacDonald, Blott, Gordon, Spiegal, & Hartmann, 1974), and the end result may be an increase in the overall stress levels of the family (cf. Doernberg, 1978). This is an unnecessary situation. Instead, parents could also use informal modes of instruction (Baker, Heifetz, & Murphy, 1980; Culatta & Horn, 1981). There is also evidence to suggest that keeping parents involved as trainers and having them participate in their child's education can have positive effects (Baker, 1976; MacDonald et al., 1974). These positive effects on the parents could benefit all family members and help reduce their stress.

Teaching parents to use naturalistic training techniques may be an alternative that would overcome problems encountered with more formal modes of teaching. Naturalistic training techniques are less formal because they are based on teaching interactions that occur naturally between the parent and child (Hart, 1985). For parents of children with handicaps, these natural training episodes need to become more consistent and systematic (Wulz, Myers, Klein, Hall, & Waldo, 1982). Naturalistic training techniques meet this requirement.

There are many potential advantages when parents are taught to use naturalistic training techniques for functional skills. The skills taught are relevant to the parents because of their functional nature. For example, teaching parents to focus on increasing their child's length of utterance has more social validity than teaching the child to sort objects. Because the training occurs in the natural context, the probability of the parents actually training skills increases (Culatta & Horn, 1981; MacDonald et al., 1974). By involving the entire family in training, family stress can potentially be decreased (cf. Doernberg, 1978). The training of skills in more than one setting (e.g., school, home) with multiple trainers (e.g., teachers, family members) increases the probability of skills generalizing and becoming functional once acquired (cf. Stokes & Baer, 1977). Parents, when taught to use techniques that are part of natural training, have generalized their skills to new settings (Culatta & Horn, 1981; Salzberg & Villani, 1983). These factors, combined with the advantages of naturalistic training techniques (i.e., naturally occurring stimuli, natural consequences), suggest a powerful and valid training strategy.

Strategies for Training Parents

Wulz et al. (1982) described a home-centered model for communication training that makes use of naturalistic training techniques. This model, called unobtrusive training, consisted of the following two components: 1) *environmental interactions* and 2) *teaching interactions*. During environmental interaction training, parents learn how to recognize communicative behavior and potential training opportunities. Parents receive environmental interaction training during an interview, when the parent and trainer discuss the child's behavior in different situations and identify examples of different communicative responses along with alternative, more appropriate responses. Parents learn to identify communicative contexts and observe the child for spontaneous target responses.

Parents also learn teaching interactions to use when the target responses do not occur spontaneously. They learn how to provide reinforcement for appropriate behavior, to model desired actions, and to use incidental teaching techniques. The training focuses on using these techniques in brief teaching interactions.

In another approach for teaching parents to use naturalistic training techniques, Innocenti, Rule, Killoran, and Stowitschek (1983) developed a curriculum for parents to teach social skills based on the coincidental teaching model (Stowitschek et al., 1985). During a workshop, parents are trained to use prompting strategies for engaging their children in appropriate behaviors and to deliver praise. Parents then learn how to identify appropriate occasions for teaching social skills.

The curriculum consists of three teaching strategies that parents can use with lessons that cover 26 different social skills. These teaching strategies include home lessons, home rehearsals, and coincidental teaching. Home lessons are short, didactic interchanges between parent and child where they discuss the use of a social skill. These exchanges involve the entire family and make all family members aware of the skill being taught. Home rehearsals are brief sessions where the parent, child, and siblings model and practice the appropriate use of a social skill. Coincidental teaching is the use of the naturalistic training technique at times appropriate for the social skill to be practiced. Parents receive home social opportunity cards that provide examples of situations where the skill might be coincidentally taught and implementation strategies for doing so.

Unfortunately, neither Wulz et al. (1982) nor Innocenti et al. (1983) present any data on changes in child or parent behavior as a result of implementing their respective parent training packages. However, the results of some empirical studies suggest that the techniques used in these training packages are valid approaches to parent training.

Empirical Support for Parents as Intervenors

Very little research has focused on the effects of parent and child behavior after teaching parents to use a variety of naturalistic training techniques. Instead, most of the research has been aimed at teaching parents specific skills that could be used in the natural environment, and the results of this training on parent and child behavior have been reviewed. One study that focused specifically on training parents in the use of a naturalistic training technique (incidental training) was conducted by Albert and Rogers-Warren (1983, March). They taught parents to use incidental teaching with their language-delayed children in the home setting. Mothers successfully learned how to use incidental teaching and observed improvements in their child's language skills.

Matson (1981) taught a group of mothers to reduce a clinical fear of strangers in their young mentally retarded children. The mothers received training to implement a variety of procedures with their children in a clinic setting. Each mother learned how to rehearse the appropriate skill prior to a planned meeting with a stranger. She also learned how to implement procedures at home. In addition, she learned how to prompt the desired behavior in the appropriate setting if it did not spontaneously occur. The mothers were successful intervenors. The dependent measures used in the study (approaching strangers, number of words spoken to strangers, and self-ratings of fear) changed in the desired direction and were similar to responses of matched nonfearful children. Treatment gains generalized to the home setting and were maintained at a 6-month follow-up.

Salzberg and Villani (1983) studied the acquisition and generalization of vocal imitation training skills by parents of preschoolers with Down syndrome. Parents were taught to use modeling, prompting, and feedback techniques in a preschool setting. They acquired the skills, and concurrent improvements in vocal imitation occurred, but the parent skills did not generalize to a home freeplay setting. Parents then learned how to use their new skills in the home setting and were given feedback based on audiotapes of the parent and child at home. The parents then demonstrated the use of the skills in the home environment, and concomitant increases occurred in the children's vocal imitation and spontaneous verbalization.

Powell, Salzberg, Rule, Levy, and Itzkowitz (1983) evaluated a training package to increase appropriate play behaviors in children, using parents as trainers. The play behavior of four children with handicaps and their siblings served as the dependent variable. Parents attended a workshop where they received instruction on how to: 1) identify, prompt, and praise appropriate play behavior; 2) select toys and activities that promote play; 3) manage inappropriate behavior; and 4) sequence training using their new skills. Following the workshop, parents conducted short teaching sessions with their children 3 times per week. Parents used prompting and praising skills appropriately. All of the children in the families increased appropriate play behavior. This increase generalized for three of the four families to a setting where the parents were absent.

This brief review of empirical research using parents as intervenors demonstrates that parents can successfully learn and implement the skills necessary for naturalistic training in the home environment. More research is needed to determine which are the best training practices, how to maintain these parent skills, and how to use the skills after the training period ends. The research reviewed on this topic is positive.

SUMMARY

The use of naturalistic training techniques appears to be an effective strategy for teaching certain skills in school and at home. Language, social, and self-help skills have all been taught successfully at school since teachers are able to learn naturalistic training techniques without difficulty. Parents are able to utilize the teaching strategies involved in naturalistic training techniques. For the child, the skills acquired through these techniques are functional, generalizable, and maintained after training. In addition to these advantages, the naturalistic teaching strategies are a logical method to manage behavior and teach at the same time. The interactions are brief, capitalizing on a preschool child's attentional skills, and are an effective one-to-one way to teach.

Although naturalistic training techniques have been proven effective, there are questions that remain to be addressed. Educators have not yet determined what skills are best taught through naturalistic training techniques, through more traditional techniques, or through a combination of both. No information is available on children's handicaps as they relate to the efficacy of learning in the natural environment. The best practices for teaching parents to use these techniques must be elucidated. Empirical studies are needed to address these and other issues.

At present, though, naturalistic training techniques have been used successfully with many different skills, with a variety of children with different handicapping conditions. These techniques have been adapted for many different environments. For working with developmentally young children, the advantages of naturalistic training techniques are especially evident and warrant their implementation.

STUDY QUESTIONS

1. Observe in a center-based early intervention program during snack time and list the skills with which teachers assist children.

2. Go on a field trip with a preschool group and note the number of times that the teacher takes the children to the restroom.

3. Observe the greeting of each child to determine how the teacher simultaneously greets the child, how he or she handles the removal of clothing, and how he or she handles the separation anxiety displayed by the child (or parent).

4. Observe a teacher as he or she interacts with different children concerning various goals or problems. Note the difference in facial expression and tone of voice.

REFERENCES

Alpert, C. L., & Rogers-Warren, A. (1983, March). *Mothers as incidental language trainers of their language-disordered children.* Paper presented at the Annual Gatlinburg Conference on Research in Mental Retardation and Developmental Disabilities, Gatlinburg, TN. (ERIC Document Reproduction Service No. ED 247 675).

Baker, B. B. (1976). Parent involvement in programming for developmentally disabled children. In L. L. Lloyd (Ed.), *Communication assessment and intervention strategies* (pp.691–733). Baltimore: University Park Press.

Baker, B. L., Heifetz, L. J., & Murphy, D. M. (1980). Behavioral training for parents of mentally retarded children: One-year follow-up. *American Journal of Mental Deficiency, 85,* 31–38.

Berler, E. S., Gross, A. M., & Drabman, R. S. (1982). Social skills training with children: Proceed with caution. *Journal of Applied Behavior Analysis, 15,* 41–53.

Blank, M., & Solomon, F. (1968). A tutorial language program to develop abstract thinking in socially disadvantaged preschool children. *Child Development, 39,* 379–389.

Campbell, C. R., & Stremel-Campbell, K. (1982). Programming "loose training" as a strategy to facilitate language generalization. *Journal of Applied Behavior Analysis, 15,* 295–301.

Casto, G., & Mastropieri, M. A. (1986). The efficacy of early intervention: A meta-analysis. *Exceptional Children, 52,* 417–424.

Casto, G., & White, K. (1985). The efficacy of early intervention programs with environmentally at-risk infants. *Journal of Children in Contemporary Society, 17,* 37–50.

Cavallaro, C. C., & Poulson, C. L. (1985). Teaching language to handicapped children in natural settings. *Education and Treatment of Children, 8,* 1–24.

Cruickshank, W. M., Bentzen, L. A., Ratzeborg, F. H., & Tannhauser, M. (1961). *Teaching methodology for brain-injured and hyperactive children.* Syracuse, NY: Syracuse University Press.

Culatta, B., & Horn, D. (1981). Systematic modification of parental input to train language symbols. *Language, Speech, and Hearing Services in the Schools, 12,* 4–12.

Doernberg, N. L. (1978). Some negative effects on family integration of health and educational services for young handicapped children. *Rehabilitation Literature, 39,* 107–110.

Fabry, B. D., Mayhew, G. L., & Hanson, A. (1984). Incidental teaching of mentally retarded students within a token system. *American Journal of Mental Deficiency, 89,* 29–36.

Fiechtl, B., Bonem, M., Morgan, J. T., Innocenti, M. S., Rule, S., & Stowitschek, J. J. (1986). *Coincidental teaching: A packet for trainers of preschool and day care staff.* Logan: Outreach, Development, and Dissemination Division, Utah State University Affiliated Developmental Center for Handicapped Persons.

Gresham, F. M. (1981). Social skills training with handicapped children: A review. *Review of Educational Research, 51,* 139–176.

Guess, D., Keogh, W., & Sailor, W. (1978). Generalization of speech and language behavior: Measurement and training tactics. In R. L. Schiefelbusch (Ed.), *Bases of language intervention* (pp. 373–395). Baltimore: University Park Press.

Halle, J. W. (1982). Teaching functional language to the handicapped: An integrative model of natural environment teaching techniques. *Journal of The Association for the Severely Handicapped, 7,* 29–37.

Halle, J. W. (1987). Teaching language in the natural environment: An analysis of spontaneity. *Journal of The Association for Persons with Severe Handicaps, 12,* 28–37.

Halle, J. W., Alpert, C. L., & Anderson, S. R. (1984). Natural environment language assessment and intervention with severely impaired preschoolers. *Topics in Early Childhood Special Education, 4*(2), 36–56.

Halle, J. W., Baer, D. M., & Spradlin, J. E. (1981). Teachers' generalized use of delay as a stimulus control procedure to increase language use in handicapped children. *Journal of Applied Behavior Analysis, 14,* 389–409.

Halle, J. W., Marshall, A. M., & Spradlin, J. E. (1979). Time delay: A technique to increase language use and facilitate generalization in retarded children. *Journal of Applied Behavior Analysis, 12,* 431–439.

Haring, N. G. (in press). A technology of generalization. In N. G. Haring (Ed.), *Generalization: Strategies and solutions for severely handicapped students.* Seattle: University of Washington.

Haring, N. G., & Phillips, L. L. (1962). *Educating emotionally disturbed children.* New York: McGraw-Hill.

Hart, B. (1985). Naturalistic language training techniques. In S. F. Warren & A. K. Rogers-Warren (Eds.), *Teaching functional language: Generalization and maintenance of language skills* (pp. 133–148). Baltimore: University Park Press.

Hart, B., & Risley, T. (1968). Establishing use of descriptive adjectives in the spontaneous speech of disadvantaged preschool children. *Journal of Applied Behavior Analysis, 1,* 109–120.

Hart, B., & Risley, T. (1974). Using preschool materials to modify the language of disadvantaged children. *Journal of Applied Behavior Analysis, 7,* 243–256.

Hart, B., & Risley, T. (1975). Incidental teaching of language in the preschool. *Journal of Applied Behavior Analysis, 8,* 411–420.

Hoyson, M., Jamieson, B., & Strain, P. S. (1984). Individualized group instruction of normally developing and autistic-like children: The LEAP curriculum model. *Journal of the Division for Early Childhood, 8,* 157–172.

Innocenti, M. S., Rule, S., Killoran, J., & Stowitschek, J. J. (1983). *The Let's Be Social home program.* Logan: Outreach, Development, and Dissemination Division, Utah State University Affiliated Developmental Center for Handicapped Persons.

Innocenti, M. S., Stowitschek, J. J., Rule, S., Killoran, J., Striefel, S., & Boswell, C. (1986). A naturalistic study of the relation between preschool setting events and peer interaction in four activity contexts. *Early Childhood Research Quarterly, 1,* 141–153.

Kayser, J. E., Billingsley, F. F., & Neel, R. S. (1986). A comparison of in-context and traditional instructional approaches: Total task, single trial versus backward chaining, multiple trials. *Journal of The Association for Persons With Severe Handicaps, 11,* 28–38.

Lehane, S., & Goldman, R. (1976). An adaptive model for individualizing young children's learning in school and at home. *The Elementary School Journal, 6,* 373–380.

MacDonald, J. D., Blott, J. P., Gordon, K., Spiegal, B., & Hartmann, M. (1974). An experimental parent-assisted treatment program for preschool language-delayed children. *Journal of Speech and Hearing Disorders, 39,* 395–415.

Matson, J. L. (1981). Assessment and treatment of clinical fears in mentally retarded children. *Journal of Applied Behavior Analysis, 14,* 287–294.

McConnell, S. R. (1987). Entrapment effects and the generalization and maintenance of social skills training for elementary school students with behavioral disorders. *Behavioral Disorders, 12,* 252–263.

McEvoy, M. A., & Odom, S. L. (1987). Social interaction training for preschool children with behavioral disorders. *Behavioral Disorders, 12,* 242–251.

McGee, G. G., Krantz, P. J., Mason, D., & McClannahan, L. E. (1983). A modified incidental-teaching procedure for autistic youth: Acquisition and generalization of receptive object labels. *Journal of Applied Behavior Analysis, 16,* 329–338.

Mudd, J. M., & Wolery, M. (1987). Training Head Start teachers to use incidental teaching. *Journal of the Division for Early Childhood, 11,* 124–134.

Neef, N. A., Walters, J., & Egel, A. L. (1984). Establishing generative yes/no responses in developmentally disabled children. *Journal of Applied Behavior Analysis, 17,* 453–460.

Oliver, C. B., & Halle, J. W. (1982). Language training in the everyday environment:

Teaching functional sign use to a retarded child. *Journal of The Association for the Severely Handicapped, 7*(3), 50–62.

Peck, C. A. (1985). Increasing opportunities for social control by children with autism and severe handicaps: Effects on student behavior and perceived classroom climate. *Journal of The Association for Persons with Severe Handicaps, 10,* 183–193.

Powell, T. H., Salzberg, C. L., Rule, S., Levy, S., & Itzkowitz, J. S. (1983). Teaching mentally retarded children to play with their siblings using parents as trainers. *Education and Treatment of Children, 6,* 343–362.

Rogers-Warren, A., & Warren, S. F. (1980). Mands for verbalization: Facilitating the display of newly trained language in children. *Behavior Modification, 4,* 361–382.

Rule, S., Killoran, J., Stowitschek, J. J., & Innocenti, M. S. (in press). *Let's be social.* Los Angeles: Communication Skill Builders

Rule, S., Killoran, J., Stowitschek, J. J., Innocenti, M. S., & Striefel, S. (1985). Training and support for mainstream day care staff. *Early Childhood Development and Care, 20,* 99–113.

Rule, S., Stowitschek, J. J., Innocenti, M. S., Striefel, S., Killoran, J., Swezey, K., & Boswell, C. (1987). The Social Integration Program: An analysis of the effects of mainstreaming handicapped children into day care centers. *Education and Treatment of Children, 10,* 175–192.

Salzberg, C. L., & Villani, T. V. (1983). Speech training by parents of Down syndrome toddlers: Generalization across settings and instructional contexts. *American Journal of Mental Deficiency, 87,* 403–413.

Schepis, M. M., Reid, D. H., Fitzgerald, J. R., Faw, G. D., van den Pol, R. A., & Welty, P. A. (1982). A program for increasing manual signing by autistic and profoundly retarded youth within the daily environment. *Journal of Applied Behavior Analysis, 15,* 363–379.

Simpson, R. L. (1987). Social interactions of behaviorally disordered children and youth: Where are we and where do we need to go? *Behavioral Disorders, 12,* 292–298.

Stokes, T. F., & Baer, D. M. (1977). An implicit technology of generalization. *Journal of Applied Behavior Analysis, 10,* 349–367.

Stowitschek, J. J., Czajkowski, L., Rule, S., Striefel, S., Innocenti, M. S., & Boswell, C. (1985). *Systematic programming of social interaction through coincidental teaching.* Logan: Outreach, Development, and Dissemination Division, Utah State University Affiliated Developmental Center for Handicapped Persons.

Stowitschek, J. J., Stowitschek, C. E., Hendrickson, J. M., & Day, R. M. (1984). *Direct teaching tactics for exceptional children.* Rockville, MD: Aspen Systems.

Strain, P. S., & Odom, S. L. (1986). Peer-social initiations: Effective intervention for social skill development of exceptional children. *Exceptional Children, 52,* 543–552.

Tingey-Michaelis, C. (1986). The importance of structure in early education programs for disadvantaged and handicapped children. *Early Child Development and Care, 23*(10), 283–297.

Warren, S. F., McQuarter, R. J., & Rogers-Warren, A. (1984). The effects of mands and models on the speech of unresponsive socially isolated children. *Journal of Speech and Hearing Disorders, 49,* 43–52.

Warren, S. F., & Rogers-Warren, A. (1980). Current perspectives in language remediation. *Education and Treatment of Children, 3,* 133–152.

Wolery, M., Ault, M. J., Doyle, P. M., & Gast, D. L. (1987). *Comparison of instructional strategies: A literature review.* Paper submitted for publication.

Wulz, S. V., Myers, S. P., Klein, M. D., Hall, M. K., & Waldo, L. J. (1982). Unobtrusive training: A home-centered model for communication training. *Journal of The Association for the Severely Handicapped, 7,* 36–47.

Chapter 16

Working with Families in Early Intervention

Nancy M. Johnson-Martin,
Barbara Davis Goldman, and Jean W. Gowen

———————————— ● ————————————

Early interventionists primarily work with parents since, obviously, an infant or young child does not identify him- or herself as handicapped and does not seek intervention services. However, whether those services are sought and the extent to which they are used effectively depends upon the parent and the relationship of the parent with the serviceproviders. This chapter highlights the various roles of the parents and the family in the early intervention process and addresses topics of interest to all persons involved.

ATTITUDES TOWARD PARENTS

In the past 2 decades, there has been a marked shift in attitudes toward the involvement of parents in the educational programs of their handicapped children. Prior to the passage of Public Law 99-142, the Education for All Handicapped Children Act of 1975, parents tended to be viewed as part of the problem and, to some extent, as passive recipients of training or therapeutic efforts by those intending to help the children. The requirements of Public Law 94-142, however, indicated that parents were viewed as part of the solution to the problem: they were invited, indeed required, to some extent, to become active in the development of Individualized Education Programs (IEPs) for their children (Turnbull & Turnbull, 1982). It was recognized that much of the learning in childhood takes place within the family context. Parental involvement was sought specifically to improve the parents' ability to teach their children and support the efforts of others who teach their children. This, in turn, would improve the developmental outcome of handicapped children.

In Public Law 99-457, the Education of the Handicapped Act Amendments of 1986, another shift in attitude is evident. This law established incentives for states to provide special education services to handicapped infants and preschoolers and to enhance the capacity of families to meet the special needs of these children. Rather than implementing only IEPs for handicapped infants or children under the age of 3, interventionists are required to develop Individualized Family Service Plans (IFSPs) for families. In this requirement, there is both the recognition that the child's development and well-being is affected by the functioning of a family system and the acknowledgment that different families may have different service needs.

Family Systems

A recognition of the importance of the family system is a major step forward. It is generally acknowledged that it is stressful to a family to raise a handicapped child. Although many of these families function well, there is evidence of the effects of stress in a number of areas. For instance: 1) even when social class and other factors are controlled, marital satisfaction is lower (Friedrich & Friedrich, 1981) and the divorce rate is higher (Bristol, 1985) among families of handicapped children than among families of nonhandicapped children; and 2) mothers and fathers of handicapped children have been found to be more depressed, to feel less competent, and to enjoy their children less than parents of normal children (Cummings, 1976; Cummings, Bayley, & Rie, 1966).

There is also evidence, however, that good support systems lead to more positive attitudes and outcomes for both parents and their handicapped children (Dunst, Trivette, & Cross, 1986).

These findings indicate that when the demands on the family system exceed its resources, not only may the child not receive optimal parenting, but the whole system may become dysfunctional. Siblings and extended family members may have strengths to offer the family, but they also have needs that must be met. If additional resources are provided to the family, the program can meet the increased demands without dysfunction.

Family Support

Clearly, those working with families of young handicapped children should direct some of their efforts to ensuring better support systems for families. Not as clear are the most effective ways to do that. One place to begin, however, is with the part of the support network that is made up of the professionals who serve these children and families. There is evidence that doctors, therapists, interventionists, and other members of the helping community are more prominent in the support systems of families of handicapped children than in the families of nonhandicapped children (Bristol, 1988; Gowen, Johnson-Martin, & Appelbaum, 1987). The participation of these professionals in the support network is necessary to assure services for the child, but there is always a danger that their efforts will *increase* rather than decrease stress on the family because they misunderstand the family's needs. Before designing program components to help families of handicapped children, it is imperative to look carefully at the kinds of pressures that are exerted on these families. Once these pressures are understood, it is possible to develop parent programs that are supportive to the functioning of the whole family.

PRESSURES ON FAMILIES OF HANDICAPPED CHILDREN

Parental Responsibility

Parenting a child is not an easy task. In our culture, the job is made more difficult by the prevailing tendency to hold parents responsible not only for the physical care and safety of their children, but also for the formation of their personalities and the height of their achievements. Although scientific literature emphasizes the transactional nature of development, which gives some responsibility for outcome to the innate characteristics of the child, mental health professionals continue to attribute most unfavorable outcomes to poor parenting (Caplan & Hall-McCorquodale, 1985). Likewise, teachers, interventionists, and the lay public tend to blame parents for poor child behavior and developmental progress. Many times parents internalize this blame.

Time Demands and Parental Participation

When a child is handicapped, the demands on the parents often increase dramatically. Many of these children have physical problems that require careful monitoring and many trips to physicians, therapists, and other health care providers. Early intervention programs require that time be available to work with the early interventionist who comes to the home, or to transport the child to and from the center-based services. Therapy and/or educational interventions for young children are usually more effective if done daily. Thus, parents may be asked to do specific teaching tasks or therapy at home daily in addition to the weekly therapy sessions and other normal parenting activities. In addition, parents remain responsible for the social and emotional well-being of their children, often while feeling uncertain about what they should expect of them in these realms.

Families frequently find that there are too few hours in the day to meet the needs of the handicapped child and the general maintenance needs of the family (e.g., shopping, cooking, cleaning). There is little or no time for leisure or other regenerating activities (Gowen & Schoen, 1985). Furthermore, depend-

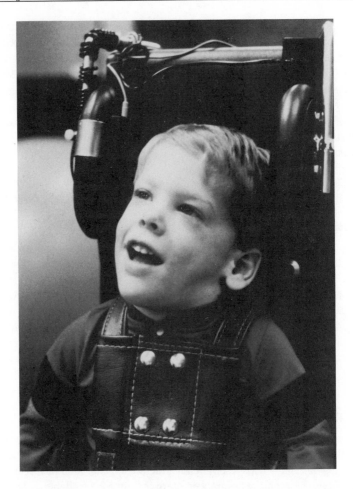

ing on the nature of the child's problems, it may be difficult to find babysitters who feel comfortable providing care. This makes it impossible for the parents to have time together or time to devote to their nonhandicapped children.

It is thus not hard to understand why families might react negatively to requests to participate in program activities that require additional time. What appears to be a lack of interest may indeed be a lack of time and/or energy. Yet, many families do find time to participate and are refreshed and helped by that participation. The issues for programs are: 1) to be responsive to the needs and interests of individual families, 2) to identify ways to help relieve some of the pressures within time-stressed families so as to free time for participation in group activities, or 3) to identify means of participation that are meaningful to the family and not time and energy intensive.

Psychological Pressures

There are many psychological pressures upon families of handicapped children. Much has been written about the grief that is experienced by families as they learn of their children's handicapping condition. Later, even though they may appear to function well, there is evidence that families often suffer a chronic sorrow, characterized by peaks and valleys of adjustment, as they care for their children over the years (Wikler, Wasow, & Hatfield, 1983). It is reasonable to believe that some of these highs and lows in coping ability are directly attributable to the nature of interactions with the service system (or lack thereof) and with the community at large, as the parents attempt to care for their children. There are three psychological pressures frequently reported by parents: frustration, hurt, and anxiety.

The Frustration of "Not Being Heard" One common complaint of parents of handicapped children is that it is difficult to get people to take them seriously or to hear what they have to say about their children (Gorham, Des Jardins, Page, Pettis, & Scheiber, 1975). This is often first evidenced in parents' early contacts with their pediatricians. Despite the growth and acceptance of early intervention programs, physicians continue to be reluctant to refer children for help, preferring to take a "wait and see" attitude. Mothers frequently report *knowing* that something was wrong with their child for many months before confirmation and referral to a program by their physicians (Bernheimer, Young, & Winton, 1983). During this period, they are often troubled by self-doubt, wondering if something is wrong with them for suspecting something is wrong with their child. Afterward, they are angry that they were "kept in the dark" so long as well as sad that their suspicions have been confirmed.

Another common situation in which parents may not feel heard is in the diagnostic process after the problem is finally recognized. Parents may observe their children taking tests and failing items they are able to do at home or that they could do if the items were administered in another way. Parents have frequently reported that professionals rarely asked what their children could do under other circumstances. When the parents did offer this information, it was often discounted (Gowen, Johnson-Martin, & Goldman, 1987).

Parents also report feeling that they are not heard when the information they have about their child is at odds with professionals' views about the general disorder. This is particularly apt to happen when the child has a relatively common disorder such as Down syndrome. One mother reported that the pediatrician described her child as "severely retarded" to a medical resident without either evaluating the child's current functioning or asking the mother about it. Yet, this child with Down syndrome was functioning within the low-normal range. Another reported the neurologist describing her severely spastic quadriplegic son as a "vegetable" without inquiring about evidence of learning ability observed at home and by the interventionists who worked with him (Gowen, Johnson-Martin, & Goldman, 1987).

The "Hurt" of Others' Reactions   It is difficult enough for parents to come to grips with their own feelings about their child's disabilities. Most of them are able to love and value their children, regardless of the nature or extent of the handicaps. Like all parents, they also want other people to value their children. They want to hear comments about their children's positive attributes. Instead, they may find their children treated with pity, curiosity, disapproval, or discomfort by friends, strangers, and professionals. Their need to protect their children and themselves from hurt may lead to social isolation.

Anxiety of Making Decisions without Adequate Information   Throughout the professional literature, there is consensus that one of the major needs of parents of handicapped children is a need for adequate information. Yet, it is often difficult for the parents to get access to the information they need. Sometimes the information is simply not available. Much remains unknown about most handicapping conditions—for example, which factors affect the outcome, which therapies are best, and so on (see Chapter 1). At other times, the information is available but not provided either because of a professional judgment that the parent will misuse the information (e.g., a child who is retarded may not be described as retarded for fear that the parents will treat him differently) or because the professional is ignorant of the information (see In-service in Chapter 5). Parents report having to "beat the bushes" to get a diagnosis and to find adequate resources (Bernheimer et al., 1983). There are also times when information is shared inadequately because of communication barriers (e.g., the professional uses jargon the parent cannot understand [Michaelis, 1980]), and times when the parent must cope with conflicting information presented by two or more professionals with different (and sometimes adamant) opinions about the meaning of available facts.

Despite this limited or confusing information, parents are required to make decisions about their children: major health decisions (e.g., surgery now or later) as well as a multitude of therapeutic and educational decisions (e.g., home- or center-based program, this or that therapist, a mainstreamed or self-contained setting, day care or home care, the adequacy of the current IEP) and more. It is not surprising that they sometimes cry, become belligerent, or simply acquiesce to whatever is suggested.

APPROACHES TO WORKING EFFECTIVELY WITH PARENTS

The primary goals of preschool programs for handicapped children should be to enhance their development and to support families in their care of these children. As noted earlier in this chapter, professionals are more frequently represented in the support networks of families who have handicapped children than in the support networks of families with nonhandicapped children. This places a special responsibility on professionals to provide the appropriate kind of support. Some of that support is provided through requisite services such as supplying information or providing therapy or education for the child. The helping professions are organized to supply this kind of support. With an over-representation of professionals in their support networks, however, families also need these professionals to provide *affective* support, that is, support that is derived through the *quality* of the *relationship* between the professional and the family members.

Unfortunately, this aspect of professional responsibility has been neglected in most training programs for professionals. Many families report that diagnostic information was shared with them in an unfeeling and insensitive fashion, greatly increasing the basic stress created by that information (Ries, 1983). While it is true that professionals must maintain some degree of objectivity in order to avoid burnout (see Chapter 5), as well as to help families make difficult decisions, "objectivity" sometimes is little more than a mask the professional hides behind in order to protect his or her feelings. Too much objectivity may produce professionals who are aloof and unfeeling when families desperately need someone who both understands and cares.

Effective Caring Relationship

Parents would be the first to say that they need professionals who will be completely honest with them. A caring relationship is not one in which information is withheld or distorted for fear of distressing a parent. Rather, it is a relationship in which information is honestly provided, grief and hurt are both acknowledged and shared, and efforts are made to help the family get on about the business of caring for the child and other members of the family.

Support through Respect

Interviews with parents indicate that one of the attributes they value most in professionals is respect for the parent (Gowen, Johnson-Martin, & Goldman, 1987). One major way this respect is expressed is by the professional not only listening to, but "hearing what the parent has to say" and treating that information as important (Gorham et al., 1975). Respect is further demonstrated by soliciting information and opinions about the child from the parent (see form for parent observation of child in Chapter 2 and for parent input in IEP in Chapter 8) and giving positive feedback about good parenting skills.

Parents ask not only for respect for themselves but also for respect for their children. In interviews, parents have described the difference it has made when a professional has interacted with their child in a way that indicates the child is accepted and valued as a unique individual, not as a representative of a syndrome or a condition. This involves interacting with the child in a natural way: 1) touching, holding, and playing with him or her; and 2) noticing and commenting on special characteristics or achievements. Parents want to know that

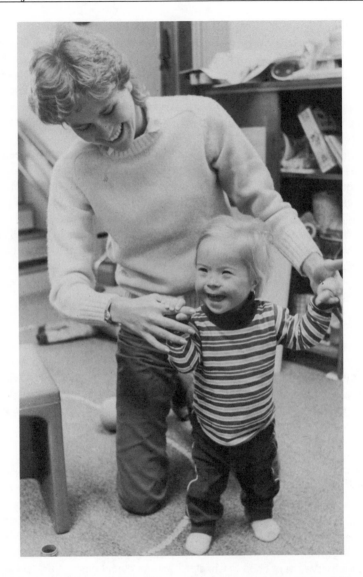

other people like their children. Respect for and appreciation of the child communicates respect for and appreciation of the parent as well (Gowen, Johnson-Martin, & Goldman, 1987).

Acceptance of Complaints

One of the things parents like about the teachers and therapists who choose to work with handicapped children is that they usually have a positive outlook toward the children. Often the outlook is a much more positive one than that of neighbors or members of the medical community. Insistence on an upbeat attitude may not be appropriate all the time, however. As key members of a social support system, it is also important for professionals to give parents permission to complain and express negative feelings. Because parents of handicapped children are prone to feeling guilt over negative feelings, it is often helpful to be sensitive to signs of stress and to indicate that negative reactions to the situation would be both normal and acceptable. An example of this would be, "Boy, it must be hard to know when to push and when to protect Billy!" or "I find it frustrating not to be able to figure out what he wants. Doesn't it get to you sometimes?"

Pitfalls to Avoid

There are at least two situations that should be avoided if one is to be an effective member of a parent's support network. First, it is important not to give parents additional "emotional baggage" by introducing one's own philosophical stances, which may run counter to those of the parent. Examples of this might include: "You are fortunate to have this child"; "Handicapped children are God's special gifts to special people"; or "You are such good parents, you should have more children." One can be positive in a more constructive way by focusing comments on positive behaviors of the parent or child; for example: "I am impressed with how sensitive you are to Johnny's communicative signals"; "You can be proud of how well you've managed the toileting"; "Johnny is smiling so much more now. It is wonderful to know when he really likes something!"

The second major interpersonal situation to avoid is that of creating too much dependency on the part of parents. It is easy for a professional, responding to genuine stress and feelings of helplessness on the part of parents, to assume too much responsibility, to "teach" the parent that they are not competent to cope without the professional. This may, in fact, be an ego boost to the professional who enjoys being needed. However, it is highly detrimental to a family in the long run. The goal of the professional should be to support the development of skills in the parent that eventually make professional help superfluous. Throughout their interactions, professionals should direct their efforts toward making parents be and feel competent with the task of raising their handicapped child.

Providing for Continuity

A major problem for most families of handicapped children is the necessity of dealing with a multitude of professionals. Often, these professionals are not aware of each others' services and may sometimes have opposing opinions. Probably the most effective way to deal with this problem is to identify a *case manager*, one person in the professional network with whom the parent is comfortable. He or she should be willing to serve as an advocate for the family and assume responsibility for helping the parent negotiate the service system (see staffing patterns in Chapter 8).

Transition between Programs

Often the most appropriate case manager is a staff member of an early intervention program (for infants) or a preschool (for 3–5-year-olds). However, this arrangement can create major problems for the family when the child leaves one program to enter another. Each "graduation" involves a shift to greater independence for the child and less intense involvement for the parents. Such a period of transition has been described by many parents as particularly stressful (Bernheimer et al., 1983). The transition may be made even more stressful by a change in case managers. An effective system of intervention provides for a gradual transition between programs and an overlap between case managers when changes must occur.

FAMILY INVOLVEMENT AND INDIVIDUALIZED FAMILY SERVICE PLANS

Under the conditions of Public Law 99-457, programs serving handicapped children under the age of 3 years are required to develop Individualized Family Service Plans (IFSPs). Those serving handicapped children 3 to 5 years old are required to have specific plans for family involvement. Guidelines and procedures for meeting these requirements, however, will need years of implementation before best practices are established.

It is not difficult to imagine some programs trying to develop plans in much the same way that they develop Individualized Education Programs (IEPs) for children. That is, they might identify or develop a "test" of family functioning that would be administered to all families in the program. Families would be assessed, those items they are not doing would become goals, and activities would be prepared to help families meet those goals.

Such an approach is fraught with enormous problems, however, particularly in a culturally diverse society. Optimal family functioning is difficult to define in such a way that it can be measured. Experienced early interventionists may be able to identify situations within a family that are not optimal for the development of the handicapped child or for other members. They may wish to alter those situations but can only do so with the family's assent and assistance. Compliance with intervention plans cannot be expected if they are not focused on problems mutually identified by the family and the interventionist. Collaboration between parents and professionals is the cornerstone of the new intervention efforts.

Models for Families

It becomes necessary, therefore, to leave our assessment and curriculum models designed for children to the needs of children, and take a fresh approach for families. Early interventionists need to identify different models of assessment, different models for the development of intervention plans, and different services to be responsive to the diversity of families and their needs.

Assessment Models   Because a family focus for educational intervention is relatively new, little has been written about how one should proceed, and few assessment instruments are available. One promising approach is included in the Family-Focused Intervention model described by Bailey et al. (1986). They suggest a three-phase process of assessment: 1) the completion of observations, rating scales, and questionnaires by the family and the interventionist, including both objective ratings and self-reports of the family's needs and resources; 2) a compilation of the data by the interventionist and an identification of initial family goals; and 3) a focused interview with the family in which the family verifies the needs indicated by the initial goals, identifies further needs, assigns priorities to the goals, and discusses strategies for meeting the goals. At the end of this process, all of the information that is necessary for the development of an individualized intervention plan for the family is available.

Families Identify their Needs   Because few assessment instruments are available to aid in the first phase of this process, Bailey and Simeonsson (1985) developed the Family Needs Survey. This instrument has been used effectively by the authors in a number of home-based early intervention programs. It consists of 35 items, each of which begins with a phrase such as "I need more. . . ." For example, one item reads, "I need to have more opportunities to meet and talk with other parents of handicapped children." The parent is asked to rate each item on a scale from 1 to 3, 1 indicating that he or she definitely does not need help with it and 3 indicating that help is definitely needed. Six categories of items are included and relate to: 1) information needs, 2) support needs, 3) financial needs, 4) needs related to explaining the child's condition or behavior to others, 5) need for help in gaining access to community services, and 6) needs related to family function.

At the Family Infant and Preschool Program, Dunst, Trivette, and Deal (1988) have also been working with an ecological model of intervention in which family members are collaborators in the assessment process and in the identification of family goals. Among the instruments that they have developed are: 1) the Family Functioning Style Scale, 2) the Assessment of Coping with Positive and Negative Events, 3) the Support Functions Scale, 4) the Family Enablement Scale, and 5) the Family Resource Scale. These efforts indicate the breadth of areas of concern in assessing families and give some idea of the complexity of the assessment process.

Individualized Family Service Plans (IFSPs)   The only models currently available for IFSPs are the IEPs that have been used in special education settings for the past 10 to 15 years. These models vary in format but share basic content: 1) broadly stated goals, 2) specific behavioral objectives, 3) means and timelines for meeting those objectives, and 4) evaluation procedures. One of the major problems for the development of IFSPs is specifying behavioral outcomes. It is much easier to make behavioral statements about goals related to developmental progress (e.g., the child will combine two objects in a functional manner) than about family interactions (e.g., the father will handle the infant in a sensitive way).

Bailey et al. (1986) suggest that one solution may be the use of Goal Attainment Scaling in which outcomes for a particular goal are specified on a 5-step continuum from best expected outcome to worst expected outcome. The Bailey et al. example used for the goal of greater positive sibling involvement states: 1) the worst expected outcome would be no progress (i.e., the sibling almost always interferes with parent-child interactions), 2) the expected outcome would be moderate progress (i.e., the sibling will not interfere with interactions between the handicapped child and the parent), and 3) the best expected outcome would be that the sibling often participates positively in interactions between the handicapped child and the parent. Such a procedure allows a complex goal to be rated along a behavioral continuum that both the interventionist and the parents can understand. It also lends itself to a reasonably objective evaluation of progress.

Services Responsive to Families   Through the development of *individualized* family service plans, programs should be able to identify *common* service needs among families that should be addressed programmatically. Although the needs and the ways in which it is feasible to meet them vary according to environmental circumstances (e.g., urban or rural settings, ethnic makeup of the community, patterns of child care), there are some needs that have been identified consistently throughout the years by families of young handicapped children. These needs should be anticipated, and ways to address them should be built into most, if not all, early intervention and preschool programs. Such things as parent support groups, respite care, and resource materials are needed by most families.

Parent Support Groups   Having a handicapped child often makes parents feel unique and separate from other parents. Many report that they do not feel that anyone really understands their situation without having been in it themselves. Thus, the opportunity to share with other parents becomes particularly important.

Parent groups function somewhat differently depending on who is involved with them. Mother groups tend to be different from father groups and from two-parent groups. Cultural norms about the expression of feelings and the characteristics of the group leader are other factors that affect group functioning.

The authors have observed one model to be very effective with a group of mothers of handicapped children in a center-based infant program and suspect that it would be useful with other groups in other settings as well. This group was composed of approximately 10 mothers who met weekly. At the first meeting, the leader described the basic format: 1) the purpose of the group was for sharing and learning; and 2) three meetings each month were designated as "program" meetings and the fourth as purely a "sharing of experiences" meeting, although any member with an important issue to share could preempt part of a program meeting. Group members identified individual improvement and educational goals to be worked on in the program meetings. The leader was responsible for arranging programs to assist in meeting the goals. For example, many mothers wanted to become more assertive in dealing with professionals. Assertiveness training, with specific role playing in situations with professionals, was arranged as the program for several meetings.

Other programs were arranged to provide the mothers with more information about the kinds of tests used with their children, to provide information on wills and trusts for handicapped children, to promote discussion of the rights of parents in the education of handicapped children, and so on. Mothers reported that this particular combination of information and emotional support through sharing experiences was a major help to them. Many of the mothers remained friends and provided respite care for one another long after their children had outgrown the program. Furthermore, the professionals who worked with both the infants and mothers observed marked progress in the mothers' interactions with their babies and with the staff (Eastman & Johnson, 1981).

Respite Care   For many families of handicapped children, the biggest issue is time. Very little time is left for parents to devote to each other or to their nonhandicapped children. Frequently, respite care has been seen as help for families in the event of a crisis rather than an ongoing service provided to release routine pressure or to provide for a regular period of relaxation for parents. Reliable and regular respite care is essential to the well-being and survival of families with handicapped infants and toddlers. If respite is not available to the parents from the extended family, it is critical to have it available from the community.

An early intervention or preschool program can assist in the development of respite programs in a variety of ways: 1) providing "flex time" for staff members so that they can be available for respite care on occasion, 2) holding training sessions for individuals in the community who are interested in providing respite care but unsure of their ability to do so, 3) helping volunteer agencies set up a respite care program (see Chapter 4), and 4) helping parents organize a system of trading respite care services among themselves and other community members. The choice of ways to assist in respite care must necessarily vary with the resources of the program, the makeup of the clientele, and the nature of the community. Plans for some sort of respite care program should be a priority for every program, however.

Library or Resource Room   Parents frequently cite information as a major need (Gowen & Schoen, 1985). Books, pamphlets, newsletters, addresses, and telephone numbers of both national and local parent organizations, as well as materials on normal and atypical child development, are all useful to parents in a setting where they can browse and read at their leisure. Parents are the best ones to determine when they are ready to study particular information, and they are often more comfortable seeking it out on their own rather than asking questions, although they may need to be directed to the information. Some programs have found it helpful to periodically publish an annotated bibliography of materials in the parent library, thereby making different kinds of information more apparent to parents.

It is also very helpful to include a toy library in such resource rooms so that parents can check out toys and try them with their children before making expensive purchases. Parents may enjoy developing such a library on their own, pooling the toys their children have outgrown, and raising money to buy additional ones.

SUMMARY

Parents of handicapped children have a particularly challenging role. In addition to the time, energy, and emotional demands of raising any child, they must deal with the additional demands on time and energy that are created by health and intervention services and they must cope both with their own grief and with emotional stress created by the reactions of others to their children. Members of the professional community play an important role in providing much needed services to these families. They are also in a position to either add to the families' stresses or reduce them through the ways they provide services and interact with the parents. It is critical that early intervention and preschool programs develop services that support families with handicapped children in both *being* and *feeling* competent in their roles as parents and advocates. In developing Individualized Family Service Plans and Plans for Family Involvement, care must be taken to avoid the imposition of goals set by professionals. Rather, parents should be viewed as the senior members of a partnership in which their needs, perceptions, and opinions are crucial to the common goal: the welfare of the child and the family.

STUDY QUESTIONS

1. Obtain permission from parents and staff and attend a group therapy or group sharing session with parents.
2. Go to a meeting of a local organization run by parents and offer to assist the group in the collection of funds or the organization of an activity or any other group projects.
3. Interview a parent who is presently being served by an early intervention program concerning his or her needs and attitudes about the program.
4. Interview a parent of a child who has graduated from an early intervention

program concerning his or her needs and attitudes about the program that served their child and about early intervention programming, in general.

REFERENCES

Bailey, D. B., & Simeonsson, R. J. (1985). *Assessing needs of families with handicapped infants: The family needs survey.* Unpublished document, University of North Carolina, Chapel Hill.

Bailey, D. B., Simeonsson, R. J., Winton, P. J., Huntington, G. S., Comfort, M., Isbell, P., O'Donnell, K. J., & Helm, J. M. (1986). Family focused intervention: A functional model for planning, implementing, and evaluating individualized family services in early intervention. *Journal of the Division for Early Childhood, 10,* 156–171.

Bernheimer, L. P., Young, M. S., & Winton, P. J. (1983). Stress over time: Parents with young handicapped children. *Developmental and Behavioral Pediatrics, 4*(3), 177–181.

Bristol, M. M. (1985, March). *Research with families of young handicapped children.* Paper presented at the Indiana State Leadership Training Conference, Indianapolis.

Bristol, M. M. (1987). Mothers of autistic and communication impaired children: Successful adaptation and the Double ABCX model. *Journal of Autism and Developmental Disorders, 17,* 469–486.

Caplan, P. J., & Hall-McCorquodale, I. (1985). Mother-blaming in major clinical journals. *American Journal of Orthopsychiatry, 55*(3), 345–353.

Cummings, S. T. (1976). The impact of the child's deficiency on the father: A study of fathers of mentally retarded and of chronically ill children. *American Journal of Orthopsychiatry, 46*(2), 246–255.

Cummings, S. T., Bayley, H. C., & Rie, H. E. (1966). Effects of the child's deficiency on the mother: A study of mothers of mentally retarded, chronically ill, and neurotic children. *American Journal of Orthopsychiatry, 36,* 595–608.

Dunst, C. J., Trivette, C. M., & Cross, A. H. (1986). Mediating influences of social support: Personal, family, and child outcomes. *American Journal of Mental Deficiency, 90*(4), 407–417.

Dunst, C. J., Trivette, C. M., & Deal, A. G. (1988). *Enabling and empowering families: Principles and guidelines for practice.* Cambridge, MA: Brookline Books.

Eastman, J., & Johnson, N. (1981, June). *Working with parents of handicapped persons.* Workshop for directors of developmental disabilities programs, North Central Region, Burlington, NC.

Friedrich, W. N., & Friedrich, W. L. (1981). Psychological assets of parents of handicapped and nonhandicapped children. *American Journal of Mental Deficiency, 85,* 551–553.

Gorham, K. A., Des Jardins, C., Page, R., Pettis, E., & Scheiber, B. (1975). Effects on parents. In N. Hobbs (Ed.), *Issues in the classification of children: Vol. 2. A source book on categories, labels, and their consequences* (pp. 154–188). San Francisco: Jossey-Bass.

Gowen, J. W., Johnson-Martin, N. M., & Appelbaum, M. (1987, April). *Predictors of distress and feelings of parenting competence in mothers of delayed and nondelayed infants.* Poster session at the biennial meeting of the Society for Research in Child Development, Baltimore.

Gowen, J. W., Johnson-Martin, N. M., & Goldman, B. D. (1987, April). Facilitating parent-child réciprocity. In P. Strain (Chair), *Report from the Early Childhood Research Institutes.* Symposium conducted at the 65th Annual Conference of the Council for Exceptional Children, Early Childhood Division, Chicago.

Gowen, J. W., & Schoen, D. (1985, December). *Information needs of parents of young special needs children.* Paper presented at 4th Biennial National Training Institute of the National Center for Clinical Infant Programs, Washington, DC.

Michaelis, C. T. (1980). *Home and school partnership in exceptional education.* Rockville, MD: Aspen Systems.

Ries, S. J. (1983). Families' perceptions for services of handicapped children. Brief research report. *Journal of Rehabilitation Research, 6*(4), 475–476.

Turnbull, A. P., & Turnbull, H. R. (1982). Parent involvement in the education of handicapped children: A critique. *Mental Retardation, 20*(3), 115–122.

Wikler, L., Wasow, M., & Hatfield, E. (1983). Seeking strengths in families of developmentally disabled children. *Social Work,* July-August, *28*(4), 313–315.

Index